# Headache: Assessment and Pain Management

# Headache: Assessment and Pain Management

Editor: Arabella Cross

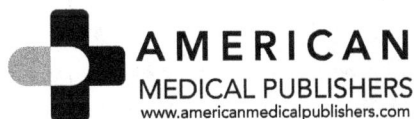

**AMERICAN**
MEDICAL PUBLISHERS
www.americanmedicalpublishers.com

AMERICAN
MEDICAL PUBLISHERS
www.americanmedicalpublishers.com

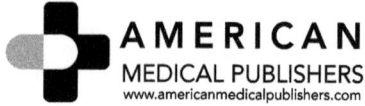

**Cataloging-in-Publication Data**

Headache : assessment and pain management / edited by Arabella Cross.
    p. cm.
Includes bibliographical references and index.
ISBN 978-1-63927-300-3
1. Headache. 2. Headache--Diagnosis. 3. Headache--Treatment. 4. Head--Diseases.
5. Pain--Treatment. I. Cross, Arabella.
RC392 .H43 2022
616.849 1--dc23

American Medical Publishers,
41 Flatbush Avenue,
1st Floor, New York,
NY 11217, USA

ISBN 978-1-63927-300-3 (Hardback)

# Contents

**Preface**.................................................................................................................................................IX

Chapter 1    **Efficacy of frovatriptan as compared to other triptans in migraine with aura** ...................................1
Stefan Evers, Lidia Savi, Stefano Omboni, Carlo Lisotto, Giorgio Zanchin and
Lorenzo Pinessi

Chapter 2    **Structured education can improve primary-care management of headache: the first
empirical evidence, from a controlled interventional study** ...................................................... 6
Mark Braschinsky, Sulev Haldre, Mart Kals, Anna Iofik, Ave Kivisild, Jaanus Korjas,
Silvia Koljal, Zaza Katsarava and Timothy J. Steiner

Chapter 3    **The efficiency of botulinum toxin type A for the treatment of masseter muscle
pain in patients with temporomandibular joint dysfunction and tension-type
headache** ............................................................................................................................... 13
Malgorzata Pihut, Ewa Ferendiuk, Michal Szewczyk, Katarzyna Kasprzyk and
Mieszko Wieckiewicz

Chapter 4    **The associations between psychosocial aspects and TMD-pain related aspects
in children and adolescents** ................................................................................................. 19
Amal Al-Khotani, Aron Naimi-Akbar, Mattias Gjelset, Emad Albadawi, Lanre Bello,
Britt Hedenberg-Magnusson and Nikolaos Christidis

Chapter 5    **Plasma urotensin-2 level and Thr21Met but not Ser89Asn polymorphisms of the
urotensin-2 gene are associated with migraines** ................................................................. 29
Sırma Geyik, Sercan Ergun, Samiye Kuzudişli, Figen Şensoy, Ebru Temiz,
Erman Altunışık, Murat Korkmaz, Hasan Dağlı, Seval Kul, Aylin Akçalı and
Ayşe Münife Neyal

Chapter 6    **Cost-effectiveness analysis of non-invasive vagus nerve stimulation for the
treatment of chronic cluster headache** ................................................................................ 37
James Morris, Andreas Straube, Hans-Christoph Diener, Fayyaz Ahmed,
Nicholas Silver, Simon Walker, Eric Liebler and Charly Gaul

Chapter 7    **Onabotulinumtoxin-A treatment in Greek patients with chronic migraine** ...................... 46
Michail Vikelis, Andreas A. Argyriou, Emmanouil V. Dermitzakis,
Konstantinos C. Spingos and Dimos D. Mitsikostas

Chapter 8    **Risk of medication overuse headache across classes of treatments for acute
migraine** ............................................................................................................................... 51
Kristian Thorlund, Christina Sun-Edelstein, Eric Druyts, Steve Kanters,
Shanil Ebrahim, Rahul Bhambri, Elodie Ramos, Edward J. Mills,
Michel Lanteri-Minet and Stewart Tepper

Chapter 9    **Real-life data in 115 chronic migraine patients treated with Onabotulinumtoxin
A during more than one year** ............................................................................................... 60
I. Aicua-Rapun, E. Martínez-Velasco, A. Rojo, A. Hernando, M. Ruiz,
A. Carreres, E. Porqueres, S. Herrero, F. Iglesias and A. L. Guerrero

Chapter 10    **Texture features of periaqueductal gray in the patients with medication-overuse headache** ....................................................................................................................... **64**
Zhiye Chen, Xiaoyan Chen, Mengqi Liu, Shuangfeng Liu, Lin Ma and Shengyuan Yu

Chapter 11    **Increased levels of intramuscular cytokines in patients with jaw muscle pain** ........................... **70**
S. Louca Jounger, N. Christidis, P. Svensson, T. List and M. Ernberg

Chapter 12    **A multicenter, open-label, long-term safety and tolerability study of DFN-02, an intranasal spray of sumatriptan 10 mg plus permeation enhancer DDM, for the acute treatment of episodic migraine** ................................................................ **79**
Sagar Munjal, Elimor Brand-Schieber, Kent Allenby, Egilius L. H. Spierings, Roger K. Cady and Alan M. Rapoport

Chapter 13    **Validation of the Social support and Pain Questionnaire (SPQ) in patients with painful temporomandibular disorders** ........................................................... **87**
Songlin He and Jinhua Wang

Chapter 14    **Onabotulinumtoxin A for the management of chronic migraine in current clinical practice: results of a survey of sixty-three Italian headache centers** .................................. **92**
Cristina Tassorelli, Marco Aguggia, Marina De Tommaso, Pierangelo Geppetti, Licia Grazzi, Luigi Alberto Pini, Paola Sarchielli, Gioacchino Tedeschi, Paolo Martelletti and Pietro Cortelli

Chapter 15    **Is topiramate effective for migraine prevention in patients less than 18 years of age?** .................................................................................................................................... **103**
Kai Le, Dafan Yu, Jiamin Wang, Abdoulaye Idriss Ali and Yijing Guo

Chapter 16    **The impact of onabotulinumtoxinA on severe headache days: PREEMPT 56-week pooled analysis** ....................................................................................................... **113**
Manjit Matharu, Rashmi Halker, Patricia Pozo-Rosich, Ronald DeGryse, Aubrey Manack Adams and Sheena K. Aurora

Chapter 17    **Therapeutical approaches to paroxysmal hemicrania, hemicrania continua and short lasting unilateral neuralgiform headache attacks: a critical appraisal** ............................... **121**
Carlo Baraldi, Lanfranco Pellesi, Simona Guerzoni, Maria Michela Cainazzo and Luigi Alberto Pini

Chapter 18    **Treatment of disabling headache with greater occipital nerve injections in a large population of childhood and adolescent patients** ................................................ **139**
Francesca Puledda, Peter J. Goadsby and Prab Prabhakar

Chapter 19    **OnabotulinumtoxinA in the treatment of refractory chronic cluster headache** ........................... **145**
Christian Lampl, Mirjam Rudolph and Elisabeth Bräutigam

Chapter 20    **Oxygen treatment for cluster headache attacks at different flow rates** ........................................... **151**
Thijs H. T. Dirkx, Danielle Y. P. Haane and Peter J. Koehler

Chapter 21    **Evaluation of ADMA-DDAH-NOS axis in specific brain areas following**
**nitroglycerin administration: study in an animal model of migraine** ........................................... 160
Rosaria Greco, Andrea Ferrigno, Chiara Demartini, Annamaria Zanaboni,
Antonina Stefania Mangione, Fabio Blandini, Giuseppe Nappi,
Mariapia Vairetti and Cristina Tassorelli

Chapter 22    **Single-pulse transcranial magnetic stimulation (sTMS) for the acute treatment**
**of migraine: evaluation of outcome data for the UK post market pilot program** ........................ 168
Ria Bhola, Evelyn Kinsella, Nicola Giffin, Sue Lipscombe, Fayyaz Ahmed,
Mark Weatherall and Peter J Goadsby

Chapter 23    **Validation of potential candidate biomarkers of drug-induced nephrotoxicity and**
**allodynia in medication-overuse headache** ........................................................................................ 176
Elisa Bellei, Emanuela Monari, Stefania Bergamini, Aurora Cuoghi, Aldo Tomasi,
Simona Guerzoni, Michela Ciccarese and Luigi Alberto Pini

Chapter 24    **The effects of acupuncture treatment on the right frontoparietal network in**
**migraine without aura patients** ........................................................................................................... 185
Kuangshi Li, Yong Zhang, Yanzhe Ning, Hua Zhang, Hongwei Liu, Caihong Fu,
Yi Ren and Yihuai Zou

**Permissions**

**List of Contributors**

**Index**

# Preface

It is often said that books are a boon to mankind. They document every progress and pass on the knowledge from one generation to the other. They play a crucial role in our lives. Thus I was both excited and nervous while editing this book. I was pleased by the thought of being able to make a mark but I was also nervous to do it right because the future of students depends upon it. Hence, I took a few months to research further into the discipline, revise my knowledge and also explore some more aspects. Post this process, I begun with the editing of this book.

Headaches are the symptoms of pain in the area of head and neck. They can be broadly classified into primary and secondary headaches. Primary headaches are recurrent headaches that are not caused by any underlying disease or structural problems. A few examples of primary headaches are migraines, cluster-type headaches and tension-type headaches. Migraine can be managed by improving the lifestyle. Tension-type headaches are treated with NSAIDs or acetaminophen. Verapamil is often recommended for the treatment of cluster headaches. They may be recurrent and may cause significant pain, but they do not pose any long term danger. Secondary headaches can be either harmless or dangerous. They may be caused by other serious conditions such as meningitis and brain tumor. Severe headaches often increase the risk of depression. The most common causes of headaches include common cold, head injury, viral infections, effects of medications, sleep deprivation, stress and dental or sinus issues. This book provides comprehensive insights into headache and pain management. It will also provide interesting topics for research which interested readers can take up. Those in search of information to further their knowledge will be greatly assisted by this book.

I thank my publisher with all my heart for considering me worthy of this unparalleled opportunity and for showing unwavering faith in my skills. I would also like to thank the editorial team who worked closely with me at every step and contributed immensely towards the successful completion of this book. Last but not the least, I wish to thank my friends and colleagues for their support.

**Editor**

# Efficacy of frovatriptan as compared to other triptans in migraine with aura

Stefan Evers[1,2]*, Lidia Savi[3], Stefano Omboni[4], Carlo Lisotto[5], Giorgio Zanchin[6] and Lorenzo Pinessi[3]

## Abstract

**Background:** The treatment of migraine attacks with aura by triptans is difficult since triptans most probably are not efficacious when taken during the aura phase. Moreover, there are insufficient data from randomised studies whether triptans are efficacious in migraine attacks with aura when taken during the headache phase. In this metaanalysis, we aimed to compare the efficacy of frovatriptan versus rizatriptan, zolmitriptan, and almotriptan.

**Methods:** Five double-blind, randomized, controlled crossover trials were pooled. All trials had an identical design. Patients were asked to treat three consecutive migraine attacks with frovatriptan 2.5 mg and three consecutive migraine attacks with a comparative triptan (rizatriptan 10 mg; zomitriptan 2.5 mg; almotriptan 12.5 mg).

**Results:** In this analysis, 117 migraine attacks with aura could be included (intention-to-treat population). The mean headache intensity after 2 hours was 1.2 +/- 1.0 for frovatriptan and 1.6 +/- 1.0 for the other triptans (p<0.05); all triptans showed significant improvement of headache. Frovatriptan resulted in significantly lower relapse rates at 24 hours and 48 hours when taken in migraine attacks with aura.

**Conclusions:** Our data suggest that frovatriptan is efficacious and even superior in some endpoints also when taken during the headache phase in migraine attacks with aura. This is of particular importance for those many patients who have migraine attacks both without and with aura.

**Keywords:** Frovatriptan; Almotriptan; Zolmitriptan; Rizatriptan; Migraine with aura; Metaanalysis

## Background

The efficacy of triptans in migraine with aura refers to different questions. First, it is of interest whether triptans are able to treat the aura symptoms [1]. Second, it has been studied whether triptans taken during the aura phase of a migraine attack are efficacious to treat the headache [1-4], which is not recommended in treatment guidelines [5]. Further, triptans are not approved to be taken during the aura phase because of their vasoconstrictive properties. Third, it is of interest whether triptans are efficacious against the headache in migraine attacks both without and with aura when taken in the headache phase. Since many patients have both types of attacks, this refers to reliability of triptan efficacy. Beside pain-free and abrupt relief from pain, this is a very important parameter for patients [6-8]. This is also expressed in

another study, when 55% of the patients would prefer a long-acting triptan versus a rapid-onset, short-acting agent [9]. The very recent guideline of the International Headache Society (IHS) for controlled trials of drugs in migraine defined consistency as one of the secondary parameters for the evaluation of results [10].

Frovatriptan is a potent 5-HT1$_{B//D}$ receptor agonist and has the highest 5-HT1$_B$ potency in the triptan class; preclinical pharmacodynamic studies demonstrated that frovatriptan is apparently cerebroselective [11]. In clinical pharmacology studies, frovatriptan was shown to have a long terminal elimination half-life time of 26 hours [11,12]. This could be an argument for better clinical consistency. However, a direct comparison of frovatriptan to different other triptans with respect to efficacy in migraine attacks with aura is still missing.

Since frovatriptan has shown advantages in some outcome parameters in a large study program comparing frovatriptan to other triptans [13], we were interested in whether this is also true when treating migraine attacks

* Correspondence: everss@uni-muenster.de
[1]Department of Neurology, University of Münster, Münster, Germany
[2]Department of Neurology, Krankenhaus Lindenbrunn, Coppenbrügge, Germany

with aura. Therefore, we performed a metaanalysis of all those trials with a head-to-head comparison of frovatriptan to another triptan in the acute treatment of migraine attacks with aura. The aim of the study was to compare the efficacy of the different triptans in the treatment of these specific attacks with respect to headache. This analysis did not aim to evaluate the efficacy of triptans when taken during the aura phase or the efficacy of triptans against the aura symptoms.

## Methods

This study is based on five trials which compared frovatriptan to rizatriptan (two trials), zolmitriptan (two trials), and almotriptan (one trial), respectively. All these trials were double-blind, randomized crossover trials. Three were Italian trials and already published [14-16]. Two were European trials not yet published as a full paper (complete data on file). All trials were approved by the local ethics committees. All patients gave written informed consent before randomization.

The trial design of these five trials was nearly identical and described previously [14-16]. In brief, patients aged ≥18 and ≤65 years with a current history of migraine with or without aura according to the IHS criteria [17] and having experienced an average of at least one but not more than six migraine attacks per month for six months prior to entry into the study were enrolled. Exclusion criteria were a history suggestive of ischaemic heart disease or any atherosclerotic disease indicating an increased risk of coronary ischaemia; symptomatic cardiac arrhythmias; history of stroke or transient ischaemic attack (TIA); uncontrolled hypertension; history of basilar, hemiplegic, or ophthalmoplegic migraine; severe liver and renal impairment; renal disease, or renal failure; known or suspected intolerance of, or hypersensitivity, or contraindications to any component of the trial medications; use of either test medication to treat any one of the last three episodes of migraine; history of intolerance or inefficacy of at least two triptans for the treatment of migraine attacks; abuse of alcohol, analgesics or psychotropic drugs; any severe concurrent medical condition that, according to the site investigator, may affect the interpretation of clinical trial results; pregnancy or breastfeeding; inability or unwillingness to issue the informed consent; more than six days per month of tension-type headache.

Patients complying with these inclusion/exclusion criteria were randomised 1 to 1 within each centre with a predetermined randomisation list in balanced blocks, to receive frovatriptan 2.5 mg or rizatriptan 10 mg, zolmitriptan 2.5 mg, and almotriptan 12.5 mg, respectively. Prior to randomisation the patients were monitored for migraine history including the MIDAS questionnaire, medical history, medications history, vital signs. If applicable, a pregnancy test was performed.

The assigned treatment was to be taken in three consecutive attacks of migraine. A patient could use up to two doses two hours apart to treat an attack, and up to two doses every 24 hours for episodes lasting more than one day. The three episodes should occur in a period not exceeding three months after randomisation. During each episode, the patient recorded on a diary the intensity of migraine pain from immediately before taking the medication up to 48 hours. The patient also recorded the use of medication, the possible relapse including time of relapse, and any possible adverse event.

After having treated three episodes, the patient switched to the alternative treatment, respectively, the other triptan or frovatriptan 2.5 mg. On this occasion, adverse events were reviewed, medication history checked and vital signs monitored. The patient treated the subsequent three consecutive attacks of migraine with the treatment received for the second period, with the same provisions as above regarding the dosing. The three episodes should also occur in a period not exceeding three months after switchover. After having treated three episodes with the second medication, the patient concluded the study. On this occasion, adverse events were reviewed, medication history checked, and vital signs monitored.

In this post-hoc analysis, we included all attacks in which an aura preceded the onset of the migraine headache (i.e. before the intake of the study drug). Patients were advised to take the study drug only when the migraine headache was beginning and not during the aura. However, it could be possible that the aura was still ongoing when the study drug was taken.

We evaluated the efficacy rate of the study drug for pain free at 2/4/24/48 hours after drug intake as primary endpoint; further we evaluated the mean headache intensity according to a grading from 0 to 3 (0 = none; 1 = mild; 2 = moderate; 3 = severe) and the 24 hour and 48 hour relapse rate. Statistical comparison among the treatments was made between the combined results from all five trials. Secondary endpoint was the mean headache intensity at different time points which was analysed by ANOVA. Percentages were compared using $Chi^2$-test. Significance level was set at p = 0.05.

## Results

The baseline characteristics including the MIDAS score [18] of all study participants (intention-to-treat population) who treated at least one migraine attack with aura are presented in Table 1. The data are pooled according to the comparative triptan. There were no significant differences in these demographic data between the five trials analysed in this study. In total, 117 migraine attacks with aura were included into this analysis (frovatriptan = 57; rizatriptan = 28; zolmitriptan = 24; almotriptan = 8).

**Table 1 Baseline characteristics of the patients included in this analysis (i.e., all patients experiencing an aura before at least one attack treated with study drug) presented separately for the four different triptans**

|  |  | Rizatriptan (n = 28) | Zolmitriptan (n = 24) | Almotriptan (n = 8) | Frovatriptan (n = 57) |
|---|---|---|---|---|---|
| Age (years) |  | 43 +/− 9 | 35 +/− 10 | 37 +/− 11 | 41 +/− 11 |
| Females |  | 89% | 88% | 100% | 91% |
| MIDAS | grade I | 4% | 0% | 0% | 4% |
|  | grade II | 4% | 0% | 0% | 6% |
|  | grade III | 36% | 55% | 38% | 43% |
|  | grade IV | 57% | 46% | 63% | 48% |
| Attack duration >2 days |  | 46% | 41% | 63% | 44% |

Data are shown as mean (+/− SD), or frequency in %. There were no significant differences.

Headache intensity when taking the study drug was not significantly different between the four triptan treatments (Table 2). The 2 hour and 4 hour pain free rate and the relapse rate for 24 hours and 48 hours are presented in Table 2. After 2 hours, more attacks were pain free after frovatriptan as compared to rizatriptan. There was a significantly lower percentage of relapse in attacks with aura treated with frovatriptan than in attacks with aura treated with the other triptans, both for the 24 and 48 hours endpoint (except for the comparison with almotriptan at 48 hours).

In Figure 1, the mean headache intensity is presented for the period covering 48 hours after intake of the study drug. There was a significantly lower mean headache intensity for frovatriptan at 4 hours as compared to all other triptans and for frovatriptan and zolmitriptan at 48 hours as compared to rizatriptan and almotriptan (but not between frovatriptan and zolmitriptan). We also pooled the data from all comparative triptans. The mean

headache intensity after 2 hours was 1.2 +/− 1.0 for frovatriptan and 1.6 +/− 1.0 for the other triptans ($p < 0.05$). After 4 hours, the mean headache intensity was 0.5 +/− 0.6 for frovatriptan and 1.2 +/− 1.1 for the other triptans ($p < 0.001$).

When analyzing the adverse events, there were no significant differences at all between the study drugs. The number and types of adverse events were quite similar to those seen in the migraine attacks without aura.

## Discussion

Our data show that frovatriptan results in a significantly lower relapse rate even when taken in acute migraine attacks with aura as compared rizatriptan, zolmitriptan, and almotriptan (the latter one not at 48 hours). This is in concordance with a previous analysis of all migraine attacks studied in a larger trial program [13]. Furthermore, this analysis confirms that triptans taken during the headache phase are in general efficacious and well

**Table 2 Pain free rate at 2 hours and headache recurrence rate at 24 hours and 48 hours for all migraine with aura attacks**

|  |  | Rizatriptan (n = 28) | zolmitriptan (n = 24) | Almotriptan (n = 8) | Frovatriptan (n = 57) | Significance |
|---|---|---|---|---|---|---|
| Baseline headache intensity[1] |  |  |  |  |  |  |
|  | mean | 2.4 +/− 0.5 | 2.2 +/− 0.6 | 2.3 +/− 0.7 | 2.1 +/− 0.7 | ns |
|  | median | 2 | 2 | 2 | 2 | ns |
| Pain free at |  |  |  |  |  |  |
|  | 2 hours | 10.7% | 25.0% | 12.5% | 29.8% | $p < 0.05$[2] |
|  | 4 hours | 35.7% | 50.0% | 25.0% | 50.9% | ns |
| Recurrence at |  |  |  |  |  |  |
|  | 24 hours | 42.9% | 37.5% | 37.5% | 26.3% | $p < 0.05$[3] |
|  | 48 hours | 89.3% | 91.7% | 87.5% | 66.7% | $p < 0.01$[4] |

[1]Headache intensity graded as 0 = none; 1 = mild; 2 = moderate; 3 = severe.
[2]$p < 0.05$ for comparison between frovatriptan and rizatriptan.
[3]only for comparison between frovatriptan and rizatriptan.
[4]post-hoc analysis: $p = 0.025$ for frovatriptan versus rizatriptan; $p = 0.019$ for frovatriptan versus zolmitriptan; $p = 0.232$ for frovatriptan versus almotriptan.
Data are shown as mean (+/− SD), or frequency in %. Statistical comparison by ANOVA or $Chi^2$-test (ns denotes not significant).

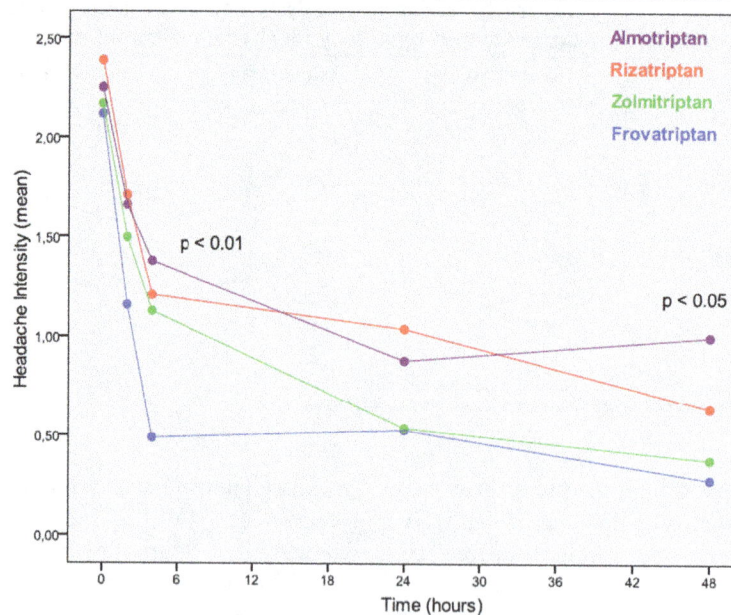

**Figure 1** Mean headache intensity[1] during attack treatment for all four different triptans. Statistical comparison by ANOVA, for post-hoc analysis see text. [1]Headache intensity graded as 0 = none; 1 = mild; 2 = moderate; 3 = severe.

tolerated in migraine with aura. This is of major importance since many patients experience migraine attacks both with and without aura; these patients do not have to change their way of acute attack treatment (e.g., the choice of a triptan) with respect to the aura.

The low recurrence rate of frovatriptan even in migraine with aura is also of interest for many patients as surveys on patients' needs have shown [6,8]. In previous trials, frovatriptan was able to decrease the overall duration of migraine attacks significantly [19], and it is more efficacious when taken during the mild, beginning phase of a migraine attack versus taken during the later severe phase [20]. The short duration of attacks and the low recurrence rate result in a significantly lower mean headache intensity in this study after 24 hours and 48 hours. The significantly lower relapse rate of frovatriptan can be explained by its pharmacological properties [21]. When comparing all triptan trials, the elimination half-life time is inversely correlated with the relapse rate ($r = -1.0$; $p = 0.0016$). Frovatriptan has by far the longest half-life time (26 hours), whereas all the other oral triptans have a half-life time between 2 and 6 hours.

Some of our findings are surprising with respect to the literature, in particular the good efficacy of frovatriptan after 2 and 4 hours as compared to rizatriptan. The baseline characteristics of the migraine attacks and the MIDAS scores show that patients with mainly severe and long-lasting migraine attacks were enrolled into this study program. This might be the reason why frovatriptan, which is normally less efficacious in the first 2 hours after drug intake, was of particular efficacy in this study.

A limitation of this study is that it is a metaanalysis of different trials which were not designed to study the efficacy in migraine with aura as their primary endpoint. However, this metaanalysis is justified, since these trials all had a nearly identical design and since the two hour pain free rates in general were not significantly different between these triptans [13], i.e. the 2 hour pain free rate was not significantly lower for frovatriptan than for rizatriptan, zolmitriptan, or almotriptan. Previous analyses had suggested that the two hour pain free rate for frovatriptan is lower than for other triptans [11]; however, this has been shown in trials with treatment at any time during the migraine attack. When reevaluating this aforementioned finding in migraine attacks treated early, there was no significant difference between frovatriptan and other triptans regarding 2 hour pain free rates [11,22]. Also in the trials analysed here, patients were advised to treat their migraine attacks early.

Another limitation is that we did not extend our comparison to the remaining triptans (sumatriptan, naratriptan, eletriptan) or to other acute migraine drugs such as NSAIDs or ergotamine derivatives. Thus, the final position of frovatriptan within all acute migraine drugs with respect to efficacy in migraine with aura cannot be determined by this study.

Finally, the number of patients/attacks with aura was quite different between the different treatment groups. In particular, the comparison to almotriptan with only 8 attacks included in this analysis is problematic due to statistical reasons (large confidence intervals etc.).

## Conclusion

In summary, frovatriptan provides an efficacious treatment for migraine attacks with aura when taken during the headache phase with respect to acute efficacy and to relapse.

### Competing interests

Stefan Evers received honoraria and research grants within the past five years by AGA Medical (now St Jude), Allergan, Almirall, AstraZeneca, BerlinChemie, CoLucid, Desitin, Eisai, GlaxoSmithKline, Ipsen Pharma, Menarini, MSD, Novartis, Pfizer, Reckitt-Benckiser, UCB.
Carlo Lisotto has occasionally served as scientific consultant for the manufacturers of frovatriptan, rizatriptan, zolmitriptan and almotriptan.
Stefano Omboni has received consultancy fees from Menarini, manufacturer of frovatriptan.
Lorenzo Pinessi has received honoraries by Almirall, Lusopharmaco, GlaxoSmithKline, Novartis, Teva, Merck Serono, Biogen Idec.
Lidia Savi has received honoraries by Almirall, Lusopharmaco, Neopharmed, Gentili.
Giorgio Zanchin received honoraries within the past five years by St Jude, Allergan, Almirall, Angelini, GlaxoSmithKline, Menarini, MSD, Pfizer, Piam.

### Authors' contributions

LS, SO, CL, GZ, and LP were responsible for patient enrolment and data collection. SE was responsible for data analysis and wrote the first draft of the manuscript. All authors read and approved the final manuscript.

### Acknowledgement

All trials analysed in this paper were sponsored by Menarini, Florence, Italy. The metaanalysis presented in this paper was supported by an unrestricted grant by Menarini, Florence, Italy.

### Author details

[1]Department of Neurology, University of Münster, Münster, Germany. [2]Department of Neurology, Krankenhaus Lindenbrunn, Coppenbrügge, Germany. [3]Department of Neurology, University of Turin, Turin, Italy. [4]Italian Institute of Telemedicine, Varese, Italy. [5]Department of Neurology, Hospital of Pordenone, Pordenone, Italy. [6]Department of Neurology, University of Padova, Padova, Italy.

### References

1. Bates D, Ashford E, Dawson R, Ensink FB, Gilhus NE, Olesen J, Pilgrim AJ, Shevlin P (1994) Subcutaneous sumatriptan during the migraine aura. Sumatriptan Aura Study Group. Neurology 44:1587–1592
2. Dowson A (1996) Can oral 311C90, a novel 5-HT1D agonist, prevent migraine headache when taken during an aura? Eur Neurol 36(Suppl 2):28–31
3. Olesen J, Diener HC, Schoenen J, Hettiarachchi J (2004) No effect of eletriptan administration during the aura phase of migraine. Eur J Neurol 11:671–677
4. Aurora SK, Barrodale PM, McDonald SA, Jakubowski M, Burstein R (2009) Revisiting the efficacy of sumatriptan therapy during the aura phase of migraine. Headache 49:1001–1004
5. Evers S, Afra J, Frese A, Goadsby PJ, Linde M, May A, Sandor P (2009) EFNS guideline on the drug treatment of migraine – revised report of an EFNS task force. Eur J Neurol 16:968–981
6. Lipton RB, Hamelsky SW, Dayno JM (2002) What do patients with migraine want from acute migraine treatment? Headache 42(Suppl 1):3–9
7. Lantéri-Minet M (2005) What do patients want from their acute migraine therapy? Eur Neurol 53(Suppl 1):3–9
8. Bigal M, Rapoport A, Aurora S, Sheftell F, Tepper S, Dahlöf C (2007) Satisfaction with current migraine therapy: experience from 3 centers in US and Sweden. Headache 47:475–9
9. Malik SN, Hopkins M, Young WB, Silberstein SD (2006) Acute migraine treatment: patterns of use and satisfaction in a clinical population. Headache 46:773–80
10. Tfelt-Hansen P, Pascual J, Ramadan N, Dahlöf C, D'Amico D, Diener HC, Møller Hansen J, Lanteri-Minet M, Loder E, McCrory D, Plancade S, Schwedt T (2012) Guidelines for controlled trials of drugs in migraine: Third edition. A guide for investigators. Cephalalgia 32:6–38
11. Comer MB (2002) Pharmacology of the selective 5-HT(IB/ID) agonist frovatriptan. Headache 42(Suppl 2):S47–53
12. Goldstein J (2003) Frovatriptan: a review. Expert Opin Pharmacother 4:83–93
13. Cortelli P, Allais G, Tullo V, Benedetto C, Zava D, Omboni S, Bussone G (2011) Frovatriptan versus other triptans in the acute treatment of migraine: pooled analysis of three double-blind, randomized, cross-over, multicenter, Italian studies. Neurol Sci 32(Suppl 1):S95–8
14. Savi L, Omboni S, Lisotto C, Zanchin G, Ferrari MD, Zava D, Pinessi L (2011) A double-blind, randomized, multicenter, Italian study of frovatriptan versus rizatriptan for the acute treatment of migraine. J Headache Pain 12:219–26
15. Tullo V, Allais G, Ferrari MD, Curone M, Mea E, Omboni S, Benedetto C, Zava D, Bussone G (2010) Frovatriptan versus zolmitriptan for the acute treatment of migraine: a double-blind, randomized, multicenter, Italian study. Neurol Sci 31(Suppl 1):S51–4
16. Bartolini M, Giamberardino MA, Lisotto C, Martelletti P, Moscato D, Panascia B, Savi L, Pini LA, Sances G, Santoro P, Zanchin G, Omboni S, Ferrari MD, Brighina F, Fierro B (2011) A double-blind, randomized, multicenter, Italian study of frovatriptan versus almotriptan for the acute treatment of migraine. J Headache Pain 12:361–8
17. Headache Classification Committee of the International Headache Society (2004) The International classification of headache disorders: 2nd edition. Cephalalgia 24(Suppl 1):9–160
18. Stewart WF, Lipton RB, Dowson AJ, Sawyer J (2001) Development and testing of the Migraine Disability Assessment (MIDAS) Questionnaire to assess headache-related disability. Neurology 56(Suppl 1):S20–28
19. Kelman L, Harper SQ, Hu X, Campbell JC (2010) Treatment response and tolerability of frovatriptan in patients reporting short- or long-duration migraines at baseline. Curr Med Res Opin 26:2097–104
20. Göbel H, Heinze A (2011) The Migraine Intervention Score - a tool to improve efficacy of triptans in acute migraine therapy: the ALADIN study. Int J Clin Pract 65:879–86
21. Géraud G, Keywood C, Senard JM (2003) Migraine headache recurrence: relationship to clinical, pharmacological, and pharmacokinetic properties of triptans. Headache 43:376–88
22. Cady R, Elkind A, Goldstein J, Keywood C (2004) Randomized, placebo-controlled comparison of early use of frovatriptan in a migraine attack versus dosing after the headache has become moderate or severe. Curr Med Res Opin 20:1465–72

# Structured education can improve primary-care management of headache: the first empirical evidence, from a controlled interventional study

Mark Braschinsky[1,2], Sulev Haldre[1,2], Mart Kals[3], Anna Iofik[4], Ave Kivisild[4], Jaanus Korjas[4], Silvia Koljal[4], Zaza Katsarava[5] and Timothy J. Steiner[6,7*]

## Abstract

**Background:** Headache disorders are under-recognized and under-diagnosed. A principal factor in their suboptimal management is lack of headache-related training among health-care providers, especially in primary care. In Estonia, general practitioners (GPs) refer many headache patients to neurological specialist services, mostly unnecessarily. GPs request "diagnostic" investigations, which are usually unhelpful and therefore wasteful. GP-made headache diagnoses are often arcane and non-specific, and treatments based on these are inappropriate.
The aim of this study was to develop, implement and test an educational model intended to improve headache-related primary health care in Estonia.

**Methods:** This was a controlled study consisting of baseline observation, intervention and follow-up observation using the same measures of effect. It involved six GPs in Põlva and the surrounding region in Southern Estonia, together with their future patients presenting consecutively with headache as their main complaint, all with their consent. The primary outcome measure was referral rate (RR) to neurological specialist services. Secondary measures included number of GP-requested investigations, GP-made headache diagnoses and how these conformed to standard terminology (ICD-10), and GP-recommended or initiated treatments.

**Results:** RR at baseline ($n = 490$) was 39.5 %, falling to 34.7 % in the post-intervention group ($n = 295$) (overall reduction 4.8 %; $p = 0.21$). In the large subgroup of patients (88 %) for whom GPs made clearly headache-related ICD-10 diagnoses, RR fell by one fifth (from 40 to 32 %; $p = 0.08$), but the only diagnosis-related RR that showed a statistically significant reduction was (pericranial) myalgia (19 to 3 %; $p = 0.03$). There was a significant increase towards use of more specific diagnoses. Use of investigations in diagnosing headache reduced from 26 to 4 % ($p < 0.0001$). Initiation of treatment by GPs increased from 58 to 81 % ($p < 0.0001$).

**Conclusions:** These were modest changes in GPs' entrenched behaviour. Nevertheless they were empirical evidence that GPs' practice in the field of headache could be improved by structured education. Furthermore, the changes were likely to be cost-saving. To our knowledge this study is the first to produce such evidence.

**Keywords:** Education, Effect measurement, Headache disorders, Management, Primary care, Global Campaign against Headache

* Correspondence: t.steiner@imperial.ac.uk
[6]Department of Neuroscience, Norwegian University of Science and Technology, Edvard Griegs Gate, Trondheim NO-7489, Norway
[7]Division of Brain Sciences, Imperial College London, London, UK
Full list of author information is available at the end of the article

# Background

Throughout Europe, and worldwide, headache disorders are highly prevalent and commonly disabling, causing heavy personal burdens and very substantial socioeconomic cost [1]. In the European Union (EU), headache disorders cost national economies well in excess of €100 billion annually [2]. Globally, headache disorders are the third cause of disability [3, 4]. Despite these compelling statistics, headache disorders are under-recognized, under-diagnosed and undertreated everywhere [1]. A principal factor in suboptimal treatment is lack of knowledge amongst health-care providers of the nature and good management of headache disorders, and this is especially so in primary care where most headache should be managed [1]. This is itself the result of very limited and wholly inadequate commitment to these disorders in medical undergraduate curricula and continuing medical education [1].

One consequence is poor outcomes. These lead in turn to patient dissatisfaction, diminished expectation, low consultation rates and persistence of these burdens largely unmitigated. Other consequences are unnecessary investigations and referrals to specialist care [1], which are wasteful of scarce health-care resources.

This spectrum of problems is encountered in Estonia, a small country of approximately 1.3 million people. Here, as elsewhere, there is a clear need for improving headache-related primary health care. Estonia is a member of the EU, but the legacy of the former Soviet health system is entrenched: purposeless over-investigation, application of arcane diagnoses, with prescription of inappropriate (often vasoactive) treatments based upon these, and very high dependence on specialist referral [5]. These behaviours are not likely easily to be changed, but the best means of doing so, with expectation of improvement in care, lies in education of health-care providers, especially in primary care [1, 6].

The aim of this study, undertaken as a project within the Global Campaign against Headache, was to develop, implement and test an educational model intended to improve headache care delivered by general practitioners (GPs) in Estonia. The primary hypothesis was that a well-structured but limited (as opposed to intensive) programme of education of GPs in headache disorders and their management would reduce referrals. We selected referral rate (RR) to specialist care as the principal outcome measure because such referrals are easily and objectively measurable. Whilst we could not, on an individual level, determine whether or not a particular referral was appropriate, we could take an informed view on whether overall RR was excessive and therefore wasteful [7]. A secondary hypothesis was that education would lessen the plethora of investigations performed by GPs in headache patients; as an outcome measure, investigation rate had the same characteristics as RR.

# Methods

## Ethics

This study was approved by the Ethics Review Committee on Human Research of the University of Tartu. Informed consent was obtained from all participants: GPs and their patients. Data-protection legislation was complied with.

## Study design

This was a controlled study, which consisted of baseline observation, intervention and outcome observation using the same measures.

## Setting and subjects

The project was conducted in the town of Põlva and the surrounding region in Southern Estonia, with a population of about 30,500. Approximately 12,500 inhabitants were registered at the only outpatients' clinic in Põlva, where seven GPs were working. GPs seeking specialist care referred their headache patients first to the single neurologist at Põlva Hospital (level two in the European model of organization of headache services [7] described by *Lifting The Burden* [LTB] and the European Headache Federation [EHF]) (summarised in Table 1). In case of need, GPs directly and the local neurologist might both send patients further, to Tartu University Hospital, for higher-level neurological consultation (level three [7]).

The intervention involved the GPs and their future patients presenting consecutively with headache as their main complaint. The GPs were the research subjects. Their future patients were not subjects directly, but were beneficiaries of the intervention, who provided data for some of the outcome measures. Additionally, the records of consecutive similar past patients (who were not excluded from becoming future patients) were scrutinised to establish baseline performance of GPs.

Age, gender and educational level of each patient were registered.

**Table 1** Headache services organised on three levels [7]

| | |
|---|---|
| Level 1. General primary care | • Frontline headache services (accessible first contact for most people with headache) |
| | • Ambulatory care delivered by primary health-care providers |
| | • Referring when necessary, and acting as gatekeeper, to: |
| Level 2. Special-interest headache care | • Ambulatory care delivered by physicians with a special interest in headache |
| | • Referring when necessary to: |
| Level 3. Headache specialist centres | • Advanced multidisciplinary care delivered by headache specialists in hospital-based centres |

## Intervention

The objective of the intervention was to provide GPs with sufficient understanding to manage, competently but not expertly, those headache disorders that are common in primary care. The intervention consisted of:

a) two educational one-day (6-h) courses to all participating GPs:
day one: didactic lectures by headache-specialists, based on the European principles of diagnosis and management of common headache disorders [8], including the recognition of important secondary headaches, and other materials in *Aids for management of common headache disorders in primary care* published jointly by LTB and EHF [9];
day two (four weeks after day one): clarifying and reinforcing discussions between the GPs and headache specialists, including analysis of clinical cases presented by the specialists and GPs from their own practices;
b) educational materials and management aids for GPs [9] translated into Estonian and (in the case only of information leaflets on headache disorders for patients) also into Russian.

## Outcome measures

Outcome measures were collected from the two groups: baseline data were collected retrospectively from past patients for the period prior to study commencement and post-intervention data were gathered prospectively from patients consulting after the intervention.

The primary outcome measure was RR: the percentage of patients referred to levels two or three. The primary analysis was the change in RR post-intervention.

Secondary outcome measures included GP-requested investigations (laboratory tests and xrays, but not CT [this and MRI are not ordered by GPs in Estonia]), GP-made headache diagnoses and GP-recommended and/or initiated treatments. Patients' comorbidities were recorded.

All these data were acquired from the electronic medical records.

In addition, past patients as well as those included prospectively were contacted during the course of the study by telephone; those who consented participated in the following enquiries in their native language (Estonian or Russian):

a) satisfaction with care, rated on a numerical rating scale (NRS) of 0–10 where 0 = "very dissatisfied" and 10 = "very satisfied";
b) adequacy of care, assessed by the Headache Under-Response to Treatment (HURT) questionnaire [10];
c) burden of headache, assessed by the Headache-Attributed Lost Time (HALT) questionnaire [11];

d) quality of life, assessed by the RAND 36-Item Health Survey 1.0 questionnaire (RAND-36) [12];
e) health satisfaction (HS) and quality of life satisfaction (QoLS) assessed by the first two questions of WHOQoL-8 [13], rated on a NRS of 1–5 where 1 was least, 3 was neutral and 5 was the highest level of satisfaction.

## Statistics

Power calculation estimated that 273 participants were required per group assuming that RR would be 25 % at baseline and fall to 15 % after intervention and using a one-sided test with 5 % significance level and 90 % power.

Data were collected and analysed using software R, version 3.0.3 for Windows. Results were adjusted for age and gender. Means ± standard deviations (SDs) were used as descriptive statistics. Pearson's chi-squared test was used to compare RRs between baseline and post-intervention groups, and the same and Fisher's exact test were used for other dichotomous variables. The relationships between NRS, QoLS and HS were tested with Spearman's correlation coefficient (CC). Student's t-test was used to evaluate differences in RAND-36. Results were considered to be statistically significant when $p < 0.05$.

## Results

Six of the seven GPs consented to participate in the study. It became evident that our assumption regarding the baseline RR was incorrect (see below): in order to achieve adequate statistical power, the baseline group included 490 patients seen during two years prior to the first day of the intervention while the post-intervention group consisted of 295 consecutive patients consulting during one year after the second day of the intervention. There was female predominance in both groups: 73 % (357/490) in the baseline and 75 % (221/295) in the post-intervention group (the difference being insignificant: $p = 0.58$). The mean age of the baseline group (43.2 ± 15.8 years) was 3.6 years lower than that of the post-intervention group (46.8 ± 17.1; $p = 0.004$). There was no apparent difference between groups in level of education ($p = 0.48$), but over two thirds of patients chose not to disclose this information.

For the primary outcome, 476/490 baseline records (data-missing rate 2.9 %) and 294/295 post-intervention records (data-missing rate 0.3 %) were included. Baseline RR was 39.5 %; with our patient numbers we had 88 % power to see a reduction of 10 % (*ie*, to 29.5 %). However the overall reduction was only 4.8 % to 34.7 %, which did not reach significance ($p = 0.21$). When RR was analysed for different diagnoses used by the GPs according to the International Classification of Diseases (ICD-10) [14], there were clear trends towards reduction (Table 2). The most frequently used ICD-10 diagnoses at

Structured education can improve primary-care management of headache: the first empirical...

9

**Table 2** Referral rates according to ICD-10 diagnoses before and after intervention

| ICD-10 diagnosis | Referral rate | | p |
| --- | --- | --- | --- |
| | Baseline | Post-intervention | |
| G44.2 Tension-type headache | 58/119 (49 %) | 50/115 (43 %) | 0.50 |
| G43 Migraine | 22/48 (46 %) | 15/45 (33 %) | 0.31 |
| G44 Other headache syndromes and R51 Headache | 79/178 (44 %) | 10/38 (26 %) | 0.06 |
| M79.1 (Pericranial) myalgia | 20/108 (19 %) | 1/36 (3 %) | 0.03 |
| Total for four headache diagnostic groups | 179/453 (40 %) | 76/234 (32 %) | 0.08 |

baseline were, in order, G44 (other headache syndromes), G44.2 (tension-type headache), M79.1 (myalgia [implying pericranial myalgia]), R51 (headache), G43 (migraine) and G43.9 (unspecified migraine). RR for patients with a diagnosis of tension-type headache decreased from 49 to 43 %, for patients with migraine from 46 to 33 % and for patients with non-specific headache diagnoses (G44 or R51) from 44 to 26 %. All these trends remained statistically insignificant, although the last was close ($p = 0.06$). The only diagnosis-related RR that showed a statistically significant reduction was that for (pericranial) myalgia (19 to 3 %; $p = 0.03$).

Within the spectrum of headache diagnoses used by GPs, there was a significant increase towards using those that were more specific (Table 3, Fig. 1).

Requests for diagnostic investigations for headache reduced from 26 % (125/490) at baseline to 4 % (13/295) post-intervention ($p < 0.0001$) (Fig. 2). Within these numbers, laboratory investigations fell from 22 to 1 % ($p < 0.0001$) and xrays from 7 to 3 % ($p = 0.038$). These changes were noted within all diagnostic groups, being most clear-cut for migraine, for which there were no investigations performed at all post-intervention (reduction from 14 to 0 %; $p = 0.01$).

Initiation of treatment by GPs increased from 58 % (286/490) at baseline to 81 % (239/295) post-intervention ($p < 0.0001$) (Fig. 2). Furthermore, use of more than one treatment option increased from 14 % (67/490) to 41 % (120/295) ($p < 0.0001$).

Proportions responding to enquiries into satisfaction with care were low: 155 patients (31.6 %) at baseline and 87 (29.5 %) post-intervention. Non-responders in the baseline group were somewhat younger (41.9 ± 15.8 *versus* 46.1 ± 15.2 years; $p = 0.006$) and included more men (31 % *versus* 19 %; $p = 0.04$). Overall satisfaction with care showed very little change in NRS mean score: from 6.4 ± 2.5 at baseline to 6.7 ± 2.3 post-intervention, which was not significant ($p = 0.36$). We found no differences by diagnostic groups, or in those in whom investigations were performed or treatments initiated, or in those referred.

There were, similarly, no significant changes in HS ($p = 0.22$) or QoLS ($p = 0.66$). The number of comorbidities was strongly correlated with lower scores in HS in both groups (baseline CC: −0.23; $p = 0.004$; post-intervention CC: −0.32; $p = 0.002$). Proportions responding to the HALT and HURT questionnaires were also low: 34.9 % in the baseline and 29.8 % in the post-intervention groups. Again, non-responders at baseline included more men (32 % *versus* 19 %; $p = 0.003$). There was no meaningful change between groups in either HURT or HALT scores (mean HALT scores were 2.8 (±1.3) at baseline and 2.9 (±1.3) post-intervention; $p = 0.49$). There were no significant overall changes in QoL measured by RAND-36, or in any of the domains.

## Discussion

This controlled intervention study has shown that GPs' behaviours were changed and practice improved by a structured educational programme, albeit not in a way that was reflected in all measures. In particular, the fall in RR (the primary outcome measure) was statistically insignificant; on the other hand, GPs made more disease-specific diagnoses while requesting far fewer investigations, and they became much more willing to initiate treatment. It should be noted that, despite the difference in their sizes, the two groups of patients on whom these comparisons were based were demographically similar. Although the age difference (43.2 *versus* 46.8 years) was significant statistically, it was not so clinically.

To our knowledge this is the first study to demonstrate empirically that GPs' practice in the field of

**Table 3** Usage of the most frequent diagnoses before and after intervention

| ICD-10 diagnosis | Baseline | Post-intervention | p |
| --- | --- | --- | --- |
| G44 Other headache syndromes | 134 (27.3 %) | 23 (7.8 %) | <0.0001 |
| G44.2 Tension-type headache | 120 (24.5 %) | 115 (39.0 %) | <0.0001 |
| M79.1 (Pericranial) myalgia | 111 (22.7 %) | 36 (12.2 %) | 0.0003 |
| R51 Headache | 55 (11.2 %) | 16 (5.4 %) | 0.009 |
| G43 Migraine and G43.9 Unspecified migraine | 46 (9.4 %) | 28 (9.5 %) | 1 |
| G43.0, G43.1, G43.2 and G43.8 Specified migraine subtypes | 4 (0.8 %) | 17 (5.8 %) | <0.0001 |

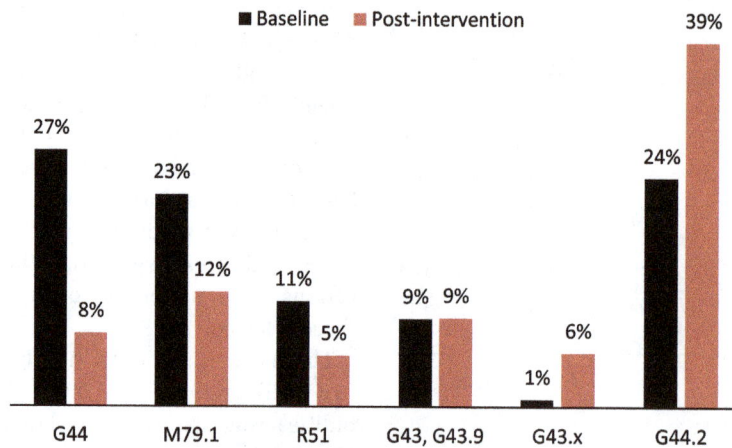

**Fig. 1** Usage of the most frequent diagnoses before and after intervention. G44: other headache syndromes; M79.1: (pericranial) myalgia; R51: headache; G43: migraine; G43.9: unspecified migraine; G43.x: specified migraine subtype; G44.2: tension-type headache. The figure depicts a clear trend, post-intervention, away from use of non-specific diagnoses towards more specific diagnoses

headache can be favourably influenced by education. The Dutch study of Smelt et al. [15], aimed specifically at migraine management and recruiting patients already on triptan therapy, failed to show a beneficial effect. This controlled trial employed clinical outcomes, and perhaps demonstrated the difficulties associated with them. The Norwegian study of Kristoffersen et al. [16], targeting medication-overuse headache only, improved outcomes in an intervention group but the essential element of the intervention was to equip GPs with a "simple and effective instrument" as a management aid; the educational element was secondary to this. Both these studies had much narrower focus than ours; we assessed the provision of

headache care to unselected patients, which was a major strength in both purpose and study design.

That there was only a small and statistically insignificant reduction in the primary outcome measure – the overall RR – was disappointing, especially since baseline RR was much higher (39 %) than anticipated (25 %). However, for patients with clearly headache-related GP-made diagnoses, RR fell by one fifth (from 40 to 32 %; $p = 0.08$), suggesting some gain in confidence in managing patients with primary headache without referral to a neurologist.

Only for patients diagnosed with (pericranial) myalgia was RR reduced significantly, but this outcome was

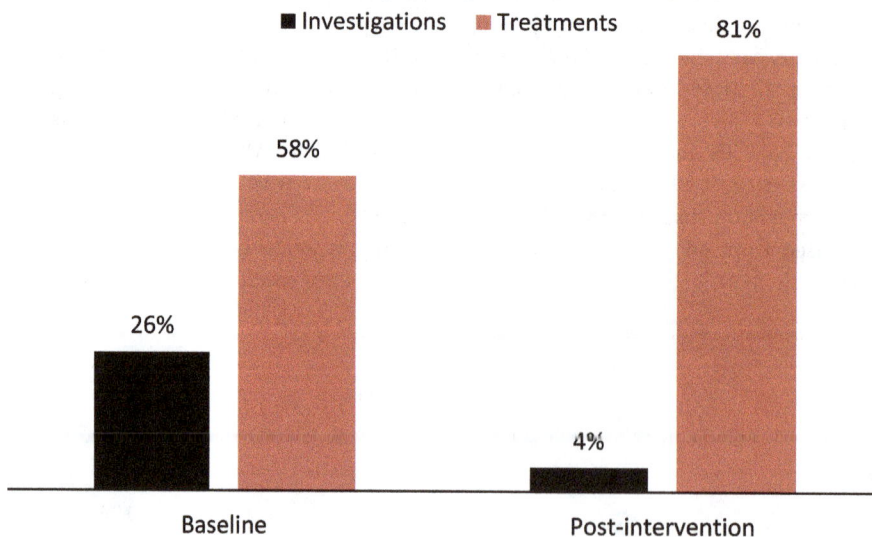

**Fig. 2** Requests for investigations and initiation of treatment before and after intervention. The figure depicts a reduction in the former and an increase in the latter post-intervention

substantially influenced by a considerable reduction in use of this diagnosis (M79.1). We did not analyse diagnostic changes case-by-case or perform quality analysis of diagnoses, but can reasonably speculate that, with better knowledge applied to recognizing and diagnosing tension-type headache, inappropriate use of M79.1 gave way to correct usage of G44.2 for this disorder. In keeping with this supposition, employment of the latter diagnosis significantly increased post-intervention. Also there was a significant reduction in diagnoses that did not specify a primary headache type. In other words, patients left their GPs' offices less frequently with diagnoses of headache as a symptom and more frequently with diagnoses naming the disease causing this symptom. GPs' practice shifted towards themselves diagnosing the most common primary headaches.

Key to this is that primary headaches are diagnosed clinically, rarely with need for investigations. Our results show that, post-intervention, GPs substantially reduced their demands for diagnostic investigations, eliminating them altogether in the case of migraine. Not only was this further evidence of learning and of confidence gained as a result, but also it produced immediate cost savings. Our study was not designed to measure cost-effectiveness, but this finding may be one of particular importance because it indicates that health-care resources can be conserved.

In line with an increased rate of specific diagnosis, the study found a greatly enhanced rate of GP-initiated treatment. At baseline, 42 % of patients appeared to receive no treatment recommendations from their GPs; post-intervention, this fell to 19 % – that is to say, 81 % of patients left their GPs' offices with clear treatment options recommended or prescribed. It was not possible in the context of the study to make any judgement of the appropriateness of treatment initiated.

Interestingly, all these changes in GPs' practice post-intervention had no discernible influence on patient-reported outcomes – satisfaction with care, satisfaction with health and quality of life, lost productive time or quality-of-life measures. It should be noted here that the instruments used, while not directly validated in the study population, had all been employed in multiple countries, cultures and languages. Where patient satisfaction is concerned, there are multiple determinants that might explain failure to indicate benefit. For example, we sought to reduce the use of investigations because these do not contribute usefully to the diagnosis of headache disorders in primary care. Similarly we aimed to reduce RR because the proportion of patients who should be referred – for diagnostic or management difficulties or for secondary headache – is much smaller than was the baseline RR [7]. Patients, however, might not agree that these reductions were in their interest.

Also we have to recognise that the study was underpowered at outset for these secondary outcome measures, added to which the proportions responding to the patient-directed enquiries were about 30 %. Realistically we should not attempt to make anything of these, because, with such low response rates, bias was also likely. Unfortunately, such response rates are not at all unusual [2] and, as was the case here, are one of the limitations of this type of study.

Other limitations here related to the scope of the study. Its aims did not include quality review of diagnoses, investigations or treatments; to do any of these would have required an entirely different approach. Also this study cannot comment on the duration of found effects, which was outside the scope of the protocol. In other words we are not able to answer the question about need for repeated interventions over time. Further studies, which are planned, are required for these purposes.

Finally it must be said that the gains achieved, at least in the principal outcome measure, were less than had been hoped for, but the fact that gains were made suggests more would be achieved with more educational input. The cost-effectiveness of this must be investigated, but is very likely to be favourable given the enormously high socioeconomic burden of headache [1, 2].

## Conclusions

GPs' practice in the field of headache can be improved by a structured yet limited educational programme. To our knowledge this study is the first to show this empirically. Improvements were modest: established practice is entrenched and change is likely to be slow. But the improvements included wider use of headache diagnoses employing accepted and more specific terminology, less demand for investigations, which are almost invariably unhelpful, less dependence on referral, which is often unnecessary, and greater willingness to initiate treatment. These changes can be expected to lead to immediate cost savings.

**Competing interests**

ZK is director and trustee of European Headache Federation and of *Lifting The Burden*. TJS is a director and trustee of *Lifting The Burden*. No other author has any competing interest.

**Authors' contributions**

The work presented here was a collaboration by all the authors. MB formulated the hypothesis, designed the study, interpreted the data and drafted the manuscript. SH designed the study, interpreted the data and made significant revisions to the manuscript. MK performed the statistical analysis, interpreted the data and revised the manuscript. AI, AK, JK and SK collected the data and revised the manuscript. ZK formulated the hypothesis, designed the study, interpreted the data and made major revisions to the manuscript. TJS formulated the hypothesis, designed the study, interpreted the data and made major revisions to the manuscript. All authors read and approved the final manuscript.

## Acknowledgements
The study was supported financially by the European Headache Federation and by *Lifting The Burden*, a UK-registered non-governmental organization conducting the Global Campaign against Headache in official relations with the World Health Organization.

## Author details
[1]Estonian Headache Society, L Puusepa str 8H, Tartu, Estonia. [2]Clinic of Neurology, University of Tartu, L Puusepa str 8H, Tartu, Estonia. [3]Estonian Genome Centre, University of Tartu, Riia 23b, Tartu, Estonia. [4]Faculty of Medicine, University of Tartu, Ravila 19, Tartu, Estonia. [5]Department of Neurology, University of Duisburg-Essen, Essen, Germany. [6]Department of Neuroscience, Norwegian University of Science and Technology, Edvard Griegs Gate, Trondheim NO-7489, Norway. [7]Division of Brain Sciences, Imperial College London, London, UK.

## References

1.  World Health Organization, Lifting The Burden (2011) Atlas of headache disorders and resources in the world 2011. WHO, Geneva
2.  Linde M, Gustavsson A, Stovner LJ, Steiner TJ, Barré J, Katsarava Z, Lainez JM, Lampl C, Lantéri-Minet M, Rastenyte D, Ruiz de la Torre E, Tassorelli C, Andrée C (2012) The cost of headache disorders in Europe: the Eurolight project. Eur J Neurol 19:703–711
3.  Vos T, Barber RM, Bell B, Bertozzi-Villa A, Biryukov S, Bolliger I, Charlson F, Davis A, Degenhardt L, Dicker D, Duan L, Erskine H, Feigin VL, Ferrari AJ, Fitzmaurice C, Fleming T, Graetz N, Guinovart C, Haagsma J, Hansen GM, Hanson SW, Heuton KR, Higashi H, Kassebaum N, Kyu H, Laurie E, Liang X, Lofgren K, Lozano R, MacIntyre MF et al. (2015) Global, regional, and national incidence, prevalence, and years lived with disability for 301 acute and chronic diseases and injuries in 188 countries, 1990–2013: a systematic analysis for the Global Burden of Disease Study 2013. Lancet 386:743–800
4.  Steiner TJ, Birbeck GL, Jensen RH, Katsarava Z, Stovner LJ, Martelletti P (2015) Headache disorders are third cause of disability worldwide. J Headache Pain 16:58
5.  Osipova VV, Azimova JE, Tabeeva GR, Tarasova SV, Amelin AV, Kutzemelov IB, Moldovanu IV, Odobescu SS, Naumova GI (2012) Headache diagnostics in Russia and post-Soviet countries: problems and solutions. Ann Clin Exper Neurol 6:16–21
6.  Martelletti P, Mitsikostas DD, Lampl C, Katsarava Z, Osipova V, Paemeleire K, Edvinsson L, Siva A, Valade D, Steiner TJ, Jensen RH (2013) Framing education on headache disorders into the Global Burden of Disease Study 2010. The European Headache Federation stands ready. J Headache Pain 14:41
7.  Steiner TJ, Antonaci F, Jensen R, Lainez JMA, Lantéri-Minet M, Valade D, on behalf of the European Headache Federation and Lifting The Burden: the Global Campaign against Headache (2011) Recommendations for headache service organisation and delivery in Europe. J Headache Pain 12:419–426
8.  Steiner TJ, Paemeleire K, Jensen R, Valade D, Savi L, Lainez JMA, Diener H-C, Martelletti P, Couturier EGM, on behalf of the European Headache Federation and Lifting The Burden: The Global Campaign to Reduce the Burden of Headache Worldwide (2007) European principles of management of common headache disorders in primary care. J Headache Pain 8(suppl 1):S3–S21
9.  Steiner TJ, Martelletti P (2007) Aids for management of common headache disorders in primary care. J Headache Pain 8(suppl 1):S2–S47, http://www.l-t-b.org/index.cfm/spKey/horizontal_activities.supporting.html. (Accessed 29 Feb 2016)
10. Buse DC, Sollars CM, Steiner TJ, Jensen RH, Al Jumah MA, Lipton RB (2012) Why HURT? A review of clinical instruments for headache management. Curr Pain Headache Rep 16:237–254
11. Steiner TJ (2007) The HALT index. J Headache Pain 8(suppl 1):S23
12. Hays RD, Morales LS (2001) The RAND-36 measure of health-related quality of life. Ann Med 33:350–357
13. Power M (2003) Development of a common instrument for quality of life. In: Nosikov A, Gudex C (eds) EUROHIS: Developing common instruments for health surveys, vol 57. IOS Press, Amsterdam, pp 145–163
14. World Health Organization (2010) International Statistical Classification of Diseases and Related Health Problems 10th Revision. At: http://apps.who.int/classifications/icd10/browse/2010/en. (Accessed 11 Sept 2015)
15. Smelt AFH, Blom JW, Dekker F, van den Akker E, Neven AK, Zitman FG, Ferrari MD, Assendelft P (2012) A proactive approach to migraine in primary care: a pragmatic randomized controlled trial. CMAJ 184:E224–E231
16. Kristoffersen ES, Straand J, Vetvik KG, Benth JS, Russell MB, Lundqvist C (2015) Brief intervention for medication-overuse headache in primary care. The BIMOH study: a double-blind pragmatic cluster randomised parallel controlled trial. J Neurol Neurosurg Psychiatry 86:505–512

# The efficiency of botulinum toxin type A for the treatment of masseter muscle pain in patients with temporomandibular joint dysfunction and tension-type headache

Malgorzata Pihut[1], Ewa Ferendiuk[1], Michal Szewczyk[1], Katarzyna Kasprzyk[2] and Mieszko Wieckiewicz[3*]

## Abstract

**Background:** Temporomandibular joint dysfunction are often accompanied by symptoms of headache such as tension-type headache which is the most frequent spontaneous primary headache. Masseter muscle pain is commonly reported in this group. The purpose of the study was to assess the efficiency of intramuscular botulinum toxin type A injections for treating masseter muscle pain in patients with temporomandibular joint dysfunction and tension-type headache.

**Methods:** This prospective outcome study consisted of 42 subjects of both genders aged 19–48 years diagnosed with masseter muscle pain related to temporomandibular joint dysfunction and tension-type headache. The subjects were treated by the intramuscular injection of 21 U (mice units) of botulinum toxin type A (Botox, Allergan) in the area of the greatest cross-section surface of both masseter bellies. Pain intensity was evaluated using visual analogue scale (VAS) and verbal numerical rating scale (VNRS) 1 week before the treatment and 24 weeks after the treatment. The obtained data were analyzed using the Wilcoxon matched pairs test ($p \leq 0{,}005$).

**Results:** The results of this study showed a decrease in the number of referred pain episodes including a decrease in pain in the temporal region bilaterally, a reduction of analgesic drugs intake as well as a decrease in reported values of VAS and VNRS after injections ($p = 0{,}000$).

**Conclusions:** The intramuscular botulinum toxin type A injections have been an efficient method of treatment for masseter muscle pain in patients with temporomandibular joint dysfunction and tension-type headache.

**Keywords:** Botulinum toxin, Masseter muscle pain, Temporomandibular joint dysfunction, Tension-type headache

## Background

Symptoms characteristic for temporomandibular joint dysfunction (TMJD) such as masticatory muscles pain, temporomandibular joint pain, derangements of the condyle-disc complex and deviations of mandible movements are often accompanied by symptoms that are not directly related to the functioning of the temporomandibular joint [1–8]. Such signs include otologic symptoms (ear pain, tinnitus, vertigo), neurovascular headaches and tension-type headaches (TTH) [9–13]. TTH are the most frequent spontaneous primary headaches. They are observed more frequently in women, and occurred in all age groups. It should be emphasized that in most cases the TTH affect middle-aged patients. This kind of headache was also observed in approximately 5–7 % of students aged 5–15 years. The American Dental Association stated that more than 15 % of American adults suffer from chronic headache pain [11–16].

Diagnostics of TTHs is based on the data collected in a screening history consisted short questions which let to analyze the background of the pain and the factors responsible for pain origin. Specialized neuroimaging modalities (magnetic resonance, angiography, positron emission tomography) are used less frequently. The

* Correspondence: m.wieckiewicz@onet.pl
[3]Department of Prosthetic Dentistry, Faculty of Dentistry, Wroclaw Medical University, 26 Krakowska St., 50-425 Wroclaw, Poland
Full list of author information is available at the end of the article

results of additional tests provide to exclude other causes of the TTH, especially migraine headache, aseptic meningitis, neuroborreliosis or pseudotumor cerebri [11, 17–18]. The following disorders should also be taken into consideration in differential diagnosis: hemicrania continua, spinal cord injury, central nervous system disorders and depression. Sinus pain, medication-induced headache and intracranial hypertension may also be important. TTH may be caused by psychoemotional factors, chronic stress, fatigue, sleep disorders and severe dehydration [17–22].

Bilateral, constant, dull ache of mild to moderate intensity without preexisting aura, vomiting, nausea is characteristic of TTH. Although TTH are not as widely recognized as migraine headaches, they constitute an important and frequent clinical problem, as they exert negative impact on the patients' quality of life. Tension-type headache is affecting the temporal and occipital region. The patient may also report the feeling of squeezing within the head. In the beginning the headache is not intensive. Later it could intensify and gain the same level of pain as the migraine headache. Moreover, the frequency at which TTH occurs is important for diagnosis: it lasts at least 30 min daily, occurs on 15 days in a month, affects the patient for more than 3 months, and is detected in all age groups, but it affects middle-aged people most frequently. TTH are frequently accompanied by sleep disorders, chronic fatigue syndrome, noise hypersensitivity and appetite loss [13, 15, 22]. Risk factors include: gender (women are affected more frequently), hormone changes, emotional stress, depression, anxiety and genetic factors. Moreover, TTH could be a result of head and neck injury, bruxism, and psychoactive and analgesic drug intake. According to the latest edition of the International Classification of Headache Disorders (ICHD-3 beta) prepared by the International Headache Society, TTH can be classified into: infrequent tension-type headaches, frequent tension-type headaches, chronic tension-type headaches, and probable tension-type headaches. Tension-type headaches accompany temporomandibular joint dysfunction with varying frequency because head and neck muscles remain in close anatomical and physiological relationship [22–26].

The aim of this prospective outcome study was to assess the efficiency of intramuscular botulinum toxin type A (BTXA) injections in a case of masseter muscle pain in patients with temporomandibular joint dysfunction and tension-type headache.

## Methods

This is a prospective outcome study which consisted of 42 subjects of both genders, aged 19–48 years (mean age was 30) with masseter muscle pain related to temporomandibular joint dysfunction and tension-type headache. Patients were recruited from the Department of Dental Prosthetics at the Jagiellonian University in Krakow during the years 2009–2014 and were included in the study if they met the following criteria: (1) presence of TMJD which include unilateral or bilateral disc displacement with or without reduction, arthralgia, degenerative joint disease, subluxation, (2) masseter muscle pain, (3) increased masticatory muscles tension, (4) TTH, (5) absence of previous neurological treatment due to headache and a head injury within 6 years and (6) patient consent to be involved in the study. The rest of patients were excluded because of general (known hypersensitivity to BTXA, myasthenia gravis, Eaton-Lambert syndrome, pregnancy or lactation and taking aminoglycosides or curare-like compounds) and/or local (infection at the proposed site of injection) contraindications for intramuscular botulinum toxin type A injections as well as absence of consent to be involved in the study.

Clinical assessment of temporomandibular joints and masticatory muscles was performed by one experienced and self-trained examiner according to the RDC/TMD recommendations [27, 28]. Further diagnostics was based on survey and clinical examination according to the International Headache Society guidelines performed by experienced physician in the Department of Neurology at the Jagiellonian University in Krakow [29]. According to the performed examination there was no indications for neuroimaging examination due to the headache in the study group. The study protocol has been approved by the Bioethical Committee of the Jagiellonian University in Krakow No: KBET/96/B/2007.

The data collected during the survey have been important for the purpose of the study: localization of the headache, pain duration, and factors responsible for pain origin. The patients were also asked whether the pain was constant, episodic, recurrent, referred, and whether it was felt as dull, sharp, burning or stinging. It was important whether the patient reported that the pain was squeezing the head as well as previous treatment due to the headache. Authors paid close attention to symptoms that accompanied pain, such as: sleep disorders, chronic fatigue, noise hypersensitivity, and pain referral within the face or other areas of the head. An important aspect was the necessity for analgesic drug administration.

After patient enrollment the treatment of masseter muscle pain consisted of intramuscular injection of 21 U (mice units) of type A botulinum toxin (Botox, Allergan), in the area of the greatest cross-section surface of both masseter bellies.

Clinical algesimetry, e.g. the evaluation of pain intensity with the use of various scales is not devoid of subjective influence. However, it is the currently indicated method of measuring pain intensity at following appointments. For the purpose of the study two scales were applied by the authors: VAS (Visual Analogue Scale) and VNRS (Verbal Numerical Rating Scale). VAS is a psychometric response scale which can be used in questionnaires [30]. It is a measurement instrument for characteristics or attitudes that cannot be directly measured. Participants specify their level of pain intensity to a statement by indicating a position along a continuous line between two end-points (0–10). VNRS comprises assessment that is based on a numerical 10–point scale (0–10) in combination with a color-coded scale in which the increase in the score is accompanied by the increase in color intensity indicated on the scale. Mean intensity of pain was evaluated by subjects 1 week before the injection (examination I) and 24 weeks after the injection because of potential absence of BTXA activity (examination II).

The results were analyzed using the Wilcoxon matched pairs test, with statistical significance at $p \leq 0,005$. The software used in the statistical analysis was STATISTICA version 8 (StatSoft Inc., Tulsa, Oklahoma, USA).

## Results

The most frequently reported complaints included: spontaneous masseter muscle pain and/or temporomandibular joint pain, clicking in the temporomandibular joint during mandible movements, impaired mastication and tension-type headaches in the anterior temporal region, medial temporal region and/or occipital region. The pain was dull, squeezing, or crushing, rarely encircling the head, and it lasted for minimum four hours daily and had been present for at least 4 months. It was unpleasant for the patients but it did not interfere with their everyday quality of life. Medication- and injury-induced migraine headache was excluded.

Table 1 presents the clinical parameters of reported headaches which have been diagnosed in the study group during examination I and II such as characteristics of pain, pain duration, accompanying symptoms of pain, referral of pain and applied analgesic drugs. The collected data have shown the valid decrease in the number of each parameter. The headache intensity which have been assessed using VAS & VNRS are presented in Fig. 1. The statistical analysis is presented in Table 2 and showed a significant decrease of reported VAS & VNRS values in examination II ($p = 0,00000$).

It is important that mean value of headache intensity during examination I was 4,86 points (maximal value 8), while the result of examination II was only 1,21 (maximal value 4). The difference between them was statistically significant because $p = 0,000$. The comparison of the examination I and II data have shown a positive changes in tension–type headache intensity. The differences mostly included: a decrease in the number of subjects with bilateral pain in the temporal region and lower number of referred pain episodes, as well as a reduction in the amount of analgesic drugs intake.

## Discussion

Independently from the results of various studies, the relationship between tension-type headaches and temporomandibular joint dysfunction can be confirmed by the decrease in headache intensity observed after the management of temporomandibular joint dysfunction. It is apparent particularly in cases in which no significant improvement in the patient's well-being is observed after conventional neurological treatment or in which a quick recurrence of the symptoms occurs if temporomandibular joint dysfunction treatment is not initiated [5, 9, 10, 13, 17].

The aim of the population-based cross-sectional study conducted by Goncalves et al. was to determine the coexistence of TTH and TMJD in adult patients [31]. The results of their study indicate that such coexistence is observed frequently and that those two entities should be discussed together. The use of intramuscular BTXA injections within the masseter muscle led to positive alterations in pain intensity and the nature of complaints related with tension-type headache. Botox is, however, routinely deposited for neurological purposes within the temporal, occipital, and quadriceps muscles [28, 32–37].

The decrease in reported the headache following pharmacotherapy of temporomandibular joint dysfunction suggests that tension-type headaches are in many cases related to excessive and long-lasting tension within the muscles of the temporomandibular joint, which remains closely interrelated within the head and neck. After the injections, the character of tension-type headache changed and its intensity decreased. Moreover, a decrease in the daily number of hours and monthly number of days during which tension-type headache affected the patient, was observed [34, 37–40].

Numerous authors in contemporary literature underline the role played by stress in the development of TTH. At the same time, for several years authors of various studies concerning etiological factors of TMJD have been underlining that stress is an increasingly important etiological factor in its development [41]. Also, the results of studies by Yancey et al., which showed that psychorelaxation treatment and behavioral techniques were effective in treating this pathology, indicate that psychogenic factors play an important role in the development of tension-type headaches [42].

Jackson et al. have shown in the meta-analysis concerning the use of BTXA in the prophylaxis of migraine and tension-type headaches that the discussed drug had a positive effect in both disorders [36]. According to them, however, one should pay attention to the possibility of complications related with the application method of the drug. Singh and Sahota stressed that Botox plays

**Table 1** The number of reported pain parameters collected in examination I and II

| Tension-type headache | | | Examination I | Examination II |
|---|---|---|---|---|
| 1. Characteristics of pain | Spontaneous headache | Unilateral | 13 | 7 |
| | | Bilateral | 29 | 20 |
| | Provoked headache | Unilateral | 8 | 3 |
| | | Bilateral | 13 | 9 |
| | Dull | | 13 | 5 |
| | Squeezing | | 9 | 4 |
| | Crushing | | 10 | 3 |
| | Encircling | | 6 | 1 |
| | Throbbing | | 4 | 2 |
| 2. Pain duration | Daily/h | | 4–6 | 2–3 |
| | Weekly/days | | 5 | 3 |
| 3. Accompanying symptoms of pain | Sleep disorders | | 19 | 5 |
| | Chronic fatigue | | 28 | 4 |
| | Noise hypersensitivity | | 5 | 1 |
| | Appetite loss | | 6 | 1 |
| 4. Referral of pain | Within the face | | 16 | 5 |
| | Within the head | | 9 | 1 |
| 5. Applied analgesic drugs | Non-steroidal anti-inflammatory drugs | | 18 | 2 |
| | Paracetamol | | 8 | 1 |

a key role in the treatment of chronic headaches, independently from essential education concerning hygiene and lifestyle modification [43].

The results of in vivo and in vitro research performed by Ashkenazi and Blumenfeld have shown that botulinum toxin type A is effective in reducing tension-type headache intensity [44]. The study has shown that this drug is effective, safe, and well tolerated in the treatment of headache. The drug is administered every 12 weeks, which is convenient for some patients when compared with taking analgesic drugs every day [45]. Mathew et al. underlined that botulinum toxin may be a good solution for the patients in whom oral medications (nonsteroidal anti-inflammatory drugs, local anesthetics and gabapentin)

have not been effective [46]. A 5-year observation of 1347 patients treated due to chronic headache using 100 mice units (MU) of botulinum toxin performed by Farinelli et al. has showed that the drug is effective and well tolerated by the patients. Absence of positive treatment outcomes were observed in only 1.6 % of the patients [47]. The study of Christidis et al. showed that other injection therapy is effective in muscle-related headaches e.g. repeated intramuscular tender-point injections with the serotonin type 3 antagonist granisetron are useful in myofascial temporomandibular disorders management [48]. It's mean that in close future physicians will be able to choose treatment option from many of injection therapies concerning temporomandibular disorders-related muscle pain.

Taking into account a positive results of the BTXA injections applied in the study, it should be noted that the dose of 21 U and used operative technique are sufficient to decrease the masseter muscle pain in patients with

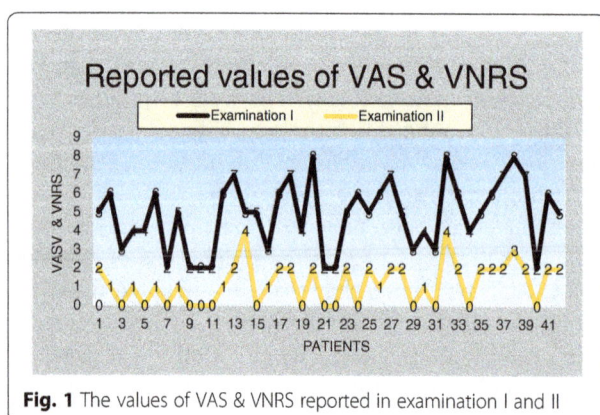

**Fig. 1** The values of VAS & VNRS reported in examination I and II

**Table 2** The results of statistical analysis concerning reported values of VAS & VNRS

| | Examination I | Examination II |
|---|---|---|
| Average ± SD | 4,86 ± 1,84 | 1,21 ± 1,12 |
| Median | 5 | 1 |
| Min - Max | 2–8 | 0–4 |
| Wilcoxon matched pairs test | $p = 0,00000$ | |

temporomandibular joint dysfunction and tension-type headache. However we don't know what happens after 6 months observations. We can assume that with the passage of time the effect of the neurotoxin goes away and the patient will begin to feel the pain again. We are able to repeat whole procedure in a case of recurrence. We have to know that current studies proofed that BTXA injections cause mandible bone loss and uncontrolled structural changes in affected and unaffected muscles [49, 50]. Therefore we have to emphasized that BTXA injections should be taken under consideration as a treatment of choice but not primary option in masseter muscle pain management and the dose should be kept as small as possible.

## Conclusion

The intramuscular botulinum toxin type A injections have been an efficient method of treatment in a case of masseter muscle pain in patients with temporomandibular joint dysfunction and tension-type headache. The authors recommend this therapy as a method of choice in a masseter muscle pain management.

### Abbreviations
TMJD: temporomandibular joint dysfunction; TTH: tension-type headache; BTXA: botulinum toxin type A; VAS: visual analogue scale; VNRS: verbal numerical rating scale.

### Competing interests
The authors declare that they have no competing interests.

### Authors' contributions
MP created research concept, performed intramuscular injections of botulinum toxin, collected data and edited the manuscript. EF selected the references. MSz wrote and edited the manuscript. KK performed neurological examination. MW wrote and edited the manuscript and finally revised it before submission. All authors read and approved the final manuscript.

### Acknowledgments
Publishing charge was supported by KNOW (Leading National Research Centre) at the Jagiellonian University in Krakow.

### Author details
[1]Department of Dental Prosthetics, Jagiellonian University in Krakow, College of Medicine, Institute of Dentistry, 4 Montelupich St., 31-155 Krakow, Poland. [2]Department of Neurology, Jagiellonian University in Krakow, College of Medicine, 3 Botaniczna St., 31-503 Krakow, Poland. [3]Department of Prosthetic Dentistry, Faculty of Dentistry, Wroclaw Medical University, 26 Krakowska St., 50-425 Wroclaw, Poland.

### References
1. Liu F, Steinkeler A (2013) Epidemiology, diagnosis, and treatment of temporomandibular disorders. Dent Clin North Am 57(3):465–479
2. Glaros A, Williams K, Lauste L (2005) The role of parafunctions, emotions and stress in predicting facial pain. J Am Dent Assoc 136:451–458
3. Nicholson RA, Houle TT, Rhudy JL et al (2007) Psychological risk factors in headache. Headache 47:413–426
4. Wu G, Chen L, Fei H, Su Y, Zhu G, Chen Y (2013) Psychological stress may contribute to temporomandibular joint disorder in rats. J Surg Res 183:223–229
5. Wieckiewicz M, Boening K, Wiland P, Shiau YY, Paradowska-Stolarz A (2015) Reported concepts for the treatment modalities and pain management of temporomandibular disorders. J Headache Pain 16(106):1–12
6. Rai B, Kaur J (2013) Association between stress, sleep quality and temporomandibular joint dysfunction: simulated Mars mission. Oman Med J 3:216–219
7. Gatchel RJ, Peng YB, Peters ML, Fuchs PN, Turk DC (2007) The biopsychosocial approach to chronic pain: scientific advances and future directions. Psychol Bull 133:581–624
8. Dahan H, Shir Y, Velly A, Allison P (2015) Specific and number of comorbidities are associated with increased levels of temporomandibular pain intensity and duration. J Headache Pain 16(528):1–10
9. Was A, Tucholska S (2011) Tension-type headache-psychological aspect. Neurologia Dziecieca 20(41):115–118
10. Rosted P, Jřrgensen A, Bundgaard M (2010) Temporomandibular dysfunction can contribute to aggravation of tension-type headache: a case report. Acupunct Med 28(3):154–155
11. Monteith T, Sprenger T (2010) Tension type headache in adolescence and childhood: where are we now? Curr Pain Headache Rep 14:424–430
12. Pihut M, Majewski P, Wisniewska G, Reron E (2011) Auriculo-vestibular symptoms related to structural and functional disorders of stomatognatic system. J Physiol Pharm 62(2):251–256
13. Branco L, Santis T, Alfaya T, Goday C, Fraqoso Y, Bussadori S (2013) Association between headache and temporomandibular joint disorders in children and addolscennts. J Oral Sci 55(1):39–43
14. Mongin F, Ciccone G, Ibertis F, Negro C (2000) Personality characteristics and accompanying symptoms in temporomandibular dysfunction, headache and facial pain. J Orofac Pain 14(1):52–58
15. Graff- Radford S, Bassiur J (2014) Temporomandibular disorders and headaches. Neurol Clin 32(2):525–527
16. Silva J, Brandão K, Faleiros B, Tavares R, Lara P, Januzzi E, Carvalho A, Carvalho E, Gomes J, Leite F, Alves B, Gómez R, Teixeira A (2014) Temporomandibular disorders are an important comorbidity of migraine and may be clinically difficult to distinguish them from tension-type headache. Arq Neuropsiquiatr 72(2):99–103
17. Blumenfeld A, Schim J, Brower J (2010) Pure tension-type headache versus tension-type headache in the migraineur. Curr Pain Headache Rep 14(6):465–469
18. Mathew P, Mathew T (2011) Taking care of the challenging tension headache patient. Curr Pain Headache Rep 15(6):444–450
19. Lebedeva ER, Kobzeva NR, Gilev DV, Olesen J (2016) Factors Associated With Primary Headache According To Diagnosis, Sex, and Social Group. Headache 56(2):341-356.
20. Freitag F (2013) Managing and treating tension-type headache. Med Clin North Am 97(2):281–292
21. Lipton R, Bigal M, Steiner T, Silberstein S, Olesen J (2004) Classification od primary headache. Neurology 63:427–435
22. Sato H, Saisu H, Muraoka W, Nakagawa T, Svensson P, Wajima K (2012) Lack of temporal summation but distinct after sensations to thermal stimulation in patients with combined tension-typeheadache and myofascial temporomandibular disorder. J Orofac Pain 26(4):288–295
23. List T, John M, Ohrbach R, Schiffman E, Truelove E, Anderson G (2012) Influence of temple headache frequency on physical functioning and emotional functioning in subjects with temporomandibular disorder. Pain 26:283–290
24. Blumenfeld A, Bender S, Glassman B, Malizia D (2011) Bruxism, temporomandibular dysfunction, tension type headache, and migraine: a comment. Headache 51(10):1549–1550
25. Evans R, Bassiur J, Schwartz A (2011) Bruxism, temporomandibular dysfunction, tension-type headache, and migraine. Headache 51(7):1169–1172
26. La Touche R, Paris-Alemany A, Gil-Martínez A, Pardo-Montero J, Angulo-Díaz-Parreño S, Fernández-Carnero J (2015) Masticatory sensory-motor changes after an experimental chewing test influenced by pain catastrophizing and neck-pain-related disability in patients with headache attributed to temporomandibular disorders. J Headache Pain 16(20):1–14
27. Vilanova LS, Garcia RC, List T, Alstergren P (2015) Diagnostic criteria for temporomandibular disorders: self-instruction or formal training and calibration? J Headache Pain 16(505):1–9
28. Dworkin SF, LeResche L (1992) Research diagnostic criteria for temporomandibular disorders: review, criteria, examinations and specifications, critique. J Craniomandibular Sleep Pract 6(4):301–355

29.  Headache Classification Subcommittee of the International Headache Society (2005) The International Classification of Headache Disorders, 2nd edn

30.  Hjermstad MJ, Fayers PM, Haugen DF, Caraceni A, Hanks GW, Loge JH, Fainsinger R, Aass N, Kaasa S (2011) Studies comparing Numerical Rating Scales, Verbal Rating Scales, and Visual Analogue Scales for assessment of pain intensity in adults: a systematic literature review. J Pain Symptom Manage 41(6):1073–1093

31.  Goncalves D, Camparis C, Speciali J, Franco A, Castanharo S, Bigal M (2011) Tmeporomandibular joint disorders are differentially associated with headache diagnoses: a controlled study. Clin J Pain 27(7):611–615

32.  Ashkenazi A, Blumenfeld A (2013) Onabotulinumtoxin A for the treatment of headache. Headache 53(2):54–61

33.  Rollnik JD, Tanneberger O, Schubert M, Schneider U, Dengler R (2000) Treatment of tension type headache with botulinum toxin type A. Headache 40:300–305

34.  Gady J, Ferneini E (2013) Botulinum toxin A and headache treatment. Conn Med 77(3):165–166

35.  Lippert-Grüner M (2012) Botulinum toxin in the treatment of post-traumatic headache - case study. Neurol Neurochir Pol 46(6):591–594

36.  Jackson J, Kuriyama A, Hayashino Y (2012) Botulinum toxin A for prophylactic treatment of migraine and tension headaches in adults: a meta-analysis. JAMA 307(16):1736–1745

37.  Levy N, Lowenthal D (2012) Application of botulinum toxin to clinical therapy: advances and cautions. Am J Ther 19(4):281–286

38.  Kaynak-Hekimhan P (2010) Noncosmetic periocular therapeutic applications of botulinum toxin. Middle East Afr J Ophthalmol 17(2):113–120

39.  Denglehem C, Maes J, Raoul G, Ferri J (2012) Botulinum toxin A: analgesic treatment for temporomandibular joint disorders. Rev Stomatol Chir Maxillofac 113(1):27–31

40.  Kotimäki J, Saarinen A (2011) Treatment of recurrent dislocation of the temporomandibular joint with botulinum toxin: an alternative approach. Duodecim 127(19):2088–2091

41.  Björling E (2009) Momentary relationship between stress and headache in adolescent girls. Headache 49:1186–1197

42.  Yancey J, Sheridan R, Koren K (2014) Chronic daily headache:diagnosis and management. Am Farm Physician 15(89):642–648

43.  Singh N, Sahota P (2013) Sleep-related headache and its management. Curr Treat Options Neurol 15(6):704–722

44.  Ashkenazi A, Blumenfeld A (2013) Onabotulinum toxin A for treatment of headache. Headache 53(Suppl. 2):54–61

45.  Persaud R, Garas G, Silva S, Stamatoglou C, Chatrath P, Patel K (2013) An evidence-based review of botulinum toxin (Botox) applications in non-cosmetic head and neck conditions. JRSM Short Rep 4(2):10

46.  Mathew N, Kailasam J, Meadors L (2008) Botulinum toxin type A for the treatment of nummular headache:four case studies. Headache 48(3):442–447

47.  Farinelli I, Coloprisco G, De Filippis S, Martelletti P (2006) Long term benefits of botulinum toxin type A (BOTOX) in chronic daily headache: a five year long experience. J Headache Pain 7(6):407–412

48.  Christidis N, Omrani S, Fredriksson L, Gjelset M, Louca S, Hedenberg-Magnusson B, Ernberg M (2015) Repeated tender point injections of granisetron alleviate chronic myofascial pain–a randomized, controlled, double-blinded trial. J Headache Pain 16(104):1–13

49.  Kün-Darbois JD, Libouban H, Chappard D (2015) Botulinum toxin in masticatory muscles of the adult rat induces bone loss at the condyle and alveolar regions of the mandible associated with a bone proliferation at a muscle enthesis. Bone 77:75–82

50.  Korfage JA, Wang J, Lie SH, Langenbach GE (2012) Influence of botulinum toxin on rabbit jaw muscle activity and anatomy. Muscle Nerve 45(5):684–691

# The associations between psychosocial aspects and TMD-pain related aspects in children and adolescents

Amal Al-Khotani[1,2*], Aron Naimi-Akbar[3], Mattias Gjelset[1], Emad Albadawi[4], Lanre Bello[5], Britt Hedenberg-Magnusson[1,2,6] and Nikolaos Christidis[1,2]

## Abstract

**Background:** Temporomandibular disorders (TMD) in children and adolescents is prevalent with pain as a common component, and has a comorbidity with psychosocial problems such as stress, depression, anxiety as well as somatic complaints. Therefore, the aim of the study was to investigate if psychosocial problems in children and adolescents are associated with TMD with pain (TMD-pain) and TMD without pain (TMD-painfree) when compared to children and adolescents without TMD.

**Methods:** This cross-sectional study consisted of 456 randomly selected children and adolescents, enrolled from 10 boy's- and 10 girl's- schools in Jeddah, between 10 and 18 years of age. On the examination day, prior to the clinical examination according to Research Diagnostic Criteria for TMD Axis I and II, the participants first answered two validated questions about TMD pain, and after that the Arabic version of the Youth Self Report scale. According to their clinical examination and diagnosis the participants were divided into three groups; non-TMD group, TMD-pain group, and TMD-painfree group.

**Results:** The TMD-pain group presents a higher frequency of the internalizing problems anxiety, depression and somatic complaints than non-TMD group ($p < 0.05$). Regarding externalizing problems the only significant association found was for aggressive behavior in the TMD-pain group ($p < 0.05$). The TMD-pain group also shows a higher frequency of social problems than the non-TMD group. However, no such difference was found when compared to the TMD-painfree group. There was also a significant association with a higher frequency of thought problems in the TMD-pain group ($p < 0.05$). The children's and adolescents' physical activities were within border line clinical range for all three groups, whereas the social competence was within the normal range. There were no significant associations between any of the groups in this respect.

**Conclusions:** TMD-pain in children and adolescents does not seem to affect the social activities. However, TMD-pain seem to have a strong association to emotional, behavior and somatic functioning, with higher frequencies of anxiety, depression, somatic problems, aggressive behavior and thought problems, than children and adolescents without TMD-pain. With respect to the biopsychosocial model the present study indicates that there are significant associations to psychosocial, somatic and behavioral comorbidities and TMD-pain in children and adolescents in the Middle East region.

**Keywords:** Temporomandibular disorders, Children, Adolescents, Psychosocial, Pain

* Correspondence: aalkhotani@yahoo.com
[1]Orofacial Pain and Jaw Function, Department of Dental Medicine, Karolinska Institutet, SE-141 04 Huddinge, Sweden
[2]Scandinavian Center for Orofacial Neurosciences (SCON), Huddinge, Sweden
Full list of author information is available at the end of the article

## Background

Temporomandibular disorders (TMD) is multifactorial broad-band term that embraces chronic pain conditions and dysfunction (both painful and painfree dysfunctions) in the orofacial region affecting the masticatory muscles, the temporomandibular joints (TMJ) and their associated structures. TMD is often associated with restricted mouth opening capacity, pain upon chewing, muscle soreness and headache. Although TMD is not life threatening, it affects quality of life considerably [1].

Recent studies indicate that the prevalence of diagnosed TMD in children and adolescents is increasing, and reaching as many as 27 % of the children and adolescents in the general population (personal communication, 2016) and approximately 30 % in a clinical setting [2, 3]. In older studies from 15 years ago the prevalence was approximately 7–14 % [4, 5]. More than 80 % of the children and adolescents diagnosed with TMD were complaining of orofacial pain (personal communication, 2016).

Further, it is well known that psychosocial problems in children and adolescents are more frequent than in the past, and also that these problems have a negative effect on children's wellbeing [6]. Further, according to the biopsychosocial theory, somatic pain is directly associated with psychological, biological as well as social perspectives. This association often continues to adulthood, consequently with a risk of extension of both somatic pain and psychosocial burdens [7, 8]. As for more general pain conditions, the biopsychosocial theory can also be applied for TMD. Several studies have shown that patients suffering from TMD also reported different psychosocial problems [9–11], somatic complaints [12], and functional impairments [13] at various intensities. Other studies have shown strong associations between TMD and emotional stress, depression, anxiety and somatic complaints [2, 14, 15]. Similarly, it has been shown that children and adolescents suffering from pain often are diagnosed with psychological conditions, including depressive disorders, and a long-term diminished quality of life [16].

Two earlier studies have investigated the relationship between TMD and behavior as well as psychosocial functioning in children and adolescents [17, 18], using the Youth Self Report scale (YSR; ASEBA School-Age Forms & Profiles) [19], or part of it. The YSR is a reliable and validated scale that evaluates competencies, psychosocial, and somatic problems in many dimensional relationships in the younger ages [20]. According to Achenbach's guidelines, YSR can be applied in children and adolescents with a mental age of 10 but not exceeding the age of 18 [19]. One of the studies presented the psychosocial functioning among patients with TMD reporting pain [17, 18], whereas in the other study, participants who reported pain (from a questionnaire) had the chance to be examined for TMD [17, 18]. None of the studies found any association between the psychosocial functioning in children and adolescents with TMD with pain and children and adolescents without TMD as well as between children and adolescents with TMD without pain and children and adolescents without TMD.

Taken together, there is a high prevalence of TMD in children and adolescents with pain as a common component with a comorbidity with psychosocial problems such as stress, depression, anxiety as well as somatic complaints. With this in mind, the hypothesis of the present study was that psychosocial problems in children and adolescents are associated with a diagnosis of TMD with pain (TMD-pain) than a diagnosis of TMD without pain (TMD-painfree). Therefore, the aim of the study was to investigate if psychosocial problems in children and adolescents are associated with TMD-pain and TMD-painfree when compared to a children and adolescents without TMD.

## Methods

The present study was a cross sectional study, carried out on children and adolescents among the general population from a major city in Saudi Arabia (Jeddah). It was approved by the local ethical committee at the Department of Medical Study and Research, Ministry of Health, Jeddah, Saudi Arabia. Prior to inclusion all participants received both written and verbal information, and gave their verbal and written consent. The study followed the guidelines of the Declaration of Helsinki.

### Participants

The education in Saudi Arabia is based on single-sex schools. Hence, in order to obtain a representative sample of the entire Jeddah city, the selection was based on a predefined set of schools, as clustered by the ministry of education. Therefore, the city of Jeddah was divided into five regions (North, South, East, West, and Central). From each region two schools with boys and two schools with girls were randomly selected. The randomization from each region was performed by a researcher (NC), who did not participate in data collection, with an internet-based application (www.randomization.com). Further, from each school one class, with an average of 30 pupils, was also randomly selected using simple sampling method; hence, the school classes' titles are drawn from a bucket by dental assistant not participating in the data collection.

In order to achieve generalizable results, all possible participants were invited, thus the present study did not have any exclusion criteria. Out of the 633 children and adolescents who were invited to participate, 509 voluntarily agreed to participate, and 456 completed all questionnaires and participated in the clinical examination, aged between 10 and 18 years, as shown in Fig. 1.

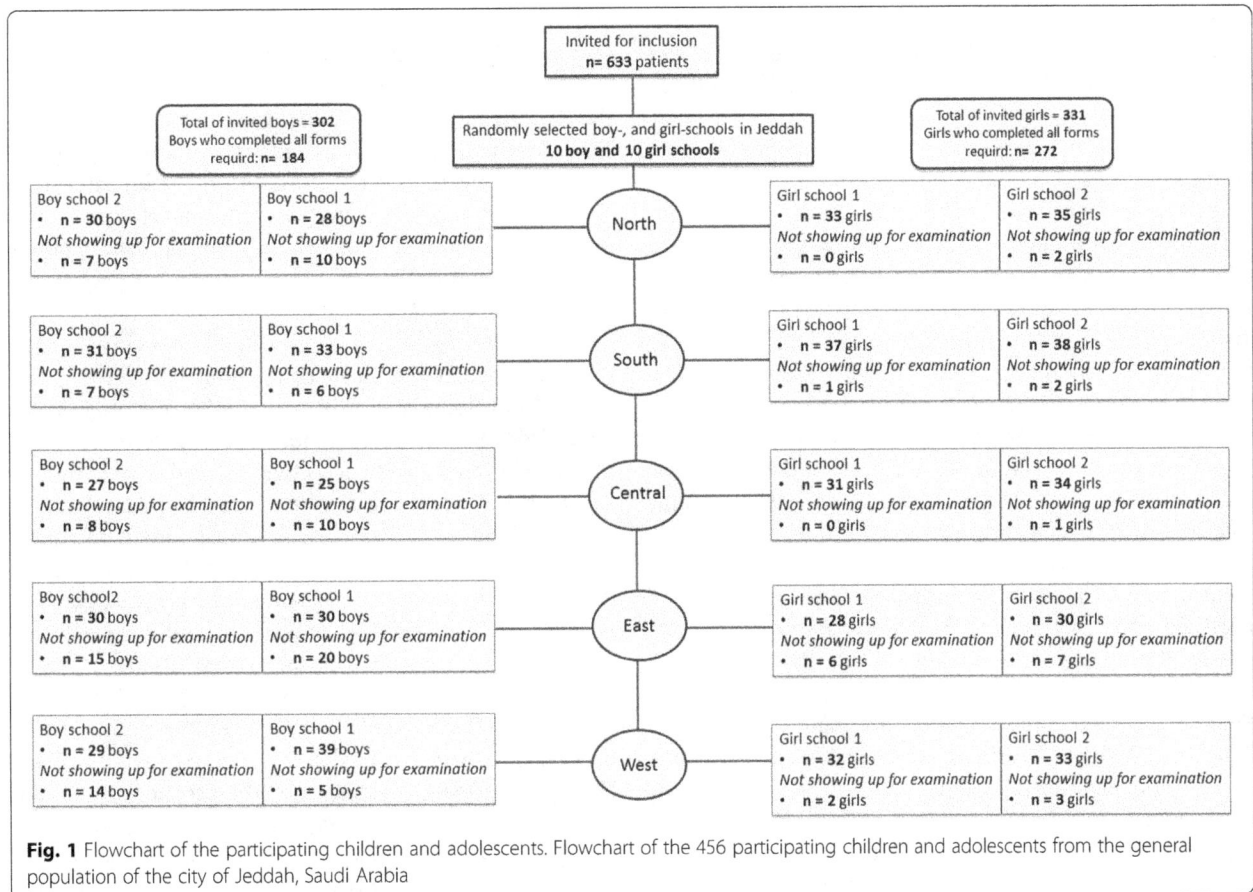

**Fig. 1** Flowchart of the participating children and adolescents. Flowchart of the 456 participating children and adolescents from the general population of the city of Jeddah, Saudi Arabia

## Study protocol

This study presents the Axis II of the Research Diagnostic Criteria for TMD (RDC/TMD). Axis I of the RDC/TMD is presented in another study (not yet published), thus, the phrase "personal communication, 2016" will be used in this study in order to refer to the previous findings from that study. According to the outcomes of the Axis I in the RDC/TMD examination (personal communication, 2016) the children and adolescents were divided into three groups; a) non-TMD which includes children and adolescents without any TMD diagnosis; b) TMD-pain which includes children and adolescents having a TMD diagnosis with pain; and c) TMD-painfree which includes children and adolescents having a TMD diagnosis without pain".

Due to cultural considerations, there was one protocol for boys and one for girls. All girls were examined in the school nurse's room using a mobile dental chair. However, all boys were invited to be examined at a dental clinic of the primary health care center for each region. In order to minimize the impact of the surroundings during the examination equal equipment were used at both examination facilities.

### Protocol for girls

One day before the clinical examination, proper information about the purpose of the study and a brief explanation of the questionnaires was presented to all girls and their parents, and the RDC/TMD history questionnaire was distributed in sealed envelopes. From the RDC/TMD questionnaire, demographic data (including ethnic and socioeconomic background information), medical history, presence of oral parafunctions, headache, previous trauma to the face, and use of oral appliances was retrieved. In addition, the scores for the Graded Chronic Pain Scale (GCPS) included in the questionnaire were also retrieved.

On the day of examination, the girls were asked to fill in the official Arabic version of the Youth Self Report (YSR), licensed from ASEBA/Research Center for Children, Youth & Families, university of Vermont, Burlington, USA. After completing this questionnaire, each participant was asked two validated questions about the presence of orofacial pain (TMD-pain) [21, 22]; 1) *"Do you have pain in the temple, face, temporomandibular joint, or jaws once a week or more?"* 2) *"Do you have pain when you open your mouth wide or chew once a week or more?"*. Finally, the clinical examination of the temporomandibular region according to the RDC/TMD Axis I protocol was performed by one examiner (A A-K), trained in this procedure by an orofacial pain specialist (Malin Ernberg; calibrated to a gold-standard examiner (Thomas List)).

### Protocol for boys

One appointment was offered to each presumable participant and proper information about the purpose of the study and a brief explanation of the questionnaires was presented to all boys and their parents. As for the girls the RDC/TMD questionnaire including the GCPS, the YSR questionnaire and the demographic data (including ethnic and socioeconomic background information), medical history, presence of oral parafunctions, headache, previous trauma to the face, and use of oral appliances was retrieved before the clinical examination. The boys were accompanied by a parent/guardian to the clinic but the parents were asked to wait outside the clinical room. However, if the parent insisted to attend together with their child, they were asked to remain passive during the entire session.

### Emotional/behavior and somatic functioning

The RDC/TMD is a widely used dual diagnostic tool (Axis I and II), also reliable to be used in children and adolescents [21]. Axis I is used in order to diagnose TMD and Axis II in order to identify psychosocial and somatic symptoms using the Symptom Checklist-90-Revised (SCL-90-R). However, the SCL-90-R is not validated for children and adolescents younger than 13 years of age [23], and was therefore replaced with YSR, which is a scale that shares the same purpose but for children and adolescents in all school ages [20].

The emotional and behavior functioning were assessed using the YSR [20]. The YSR comprises of two main domains: 1) Problem Checklist, and 2) Social competence. The Problem Checklist contains 112 problem statements. As in a previous study regarding TMD pain in adults in Saudi Arabia, 3 statements about sexual problems were removed in the current study, due to cultural considerations [24]. The statements of the Problem Checklist explicate the major clusters: anxiety, depression, somatic complain, aggressive disorders, as well as social and attention problems. The major clusters are grouped into 3 subscales; a) broad-band internalizing and externalizing, b) eight narrow-band syndromes, c) DSM-oriented scales [20]. The eight narrow band syndromes are; 1) Anxious/Depressed, 2) Withdrawn/Depressed, 3) Somatic Complaints, 4) Social problems, 5) Thought problems, 6) Attention problems, 7) Rule-breaking behavior, and 8) Aggressive behavior. The DSM-oriented scales include; I) Affective problems, II) Anxiety problems, III) Somatic problems, IV) Attention Deficit/Hyperactivity problems, V) Oppositional Defiant problems,

and VI) Conduct problems. Each statement is rated as 0 (not true), 1 (somewhat or sometimes true), or 2 (very true or often true) The YSR is reliable and valid [20]. Both for the data entry (scores) and for proper data grouping into the subscales, a licensed software scoring program (ASEBA™ version 9.1) was used. As a result, percentiles and T-scores are presented for all subscales and syndromes. The normal T-score range for all syndromes is 50–64, the border line clinical range is 65–69, while the clinical range is 70–100.

### Physical activities and social competence

The second domain of YSR, i.e., the Social competence, comprises of seven statements which cover three areas; social relations, physical activities, and the mean of self-reported academic performance [20]. Also for this domain the licensed software scoring program (ASEBA™ version 9.1) was used. As a result, percentiles and T-scores are presented for all activities and social competences. The normal T-score range is 36–65, the border line clinical range is 32–35, while the clinical range is 20–31.

The Graded Chronic Pain Scale (GCPS) [25] is included in the RDC/TMD Axis II [26]. The GCPS severity scale is divided into two parts. The first part is used to assess characteristic pain intensity and the second part limitations in physical functioning due to pain, including disability days. The disability days comprises of four grades (0–3) where 0 = 0–6 disability days, 1 = 7–14 disability days, 2 = 15–30 disability days, and 3 = 31+ disability days. However, when assessing physical functioning disability points (DP 0–6) is combined with pain intensity (0–100) as follows: Grade 0 = no TMD-pain in the previous 6 months; Grade I = low disability (<3 DP) and low intensity pain (<50); Grade II = low disability (<3 DP) and high intensity pain (>50); Grade III = high disability, moderately limiting (3–4 DP regardless of pain intensity); Grade IV = high disability, severely limiting (5–6 DP regardless of pain intensity).

### Statistics

Depending on the diagnoses that are presented in a previous study (personal communication, 2016), 456 participants were divided into three groups; non-TMD, TMD-pain and TMD-painfree. According to the power calculation 450 children and adolescents were necessary to detect true odds ratios for disease of 0.538 up to 1.860 with a power of 90 % and a significance level of 0.05, but 633 were invited due to the risk of children and adolescents not showing up for examination.

The descriptive statistics are presented as mean (SD) and median (IQR) depending on distribution of data, and also frequencies (%). To analyze differences in T-scores between the three groups the median score was modeled using quantile regression. In the model not adjusted for potential confounding factors TMD groups was included as dichotomous dummy variables with non-TMD as the reference group. The multivariate model adjusting for potential confounding factors also included sex (male/female), age (10–13 years/14–18 years), as well as Saudi Arabian nationality (yes/no) as dichotomous variables. Family income was modeled as a dichotomous dummy variables and it included 3 categories (below average/average/above average) which was based on the average income in Saudi Arabia for the year 2013 (15 000 SR/month) (www.cdsi.gov.sa). Subgroup analyzes stratified on sex and age groups separately were also performed with the stratification variable excluded from the model. $P$-values were based on 100 bootstrap samples. All analyzes were performed in STATA 12 SE. $P$-values lower than 0.05 and confidence intervals not including 0 were considered statistically significant.

## Results
### Study population
The demographic characteristics for all children and adolescents are presented in Table 1. They were categorized into one of three groups; a) the non-TMD group: all children and adolescents with no definite diagnosis, b) the TMD-painfree group: children and adolescents diagnosed with either osteoarthrosis and/or disc displacement with or without reduction, and c) TMD-pain group: children and adolescents diagnosed with either

**Table 1** Demographic data from 456 randomly selected children and adolescents in the general population of the city of Jeddah, Saudi Arabia

| | Non-TMD n (%) | TMD-painfree n (%) | TMD-pain n (%) |
|---|---|---|---|
| Individuals | 332 (72.8 %) | 26 (5.7 %) | 98 (21.5 %) |
| Age | | | |
|   Mean (SD) | 13.9 (2.3) | 14.6 (2.3) | 14.2 (2.4) |
|   Min-max | 10–18 | 12–18 | 11–18 |
|     10–13 years | 177 (53.3 %) | 10 (38.5 %) | 48 (49 %) |
|     14–18 years | 155 (46.7 %) | 16 (61.5) | 50 (51 %) |
| Sex | | | |
|   Boys | 138 (41.6 %) | 11 (42.3 %) | 35 (35.7 %) |
|   Girls | 194 (58.4 %) | 15 (57.7 %) | 63 (64.3 %) |
| Ethnic origin | | | |
|   Saudi Arabia | 217 (65.4 %) | 13 (50 %) | 61 (62.2 %) |
|   Non-Saudi[a] | 115 (34.6 %) | 13 (50 %) | 37 (37.8 %) |
| Parental income | | | |
|   Below average | 172 (53.4 %) | 11 (45.8 %) | 50 (51.6 %) |
|   Average | 109 (33.9 %) | 11 (45.8 %) | 29 (30 %) |
|   Above average | 41 (12.7 %) | 2 (8.3 %) | 18 (18.6 %) |

[a]Middle East, Gulf Area and Africa

myofascial pain with or without limited mouth opening and/or arthralgia and/or osteoarthritis. Of note, none of the children was diagnosed with disc displacement with reduction (personal communication, 2016). There were no differences among the groups in regards to demographic characteristics nor when medical and oral health were taken into consideration (personal communication, 2016). There were further no differences when taking the ethnic origin into consideration, i.e., between the Saudi and the Non-Saudi participants, neither in the background data nor in any of the outcomes.

### Emotional/behavior and somatic functioning
#### Broad band internalizing and externalizing scale and narrow-band syndrome scale
The mean and median range of T-scores were within normal range in all three groups (50–64) for all syndromes of the narrow-band syndrome scale. In the unadjusted analysis the TMD-pain group presents significant associations with an increase in T-scores of internalizing problems, i.e., Anxious/Depressed, Withdrawn/Depressed and Somatic Complaints, when compared to the non-TMD group ($p < 0.05$). In the adjusted analysis, however, the TMD-pain group presents a significant association with the internalizing problems Withdrawn/Depressed as well as with Somatic Complaints ($p < 0.05$), as shown in Table 2.

In the subgroup analyzes stratified on age there was a stronger association with increase in T-score for internalizing problems Anxious/Depressed and TMD-pain in the younger age group (10–13 years) (Coefficient = 5; 95 % CI: 0.9–9.1) compared to the older age group (14–18 years) (coefficient = 1; 95 % CI: – 3.1–5.1). Both retrieved from adjusted analyzes ($p < 0.05$).

Regarding externalizing problems the only significant association found was for Aggressive Behavior in the TMD-pain group according to the unadjusted analysis ($p < 0.05$), Table 2.

Further, the TMD-pain group showed a significant increase in Social problems than the non-TMD group both in the unadjusted and adjusted analysis ($p < 0.05$), shown in Table 2. When the internalized syndromes of the narrow-band syndrome scales were analyzed s stratified on sex, there were stronger associations with increased T-scores and TMD-pain among boys than girls, Anxious/Depressed (Coefficient = 5; 95 % CI: 0.4–9.6), Somatic Complaints (Coefficient = 10; 95 % CI: 4.9–15.1) ($p < 0.001$), and Attention Problem (Coefficient = 4; 95 % CI: 1.3–6.7) ($p < 0.05$) (presented coefficients are for boys). Further, there was more increased T-score associated with TMD-pain in the narrow-band syndrome Anxious/Depressed in the younger age group (10–13) compared to the older (10–13) (Coefficient =5; 95 % CI: 1.0–9.1) ($p < 0.05$). Finally, there was also a significant

**Table 2** Associations between TMD and internalizing problems, externalizing problems, social, thought and attention problems. Regression coefficients are presented with 95 % confidence intervals retrieved from quantile regression analysis

| | Syndromes | Non-TMD | TMD-painfree | TMD-pain |
|---|---|---|---|---|
| Internalizing problems | Anxious/Depressed | | | |
| | Unadjusted Coeff. | ref | −2 | 4[a] |
| | 95 % CI | | (−8.2)–4.2 | 1.2–6.6 |
| | Adjusted Coeff. | ref | −4 | 2 |
| | 95 % CI | | (−8.2)–0.2 | (−1)–5 |
| | Withdrawn/Depressed | | | |
| | Unadjusted Coeff. | ref | −1 | 3[a] |
| | 95 % CI | | (−4.5)–2.5 | 1.1–5 |
| | Adjusted Coeff. | ref | −1 | 3[a] |
| | 95 % CI | | (−4.4)–2.4 | 0.7–5.2 |
| | Somatic Complaints | | | |
| | Unadjusted Coeff. | ref | −1 | 5[a] |
| | 95 % CI | | (−4.1)–2.1 | 0.9–9.1 |
| | Adjusted Coeff. | ref | −1 | 5[a] |
| | 95 % CI | | (−4.4)–2.4 | 1.7–8.3 |
| | Social Problems | | | |
| | Unadjusted Coeff. | ref | −3 | 4[a] |
| | 95 % CI | | (−6.4)–0.4 | (−1.9)–6.1 |
| | Adjusted Coeff. | ref | −3 | 3[a] |
| | 95 % CI | | (−6.6)–0.6 | 0.7–5.3 |
| | Thought Problems | | | |
| | Unadjusted Coeff. | ref | 1 | 3[a] |
| | 95 % CI | | (−1.7)–3.7 | 1.3–4.7 |
| | Adjusted Coeff. | ref | 0 | 1 |
| | 95 % CI | | (−2.2)–2.2 | (−0.7)–2.7 |
| | Attention Problem | | | |
| | Unadjusted Coeff. | ref | −1 | 2 |
| | 95 % CI | | (−4.2)–2.2 | (−0.8)–4.8 |
| | Adjusted Coeff. | ref | −0.5 | 1.5 |
| | 95 % CI | | (−3.7)–2.7 | (−0.6)–3.6 |
| Externalizing problems | Rule-Breaking Behavior | | | |
| | Unadjusted Coeff. | ref | −1 | 0 |
| | 95 % CI | | (−2.8)–0.8 | (−1.5)–1.5 |
| | Adjusted Coeff. | ref | −1 | 0 |
| | 95 % CI | | (−2.8)–0.8 | (−1.3)–1.3 |
| | Aggressive Behavior | | | |
| | Unadjusted Coeff. | ref | 1 | 3[a] |
| | 95 % CI | | (−2.6)–4.6 | 0.2–5.8 |
| | Adjusted Coeff. | ref | 0 | 2 |
| | 95 % CI | | (−2.9)–2.9 | (−0.2)–4.2 |

[a] = significant difference between TMD-pain group and TMD-painfree (p < 0.05)
Both unadjusted analysis and adjusted for age, sex, ethnic origin and parental income are presented

association of Thought problems in the TMD-pain group with the unadjusted analysis (p < 0.05). This association was not found in the adjusted analysis, also Table 2.

### DSM-oriented scales

Table 3 shows that children and adolescents in the TMD-pain group reported presence of affective, anxiety, and somatic problems in the DSM-oriented scales significantly compared to non-TMD in both the unadjusted and adjusted analyses (p < 0.05). This significance was not found when compared to the TMD-painfree group.

**Table 3** Associations between TMD and DSM-Oriented scale: Regression coefficients are presented with 95 % confidence intervals retrieved from quantile regression analysis

| | Non-TMD | TMD-painfree | TMD-pain |
|---|---|---|---|
| Affective problems | | | |
| Unadjusted Coeff. | ref | 3 | 4[a] |
| 95 % CI | | (−0.1)–6.1 | 2.2–5.8 |
| Adjusted Coeff. | ref | 1 | 3[a] |
| 95 % CI | | (−2.8)–4.8 | 0.5–5.5 |
| Anxiety problems | | | |
| Unadjusted Coeff. | ref | 0 | 3[a] |
| 95 % CI | | (−2.7)–2.7 | 0.3–5.7 |
| Adjusted Coeff. | ref | −1 | 4[a] |
| 95 % CI | | (−3.9)–1.9 | 1.3–6.7 |
| Somatic problems | | | |
| Unadjusted Coeff. | ref | −1 | 5[a] |
| 95 % CI | | (−2.6)–0.6 | 3.2–6.8 |
| Adjusted Coeff. | ref | −1 | 3.5[a] |
| 95 % CI | | (−2.8)–0.8 | 1.3–5.7 |
| Attention deficit/hyperactivity problems | | | |
| Unadjusted Coeff. | ref | 0 | 1 |
| 95 % CI | | (−1.5)–1.5 | (−0.7)–2.7 |
| Adjusted Coeff. | ref | 0 | 1 |
| 95 % CI | | (−1.5)–1.5 | (−0.4)–2.4 |
| Oppositional defiant problems | | | |
| Unadjusted Coeff. | ref | 0 | 0 |
| 95 % CI | | (−1.2)–1.2 | (−1.1)–1.1 |
| Adjusted Coeff. | ref | −0.3 | 0.5 |
| 95 % CI | | (−1.5)–0.8 | (−0.4)–1.4 |
| Conduct problems | | | |
| Unadjusted Coeff. | ref | −1 | 2 |
| 95 % CI | | (−4.2)–2.2 | (−0.8)–4.8 |
| Adjusted Coeff. | ref | −0.5 | 1.5 |
| 95 % CI | | (−3.7)–2.7 | (−0.6)–3.6 |

[a] = significant difference between TMD-pain group and TMD-painfree (p < 0.05)
Both unadjusted analysis and adjusted for age, sex, ethnic origin and parental income are presented

When the DSM-oriented scales were analyzed separately for age groups and sex there was a significantly increased risk to develop Affective Problems (Coefficient = 5; 95 % CI: 1.0–9.0), and Anxiety Problems (Coefficient = 3; 95 % CI: 0.7–5.3) ($p < 0.05$) in the younger age group (10–13) compared to the older age group (14–18) with TMD-pain. Further, a significant increase in Attention Deficit/Hyperactivity Problems T-scores (Coefficient =4; 95 % CI: 1.7–6.3) and Oppositional Defiant Problems (Coefficient =2; 95 % CI: 0.3–3.7) associated with TMD-pain in boys than girls. Further, there is also an increase Oppositional Defiant Problems (Coefficient =2; 95 % CI: 0.2–3.8) ($p < 0.05$) associated with TMD-pain in older age group (14–18) than younger age group (10–13).

### Physical activities and social competence

The mean range for children's physical activities were within border line clinical range for all three groups, whereas the social competence was within the normal range (Table 4). There were no significant associations between the TMD-pain, TMD-painfree, and non-TMD groups in this respect.

According to the GCPS, the children and adolescents in the TMD-pain group scored significantly higher frequencies in the higher severity grades (Grade I, II and III) than the children and adolescents in the non-TMD and TMD-painfree groups ($p < 0.05$), as shown in Fig. 2.

### Discussion

Emotions and/or emotional influences, either pleasant or un-pleasant, play a great role in the pain experience in children and adolescents with a TMD pain condition [27]. Likewise the current study indicates that emotions have a significant association to TMD-pain in children. This since the present study showed significant associations in children and adolescents with a TMD-pain diagnosis and all internalizing problems investigated, i.e., Anxious/Depressed, Withdrawn/Depressed, Somatic Complaints. These findings are coinciding with the findings of previous studies showing that anxiety and depression frequently occur in children and adolescents having TMD signs and/or symptoms [28, 29]. The findings of the present study are also in accordance with other studies, who stated that adolescents with increased TMD-pain had significantly higher frequencies of internalizing problems (i.e., depression, anxiety and somatic complaint) and aggressive behavior compared to healthy controls [7, 18]. This was also reported in a study that showed that children and adolescents who repeatedly visited physicians for their orofacial pain also were complaining of depression in the form of sadness, anger, sleep disturbances as well as problems in school attendance. As a remark that study also reported that

**Table 4** The range for children's physical activities and their social competence in 456 randomly selected children and adolescents in the general population of the city of Jeddah, Saudi Arabia

|  | Non-TMD | TMD-painfree | TMD-pain |
|---|---|---|---|
| Activites |  |  |  |
| Mean (SD) | 32.6 (7.7) | 35.8 (8) | 33.4 (7.7) |
| Median (IQR) | 32 (11) | 35 (6) | 35 (12) |
| Min-max | 20–65 | 22–61 | 20–52 |
| Unadjusted | ref | 3 | 1 |
| 95 % CI |  | (−0.4)–6.4 | (−2.1)–4.1 |
| Adjusted | ref | 2 | 0.5 |
| 95 % CI |  | (−1.1)–5.1 | (−2.5)–3.5 |
| Social |  |  |  |
| Mean (SD) | 40.5 (7.3) | 41.3 (6.6) | 41.3 (6.7) |
| Median (IQR) | 41 (11) | 43 (10) | 41 (10) |
| Min-max | 25–62 | 28–50 | 29–59 |
| Unadjusted | ref | 2 | 0 |
| 95 % CI |  | (−2.7)–6.7 | (−2.2)–2.2 |
| Adjusted | ref | 1 | 0 |
| 95 % CI |  | (−3.4)–5.4 | (−2.5)–2.5 |

myofascial pain in the orofacial region in children and adolescents often is misdiagnosed as recurrent ear infections [30]. An explanation for the increased pain sensation might be due to the fact that anxiety exacerbates the masticatory muscle tension by clenching and grinding, which in turn leads to an increased release of pro-inflammatory cytokines followed by a sensitization of the whole pain

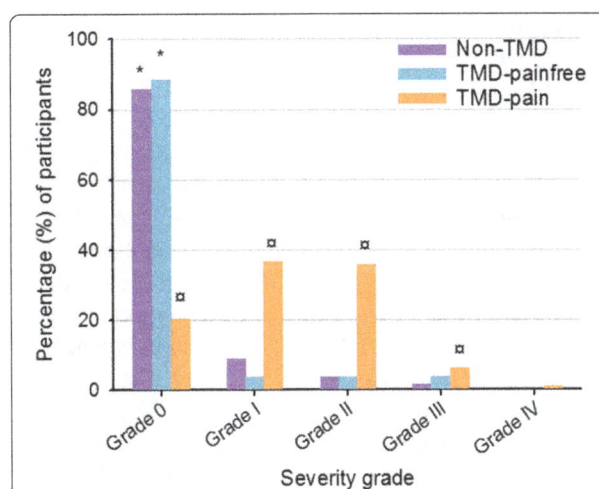

**Fig. 2** Differences in the severity grades of the Graded Chronic Pain Scale for the three different groups (non-TMD; TMD-pain; TMD-painfree). Children and adolescents in the TMD-pain group scored significantly higher frequencies in the severity grades (i.e., higher than Grade 0) of the Graded Chronic Pain Scale (GCPS) than children and adolescents in the non-TMD and TMD-painfree groups ($p < 0.05$)

pathway [31]. Furthermore, another study reported a significant association between TMD and anxiety [32]. However, in contrast to the present study, that study did not find any association between TMD and depression [32]. One explanation to this difference could be the fact that they included a younger age group (8–12 years) than the present study (10–18 years). Another could be that they have used a different scale that was not validated for children, the Hospital Anxiety and Depression Scale (HADS), to assess depression and anxiety. Concurrently, it has been shown that acute short-term TMD conditions are more frequently associated with anxiety, whereas long-term TMD conditions are more correlated to depressive disorders [33]. Finally, Hofstra and co-workers (2001) followed the same children and adolescents for 10 years and they found that all internalizing problems that children and adolescents reported remained to the adulthood [7]. This finding indicate that some problems remain during the transition stage from childhood to the adulthood and this warrants not only early diagnosis of TMD-pain in children and adolescents but also a decent management of TMD-pain in children.

As in this study, also other studies showed that children and adolescents with TMD-pain report a significantly higher degree of somatic complaints than children and adolescents without TMD pain. However, in contrast to this study they reported that the somatic complaints were more intense than emotional complaints [5, 27]. Moreover, this study also indicates that aggressive behavior and thought problems associated with TMD-pain, which is in similarity with a longitudinal study showing that aggressive behavior among these children and adolescents is passed on to adulthood [34].

The TMD-pain group showed significant associations to affective, somatic and anxiety problems according to the DSM-oriented scale in the present study. In view of this, a previous longitudinal study showed that emotional and behavioral problems in childhood continued to adulthood and met the criteria of DSM-VI [7]. Hence, these affective, somatic and anxiety problems in the TMD-pain group might go on into the adulthood and consequently have a negative impact on the individual's quality life. One explanation to why emotional and behavioral problems continue to adulthood, when they are associated with TMD-pain, could be that cognitive and nociceptive systems already affected by pain once, easily can recall these associations [27]. This, since the affective problems and their associations with TMD-pain share the pathways of the nervous system that mediate pleasant and unpleasant emotions [35]. Another explanation could be that both sensory and affective abilities share memories from early pain experiences [36]. Further, other studies found that abdominal as well as pain in the temporomandibular region contribute not only to depression and anxiety but also to general body malfunctions and/or somatization [18, 37].

The present study reported limitations in physical activities in both the TMD- and non-TMD groups. However, no significant associations were observed between the groups. However, previous studies have shown a weak relationship between TMD, headache and low incidence of sport activity [18, 38]. Furthermore, the current study shows that social activities (relations) were within the normal range in all groups. Hence, it seems that TMD-pain did not limit their social relations which is comparable to the results of List and co-workers (2001) who found that TMD-pain did not have any effect on daily activities [18].

This study indicates that the risk of developing internalizing problems, such as Anxious/Depressed, Somatic Complaints and Attention Problem, is increased in boys with TMD-pain when compared to girls. This finding is in contrast to a previous study indicating that depressive symptoms and somatic complaints co-occurred in girls more than boys with TMD pain [17]. One explanation to the finding that boys with TMD-pain have an increased risk of developing internalizing problems could be that boys in this study reported the same level of physical activity as girls, which is in contrast to previous studies in Saudi Arabia indicating that boys report a higher degree of physical activitiy than girls [39]. With this in mind, one could speculate if boys suffering from TMD-pain reported lower physical activities than normal due to the TMD-pain or if TMD-pain might lead to a decreased level of physical activity [40]. Another possible reason for this finding could be related to the drop-outs among the boys. Perhaps those boys were more physically active than the participating boys and therefore did not have the time to participate.

The same study also showed that somatic complaints increased with age. However, that finding is in contrast to the present study where no such increase was found. One explanation could be that since emotions play a great role in the pain experience in children and adolescents with a TMD-pain condition [27]. Then, repeated pain or continuous pain or longer duration of a pain condition will most likely induce un-pleasant emotions such as anxiety, depression, somatic, hyperactivity problems and also oppositional defiant problems, which this study showed to be more present in boys with TMD-pain.

One unexpected finding was the fact that the younger age group (10–13) reported a higher degree of affection problems, and a higher level of anxiety than the older age group (14–18). These significant differences between the age groups might be due to the notion that the younger children have a greater tendency to self-evaluate their pain at the extreme level on the pain scale than the older children [41]. Although the settings for boys and girls were equal, despite the fact that all girls were examined in the school nurse's room using a mobile dental chair and the boys at a dental clinic of the primary health care center, one can consider this issue as a limitation for the study, which might have led to a higher amount of dropouts among the boys. However, a strength of the current study is the randomization of the sample that allow the authors to generalize the results, since it was a representative sample for the city. Another strength is that only one examiner, trained in RDC/TMD, performed the clinical examination of all children. A final strength is that the questionnaires were filled in by the children and/or the adolescents without the influence of their parents/guardians.

## Conclusion

In conclusion, TMD-pain in children and adolescents does not seem to affect the social activities but it seems to have a strong association to emotional, behavior and somatic functioning, with higher frequencies of anxiety, depression, somatic problems, aggressive behavior and thought problems than children and adolescents without TMD-pain. With respect to the biopsychosocial model the present study indicates that there are significant associations to psychosocial, somatic and behavioral comorbidities and TMD-pain in children and adolescents in the Middle East region.

### Abbreviations

DP: Disability Points; GCPS: Graded Chronic Pain Scale; RDC/TMD: Research Diagnostic Criteria for Temporomandibular Disorders; SCL-90-R: Symptom Checklist-90-Revised; TMD: Temporomandibular Disorders; TMJ: Temporomandibular Joint; YSR: Youth Self Report scale.

### Competing interests

The authors declare that they have no competing interests. The authors alone are responsible for the content and writing of the paper.

### Authors' contributions

AAK wrote the manuscript, designed and performed the research, and analyzed the data. ANA designed the research, analyzed the data, and participated in manuscript editing. MG analyzed the data, and participated in figure editing. EA, LB and BHM participated in the design and planning of the research, and participated in manuscript editing. NC designed the research, analyzed the data, and participated in manuscript editing. All authors have read and approved the final version of the manuscript.

### Acknowledgements

The current study was financially supported by a grant from Ministry of health, Saudi Arabia. Thanks and appreciation to Dr. Abdulhamid Mohammed Khateeb and Dr. Muaaz Fadel Abdeen Dental Speciality Center, Ministry of Health, Jeddah, Saudi Arabia for their great help and assisting during the preparation for the boys' examination, and also Miss Joudi Bathallath for her kind help in paper work and the preparation of the examination of the girls.

### Author details

[1]Orofacial Pain and Jaw Function, Department of Dental Medicine, Karolinska Institutet, SE-141 04 Huddinge, Sweden. [2]Scandinavian Center for Orofacial Neurosciences (SCON), Huddinge, Sweden. [3]Cariology, Department of Dental Medicine, Karolinska Institutet, SE-141 04 Huddinge, Sweden. [4]Dental Speciality Center, Ministry of Health, Jeddah, Saudi Arabia. [5]Pediatric Dentistry and Orthodontics Department, College of Dentistry, King Saud University, Riyadh, Saudi Arabia. [6]Department of Clinical Oral Physiology at the Eastman Institute, Stockholm Public Dental Health (Folktandvården SLL AB), SE-113 24 Stockholm, Sweden.

### References

1. Suvinen TI, Reade PC, Kemppainen P, Kononen M, Dworkin SF (2005) Review of aetiological concepts of temporomandibular pain disorders: towards a biopsychosocial model for integration of physical disorder factors with psychological and psychosocial illness impact factors. Eur J Pain 9(6):613–633. doi:10.1016/j.ejpain.2005.01.012
2. Minghelli B, Cardoso I, Porfirio M, Goncalves R, Cascalheiro S, Barreto V, Soeiro A, Almeida L (2014) Prevalence of temporomandibular disorder in children and adolescents from public schools in southern portugal. N Am J Med Sci 6(3):126–132. doi:10.4103/1947-2714.128474
3. Casanova-Rosado JF, Medina-Solis CE, Vallejos-Sanchez AA, Casanova-Rosado AJ, Hernandez-Prado B, Avila-Burgos L (2006) Prevalence and associated factors for temporomandibular disorders in a group of Mexican adolescents and youth adults. Clin Oral Investig 10(1):42–49. doi:10.1007/s00784-005-0021-4
4. Alamoudi N, Farsi N, Salako NO, Feteih R (1998) Temporomandibular disorders among school children. J Clin Pediatr Dent 22(4):323–328
5. List T, Wahlund K, Wenneberg B, Dworkin SF (1999) TMD in children and adolescents: prevalence of pain, gender differences, and perceived treatment need. J Orofac Pain 13(1):9–20
6. Kelleher KJ, McInerny TK, Gardner WP, Childs GE, Wasserman RC (2000) Increasing identification of psychosocial problems: 1979–1996. Pediatrics 105(6):1313–1321
7. Hofstra MB, Van Der Ende J, Verhulst FC (2001) Adolescents' self-reported problems as predictors of psychopathology in adulthood: 10-year follow-up study. Br J Psychiatry 179:203–209
8. Hadjistavropoulos T, Craig KD, Duck S, Cano A, Goubert L, Jackson PL, Mogil JS, Rainville P, Sullivan MJ, de C Williams AC, Vervoort T, Fitzgerald TD (2011) A biopsychosocial formulation of pain communication. Psychol Bull 137(6):910–939. doi:10.1037/a0023876
9. Reissmann DR, John MT, Wassell RW, Hinz A (2008) Psychosocial profiles of diagnostic subgroups of temporomandibular disorder patients. Eur J Oral Sci 116(3):237–244. doi:10.1111/j.1600-0722.2008.00528.x
10. Manfredini D, Marini M, Pavan C, Pavan L, Guarda-Nardini L (2009) Psychosocial profiles of painful TMD patients. J Oral Rehabil 36(3):193–198. doi:10.1111/j.1365-2842.2008.01926.x
11. Rollman GB, Gillespie JM (2000) The role of psychosocial factors in temporomandibular disorders. Curr Rev Pain 4(1):71–81
12. Yap AU, Tan KB, Chua EK, Tan HH (2002) Depression and somatization in patients with temporomandibular disorders. J Prosthet Dent 88(5):479–484. doi:10.1067/mpr.2002.129375
13. Barbosa TD, Miyakoda LS, Pocztaruk RD, Rocha CP, Gaviao MBD (2008) Temporomandibular disorders and bruxism in childhood and adolescence: review of the literature. Int J Pediatr Otorhinolaryngol 72(3):299–314. doi:10.1016/j.ijporl.2007.11.006
14. Alamoudi N (2001) Correlation between oral parafunction and temporomandibular disorders and emotional status among saudi children. J Clin Pediatr Dent 26(1):71–80
15. Bertoli FM, Antoniuk SA, Bruck I, Xavier GR, Rodrigues DC, Losso EM (2007) Evaluation of the signs and symptoms of temporomandibular disorders in children with headaches. Arq Neuropsiquiatr 65(2A):251–255
16. Siegel LJ, Smith KE (1989) Children's strategies for coping with pain. Pediatrician 16(1–2):110–118
17. Nilsson IM, Drangsholt M, List T (2009) Impact of temporomandibular disorder pain in adolescents: differences by age and gender. J Orofac Pain 23(2):115–122
18. List T, Wahlund K, Larsson B (2001) Psychosocial functioning and dental factors in adolescents with temporomandibular disorders: a case–control study. J Orofac Pain 15(3):218–227
19. Achenbach T, Rescorla L (2001) The manual for the ASEBA school-age forms & profiles. University of Vermont, Research Center for Children, Youth, and Families, Burlington
20. Achenbach TM, aECS (1991) Manual for the child behaviour checklist:4–18 profile. University of Vermont Dept of Psychiatry, Burlington
21. Wahlund K, List T, Dworkin SF (1998) Temporomandibular disorders in children and adolescents: reliability of a questionnaire, clinical examination, and diagnosis. J Orofac Pain 12(1):42–51

22. Nilsson IM, List T, Drangsholt M (2005) Prevalence of temporomandibular pain and subsequent dental treatment in Swedish adolescents. J Orofac Pain 19(2):144–150

23. Goldfinger K, Pomerantz AM (2014) Psychological assessment and report writing. 2nd edition. California, USA: SAGE Publications, Inc. p.102

24. Al-Harthy M, Al-Bishri A, Ekberg E, Nilner M (2010) Temporomandibular disorder pain in adult Saudi Arabians referred for specialised dental treatment. Swed Dent J 34(3):149–158

25. Von Korff M, Ormel J, Keefe FJ, Dworkin SF (1992) Grading the severity of chronic pain. Pain 50(2):133–149

26. Dworkin SF, LeResche L (1992) Research diagnostic criteria for temporomandibular disorders: review, criteria, examinations and specifications, critique. J Craniomandib Disord 6(4):301–355

27. Wahlund K, List T, Ohrbach R (2005) The relationship between somatic and emotional stimuli: a comparison between adolescents with temporomandibular disorders (TMD) and a control group. Eur J Pain 9(2):219–227. doi:10.1016/j.ejpain.2004.06.003

28. Bonjardim LR, Gaviao MB, Pereira LJ, Castelo PM (2005) Anxiety and depression in adolescents and their relationship with signs and symptoms of temporomandibular disorders. Int J Prosthodont 18(4):347–352

29. Ferreira CL, Da Silva MA, de Felicio CM (2009) Orofacial myofunctional disorder in subjects with temporomandibular disorder. Cranio 27(4):268–274. doi:10.1179/crn.2009.038

30. Belfer ML, Kaban LB (1982) Temporomandibular joint dysfunction with facial pain in children. Pediatrics 69(5):564–567

31. McGregor NR, Zerbes M, Niblett SH, Dunstan RH, Roberts TK, Butt HL, Klineberg IJ (2003) Pain intensity, illness duration, and protein catabolism in temporomandibular disorder patients with chronic muscle pain. J Orofac Pain 17(2):112–124

32. Pizolato RA, Freitas-Fernandes FS, Gaviao MB (2013) Anxiety/depression and orofacial myofacial disorders as factors associated with TMD in children. Braz Oral Res 27(2):156–162

33. Gatchel RJ, Garofalo JP, Ellis E, Holt C (1996) Major psychological disorders in acute and chronic TMD: an initial examination. J Am Dent Assoc 127(9):1365–1370, 1372, 1374

34. Pereira LJ, Pereira-Cenci T, Pereira SM, Cury AA, Ambrosano GM, Pereira AC, Gaviao MB (2009) Psychological factors and the incidence of temporomandibular disorders in early adolescence. Braz Oral Res 23(2):155–160

35. Lane RD, Reiman EM, Bradley MM, Lang PJ, Ahern GL, Davidson RJ, Schwartz GE (1997) Neuroanatomical correlates of pleasant and unpleasant emotion. Neuropsychologia 35(11):1437–1444

36. Craig KD (1999) Emotions and psychobiology textbook of pain, 4th edn. Churchill Livingstone, Edinburgh

37. Macfarlane TV, Blinkhorn AS, Davies RM, Ryan P, Worthington HV, Macfarlane GJ (2002) Orofacial pain: just another chronic pain? Results from a population-based survey. Pain 99(3):453–458

38. Carlsson J, Larsson B, Mark A (1996) Psychosocial functioning in schoolchildren with recurrent headaches. Headache 36(2):77–82

39. Al-Nakeeb Y, Lyons M, Collins P, Al-Nuaim A, Al-Hazzaa H, Duncan MJ, Nevill A (2012) Obesity, physical activity and sedentary behavior amongst British and Saudi youth: a cross-cultural study. Int J Environ Res Public Health 9(4):1490–1506. doi:10.3390/ijerph9041490

40. Rabbitts JA, Holley AL, Groenewald CB, Palermo TM (2016) Association between widespread pain scores and functional impairment and health-related quality of life in clinical samples of children. J Pain. doi:10.1016/j.jpain.2016.02.005

41. Alwugyan I, Alroumi F, Zureiqi M (2007) Expression of pain by children and its assessment in Kuwait. Med Princ Pract 16(suppl 1):21–26. doi:10.1159/000104543

# Plasma urotensin-2 level and Thr21Met but not Ser89Asn polymorphisms of the urotensin-2 gene are associated with migraines

Sırma Geyik[1*], Sercan Ergun[2], Samiye Kuzudişli[3], Figen Şensoy[4], Ebru Temiz[5], Erman Altunışık[6], Murat Korkmaz[5], Hasan Dağlı[5], Seval Kul[7], Aylin Akçalı[1] and Ayşe Münife Neyal[1]

## Abstract

**Background:** Urotensin-II (U-II) is a peptide recognized by its potent vasoconstrictor activity in many vascular events, however the role of urotensin-II in migraine has not been considered yet. The molecular mechanisms and genetics of migraine have not been fully clarified yet, but it is well-known that vascular changes considerably contribute in pathophysiology of migraine and also its complications. The aim of this study was to analyze the plasma U-II levels along with genotype distributions and allele frequencies for UTS2 Thr21Met and Ser89Asn polymorphisms among the patients with migraine without aura (MWoA).

**Methods:** One hundred eighty-six patients with MWoA and 171 healthy individuals were included in this study. Plasma U-II levels were measured in attack free period. The genotype and allele frequencies for the Thr21Met (T21M) and Ser89Asn (S89N) polymorphisms in the UTS2 gene were analyzed.

**Results:** Plasma U-II levels were significantly higher in MWoA patients ($p = 0.002$). We detected a significant association between the T21M polymorphism in the UTS2 gene and migraine (53.8 % in patients, 40.4 % in controls, $p = 0.035$), but not with S89N polymorphism ($p = 0.620$). A significant relationship was found between U-II levels and MIDAS score ($\beta = 0.508$, $p = 0.001$).

**Conclusion:** Our study suggests that U-II may play a role in migraine pathogenesis; also Thr21Met polymorphism was associated with the risk of migraine disease. Further studies are needed for considering the role of U-II in migraine pathophysiology and for deciding if UTS2 gene may be a novel candidate gene in migraine cases.

**Keywords:** Migraine without aura, Urotensin-2, ELISA, UTS2 gene polymorphisms, Thr21Met, Ser89Asn

## Background

Migraine is a common neurological disorder that affects approximately 12 % of the population [1]. However, in recent years, it has been suggested that migraines are formed as a result of neuronal vascular event chains triggered by endogenous and/or exogenous factors in people with a genetic predisposition [2, 3]. Many first-degree relatives of migraine patients have a history of migraines, and twin studies conducted show that migraines have a strong genetic component [4–6].

Urotensin-2 (U-II) is a cyclic peptide composed of 11 amino acids that was first isolated from the goby neurosecretory system in 1969 [7]. The human receptor for U-II (hUT2R) is a G-protein coupled receptor (GPR14) [8]. U-II and its receptor (UTR) are found in different tissues such as the central nervous system, peripheral vascular tissues, the heart, and the kidneys [8, 9]. Clark et al. suggested that UII receptor mRNA and choline acetyltransferase exist together in the mesopontine tegmental area [10]. U-II is a vasoactive substance that has a similar peptide structure to somatostatin and is a more powerful vasoconstrictor than

* Correspondence: drsirmageyik@hotmail.com
[1]Department of Neurology, Faculty of Medicine, University of Gaziantep, Gaziantep, Turkey
Full list of author information is available at the end of the article

endothelin-1 (ET-1) [11]. The vasoconstrictor effect of U-II is 50 times higher on arteries and 10 times higher on veins than ET-1. U-II is thought to have endothelium-dependent vasodilator and endothelium-independent vasoconstrictor effects, and its net effect may depend on the balance between these two individual effects [12]. However, studies have shown that it plays other physiological roles beyond the regulation of vascular tone and cholinergic activity. The urotensinergic system has been shown to be associated with heart failure, hypertension, diabetes, preeclampsia, renal and liver diseases, neurological and psychiatric disorders [13, 14]. U-II is known to be expressed in the brain and spinal cord. It is recognized as a neuro-mediator in the central nervous system [15, 16].

U-II may also play a role in migraine pathogenesis, especially considering its known effects on the central and peripheral nervous system. The U-II gene (UTS2) is located at the 1p36 locus. According to data from the US National Center for Biotechnology Information, more than 60 single nucleotide polymorphisms (SNPs) have been recorded in the human UTS2 gene. Thr21Met (T21M, rs228648) and Ser89Asn (S89N, rs2890565) polymorphisms have been found at high allelic frequencies in Japanese populations [17]; these are the same polymorphisms that were selected for investigation in our study. Although many studies have shown the roles of various genetic factors and polymorphisms in migraine disease, no studies have focused on the T21M and S89N polymorphisms in the UTS2 gene in migraine patients until now.

Therefore, the purpose of this study is to examine the possible relationships between the T21M and S89N polymorphisms in the UTS2 gene and MWoA and to detect the possible role of U-II in the pathogenesis of MWoA by measuring serum U-II levels.

## Methods

### Study population

Study approval was obtained from the Ethics Committee of the Gaziantep University Faculty of Medicine. Informed consent was obtained from all subjects prior to the study. This study examined 186 consecutive patients aged 18–45 years, who were diagnosed as having migraines, had not been on prophylactic treatment for at least 3 months and had least 72 h migraine attack drug-free period before obtaining blood samples in the interictal phase. Since it is thought to have endothelium-dependent vasodilator and endothelium-independent vasoconstrictor effects, and its net effect may depend on the balance between these two individual effects and we don't know if it has an effect in migraine attacks we decided to obtain the blood samples in the interictal phase from all of the patients.

Migraines were diagnosed according to the ICHD-2 criteria [18] by experienced neurologists in our clinic and then enrolled into the study. For homogenizing the group, we selected only MWoA patients. The control group ($n$ = 171) was composed of age and gender matched healthy cases that consented to join to the control group.

Cases with history of diabetes mellitus (fasting blood glucose ≥ 120 mg/dl); hypertension (Blood pressure (BP) ≥ 140/90 mmHg); chronic renal failure; liver cirrhosis; any type of cancer; thyroid diseases; alcohol and substance abuse; chronic neurologic illnesses, including epilepsy, Parkinson's disease, Huntington's disease, Alzheimer's disease, Wilson's disease, and previous cerebrovascular and cardiovascular diseases, morbid obesity; and any existing infection were excluded from both groups. The medical histories, physical and neurologic examination findings, and body mass indices (BMI) of all cases were recorded. The migraine patients were questioned regarding the disease duration, the type of migraine, the frequency of migraine attacks (for the last 3 months), drugs used, and smoking. The Migraine Disability Assessment Scale (MIDAS) was applied to measure the extent to which migraine headaches decreased the patients' standard of living. Routine laboratory examinations, including total blood count, serum electrolytes, serum creatinine, blood urea nitrogen (BUN), fasting blood glucose levels, and liver function tests, were performed in all cases. The glomerular filtration rate (GFR) was calculated according to the Modification of Diet in Renal Disease (MDRD) guidelines [19].

### Power analysis

Sample size was estimated using a power calculation based on 0.2 ± 0.6 changes in urotensin between groups. It was estimated that at least 142 participants in each group would be required to detect a significant difference between control and migraine groups at 80 % power level and an alpha error of % 5.

### Blood samples and DNA isolation

Venous blood samples were drawn from the antecubital vein in the morning hours after 12 h of fasting and for at least 72 h without symptomatic migraine medication. The plasma was separated from the blood samples by adding EDTA and centrifuging the samples at 1000 g for 15 min. The plasma samples were then stored at -80 °C until U-II levels were measured. Plasma U-II concentrations were measured using a quantitative sandwich-type enzyme immunoassay UT2 kit (Elx 800 ELISA; Cusabio Biotech, Winooski, VT, USA). Genomic DNA extraction was performed from the plasma-free blood pellets using a standard proteinase K and salt precipitation method. The extracted DNA was stored at -20 °C.

### SNP genotyping

Samples were genotyped for the UTS2 SNPs using a validated TaqMan SNP Genotyping Assay (Applied Biosystems

Inc. (ABI), Foster City, CA, USA) that employed predesigned primers and probes for the UTS2 gene SNPs (T21M, rs228648; S89N, rs2890565) (ABI). One allelic TaqMan probe was labeled with a fluorescent FAM dye, and the other was labeled with a VIC dye. For each polymerase chain reaction (PCR), 5 μL of genomic DNA solution (5 ng/μL) was added to an aliquot of 2× TaqMan universal PCR Master Mix, resulting in primer and probe final concentrations of 180 and 40 nM, respectively. The amplification protocol consisted of the following steps: (1) an initial denaturation at 95 °C for 10 min and (2) 40 cycles of denaturation at 95 °C for 15 s and annealing and extension at 60 °C for 1 min, with amplification and fluorescence detection performed using a Qiagen Rotor-Gene Q Real-time PCR system. At least 10 % of the blood samples were run twice in separate assays with a concordance of genotype designation of 100 %.

### Statistical analysis

The results are expressed as either means ± the standard deviations (SDs) or the percentage. Statistical analysis was performed using the Statistical Package for Social Sciences (SPSS) software version 20.0 (Inc. Chicago, IL). The chi-squared test was used to calculate significant differences in the genotype and allele frequencies. The unpaired Student's t test was used to compare the differences between the mean values of the 2 groups. The effects of the genetic polymorphisms on the risk of SSc were estimated with an odds ratio (OR) and 95 % confidence interval (CI). The haplotype analysis was performed using SHEsis software (http://analysis.bio-x.cn/myAnalysis.php). All of the statistical tests and p values were two-sided, and $p < 0.05$ was considered statistically significant.

### Results

One hundred eighty-six patients diagnosed with MWoA and 171 healthy control subjects were enrolled in this study. No significant differences existed between the two groups in terms of gender distribution, age, BMI, or smoking status. A total of 101 (54.3 %) migraine patients were using migraine attack drugs (triptans, nonsteroidal anti-inflammatory drugs (NSAIDs), paracetamol and combination analgesic). The demographic and laboratory characteristics of the study group are shown in Table 1.

### Plasma urotensin-2 levels by ELISA assay

The mean U-II levels were 1.19 ± 0.69 pg/ml in the migraine group and 0.97 ± 0.7 pg/ml in the control group. U-II plasma levels were significantly higher in the migraine group ($p = 0.002$) (Fig. 1). No differences in U-II levels were found in terms of gender, smoking status, symptomatic medication history in either group (Table 2). Disease duration and attack frequency were not significantly correlated with U-II levels (β:0.48/p:0.657, β: 0.195/

**Table 1** Demographic, clinical and laboratory characteristics of the patient and control groups

| Parameters | Patients ($n = 186$) | Control ($n = 171$) | p |
|---|---|---|---|
| Mean age (years) | 29.30 ± 5.45 | 28.77 ± 5.44 | 0.360 |
| Gender (n, %) | | | |
| Female | 133 (71.5) | 124 (72.5) | 0.832 |
| Male | 53 (28.5) | 47 (27.5) | |
| BMI (kg/m$^2$) | 25.94 ± 2.84 | 26.02 ± 2.86 | 0.795 |
| Hgb (g/dL) | 12.68 ± 0.6 | 12.66 ± 0.6 | 0.538 |
| Wbc (×10$^3$/mL) | 5.9 ± 1.17 | 4.46 ± 1.17 | 0.190 |
| Urea (mg/dL) | 18.55 ± 4.91 | 18.60 ± 4.95 | 0.927 |
| GFR (ml/min) | 106 ± 7 | 101 ± 9 | 0.206 |
| ESR (mm/h) | 4.96 ± 1.44 | 4.97 ± 1.45 | 0.929 |
| CRP (mg/L) | 0.71 ± 0.3 | 0.7 ± 0.3 | 0.725 |
| Smoking (n, %) | 41 (22) | 38 (22.2) | 0.967 |
| Disease duration (years) | 6.98 ± 3.87 | | |
| Attack frequency (n, %) | | | |
| 1–5/month | 114 (61.3) | | |
| 6–10/month | 56 (30.1) | | |
| > 10/month | 16 (8.6) | | |
| MIDAS score | 2.86 ± 1.12 | | |
| Vomiting | 99 (52.3) | | |
| FF | 143 (76.8) | | |
| Mood changes | 132 (70.9) | | |

*BMI* body mass index, *ESR* erythrocyte sedimentation rate, *CRP* C-reactive protein, *GFR* glomerular, *Hgb* hemoglobin, *WBC* white blood cell *MIDAS* Migraine Disability Assessment Scale, *FF* photophobia and phonophobia

p:0.175; respectively). A significant relationship was found between U-II levels and MIDAS score. U-II levels were significantly higher in patients with higher MIDAS scores. A 1 unit increase in the MIDAS score resulted in a 0.508 unit increase in U-II levels (β = 0.508, $p = 0.001$) (Fig. 2).

### Genotyping

Genotype and allele frequencies for T21M (rs228648) and S89N (rs2890565) polymorphisms in the UTS2 gene in the patient and control groups are shown in Table 3. We detected a significant association between the T21M polymorphism in the UTS2 gene and migraine but no significant relationship between the S89N polymorphism and migraine in our study ($p = 0.620$). T21T genotype frequency was more prevalent in the control group (34.4 % in the patients compared with 42.1 % in the controls). T21M genotype frequency was more prevalent in the migraine group (53.8 % in the patients compared with 40.4 % in the controls, $p = 0.035$) and the According to these results, patients with theT21M genotype are 1.63 times more likely to become migraine patients than patients with the T21T genotype (OR = 1.63, $p = 0.035$).

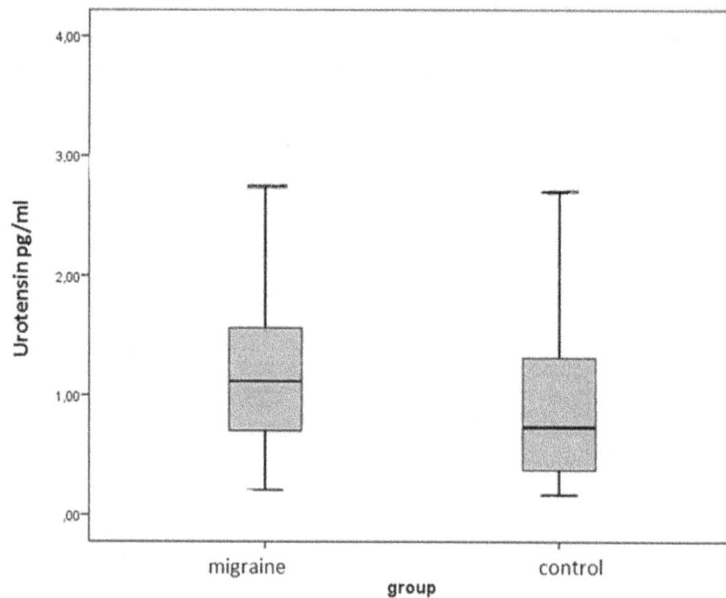

**Fig. 1** Urotensin-2 levels (pg/mL) in the migraine and control groups

**Table 2** Comparison of plasma Urotensin-II levels according to demographic and clinical variables

| Demographic and clinical variables | Urotensin (pg/ml) | | |
| --- | --- | --- | --- |
| | Migraine | Control | p value |
| Smoking | 1.15 ± 0.51 | 0.99 ± 0.52 | 0.003* |
| Non-smoking | 1.104 ± 0.6 | 0.82 ± 0.61 | 0.001* |
| p value | 0.965 | 0.854 | |
| Female | 1.19 ± 0.48 | 0.96 ± 0.62 | 0.001* |
| Male | 0.98 ± 0.45 | 0.84 ± 0.48 | 0.003* |
| p value | 0.185 | 0.832 | |
| Drugs (+) | 1,13 ± 0.4 | - | |
| Drugs (–) | 1,11 ± 0.51 | - | |
| p value | 0,981 | | |
| Vomiting (+) | 1.21 ± 0.6 | | |
| Vomiting (–) | 1.04 ± 0.51 | | |
| p value | 0.004* | | |
| FF (+) | 1.19 ± 0.5 | | |
| FF (-) | 1.17 ± 0.6 | | |
| p value | 0.967 | | |
| Mood (+) | 1.28 ± 0.7 | | |
| Mood ( ) | 0.99 ± 0.6 | | |
| p value | 0.001* | | |

Valuables are expressed as the mean ± SD
Drug (+): Using symtomatic migraine drugs
Drug (-): Not using symptomatic migraine drugs
*FF* photophobia and phonophobia
*p < 0.05

No significant differences were found in the 21 M polymorphism allele frequencies between the migraine and control groups ($p = 0.786$). Moreover, no significant relationships were found between the MIDAS scores and the T21M ($p = 0.502$) or S89N ($p = 0.300$) polymorphisms in the UTS2 gene in the migraine groups. Finally, no significant relationships were found between the smoking status and the T21M ($p = 0.885$) or S89N ($p = 0791$) polymorphisms in the UTS2 gene in the migraine group. There were insignificant increases in MN, MS and TS haplotype frequencies in migraine patients (Table 4).

### Relationship between genotypes and expression

The plasma levels of U-II were tended to be higher without statistical significance in TM and MM genotype ($p = 0.545$). The relationship between plasma U-II protein level and Thr21Met polymorphism in patients was shown in Fig. 3.

### Discussion

Our results revealed a significant elevation of serum U-II levels in migraine patients. Additionally, a significant association of migraine with T21M polymorphism but not with S89N polymorphism of urotensin gene was observed in the present study.

Several peptides have been reported in relation with migraine pathophysiology. The role of calcitonin generelated peptide (CGRP) in migraine pathogenesis is still under investigation in current researches [20, 21]. Pituitary adenylate cyclase-activating polypeptide and substance P (SP) had craniocervical vasodilatation, plasma protein

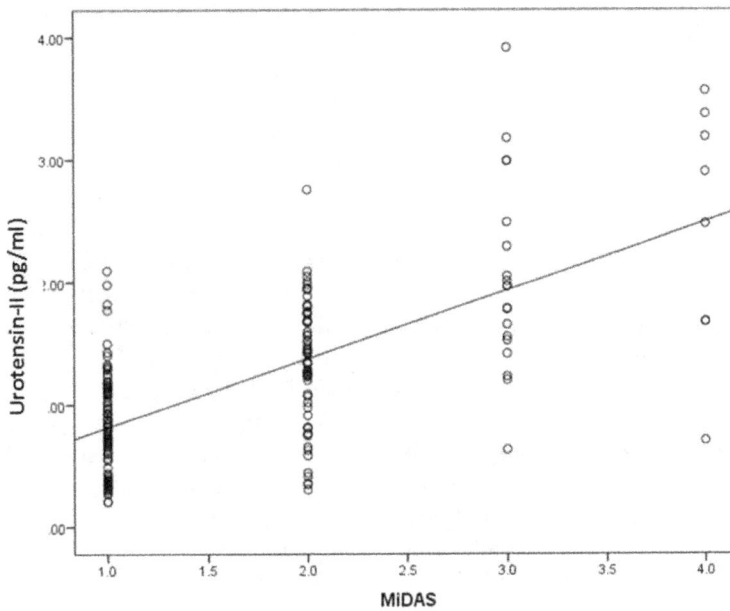

**Fig. 2** The correlation between U-II levels and MIDAS scores

extravasation, peripheral and central sensitization effects in migraine pathogenesis [22]. Serum levels of vaso-active intestinal peptide (VIP); a marker of parasympa-thetic nervous system, was found to be increased in chronic and episodic migraineurs in attack free period [23]. Diverse results for neuropeptide Y (NPY); a marker of sympathetic nervous system with long-lasting vaso-constrictor effects in cerebral circulation, was reported in migraineurs [22].

U-II and its receptor have many functions, including the regulation of behavior and neuroendocrine activities, cardiovascular tone control, motor activity, the sleep-wake cycle, and hypothalamic-pituitary-adrenal axis control [14, 24–26]. U-II plasma concentrations are low in healthy indi-viduals [13]. Previously some studies have measured higher UT2 peptide levels in various metabolic and cardiovascular diseases such as; chronic heart failure, acute myocardial infarction, hypertension and diabetes mellitus [27–29].

**Table 3** Distributions of the T21M and S89N polymorphisms among the groups

| Genotype/Allele | Control (n = 171) n (%) | Migraine (n = 186) n (%) | p | OR [95 % CI] |
|---|---|---|---|---|
| T21M | | | | |
| TT | 72 (42.1) | 64 (34.4) | Reference | |
| TM | 69 (40.4) | 100 (53.8) | 0.035 | 1.63 [1.034–2.571] |
| MM | 30 (17.5) | 22 (11.8) | 0.559 | 0.825 [0.433–1.572] |
| T | 213 (62.3) | 228 (61.3) | Reference | |
| M | 129 (37.7) | 144 (38.7) | 0.786 | 1.043 [0.771–1.411] |
| HWE | p = 0.065 | p = 0.069 | | |
| S89N | | | | |
| SS | 151 (88.3) | 161 (86.6) | Reference | |
| SN | 20 (11.7) | 25 (13.4) | 0.620 | 1.172 [0.625–2.198] |
| NN | 0 (0.0) | 0 (0.0) | - | |
| S | 322 (94.2) | 347 (93.3) | 0.632 | 0.862 [0.470–1.582] |
| N | 20 (5.8) | 25 (6.7) | Reference | |
| HWE | p =0.417 | p =0.325 | | |

*OR* odds ratio, *CI* confidence interval, and *HWE* Hardy Weinberg equilibrium
*p < 0.05

**Table 4** Haplotype distributions of UTS2 gene polymorphisms in migraine patients and controls

| Site 1 | Site 2 | Case (freq) | Control (freq) | p | Odds Ratio [95 %CI] |
|--------|--------|-------------|----------------|-------|---------------------|
| M | N | 24.99 (0.067) | 18.45 (0.054) | 0.468 | 1.257 [0.676–2.338] |
| M | S | 119.01 (0.320) | 110.55 (0.323) | 0.891 | 0.978 [0.714–1.340] |
| T | N | 0.01 (0.000)[a] | 1.55 (0.005)[a] | - | - |
| T | S | 227.99 (0.613) | 211.45 (0.618) | 0.822 | 0.966 [0.714–1.307] |

[a]Frequencies < 0.03 were ignored in the analysis

Considerably increased risk of ischemic events, in various organs including brain has already been documented in migraine [30]. Currently the exact mechanisms of that relation between migraine and stroke are not understood entirely. Distinct mechanisms were proposed for migraine-related ischemia that occurs either during the attack or attack-free periods. Additionally, it is not clear yet if stroke is a consequence of migraine or both of the conditions occur due to another shared pathological course. In this case, a genetic link may be responsible for influencing the course and variability of the consequences of migraine [31]. Nevertheless, endothelial dysfunction was proposed as one of the main paths in this association [32, 33].

U-II is a vasoactive peptide with ubiquitous effects in various human body tissues. It has been suggested to have endothelium-dependent vasodilator and endothelium-independent vasoconstrictor effects, with its net effect depending on the balance between these two individual effects [12]. Yet in general, U-II is known to have a powerful vasoconstrictor effect.

As mentioned above, since U-II has dual effect on endothelium through distinct pathways and we don't have data if it has an effect in migraine attacks or not, the blood samples were obtained in the interictal phase in all of the cases. Therefore, the significantly higher levels of plasma U-II in the present study present only the U-II status in the attack-free period that may be a limitation of the present study. Understanding the effects of U-II on the attacks is yet to be waiting for further investigation. However, we believe that the stated concerns about the dual effect of U-II should be taken under consideration also in further research that aim to investigate the plasma U-II effects in migraine attacks.

We found a significant positive relation between the MIDAS scores and plasma U-II levels in the present study. This finding may indicate that the severity of migraine may be influenced by plasma U-II and in turn it may have a bad effect in quality of life of the cases.

Many first-degree relatives of migraine patients have a history of migraine, and twin studies showed that migraine have a strong genetic component [3–5]. Genetic factors may cause a tendency (predispose) to have migraine attacks. Despite increasing number of studies suggesting a role for genetic factors in the pathogenesis of migraine, the responsible genes have not yet been determined. Despite, neuronal vascular event chains triggered by endogenous and/or exogenous factors in people with a genetic predisposition, it is now believed that neuronal dysfunction is the possible primary reason in the pathophysiology of the disease and vasodilation and vasoconstriction phases are probably epiphenomena [34, 35].

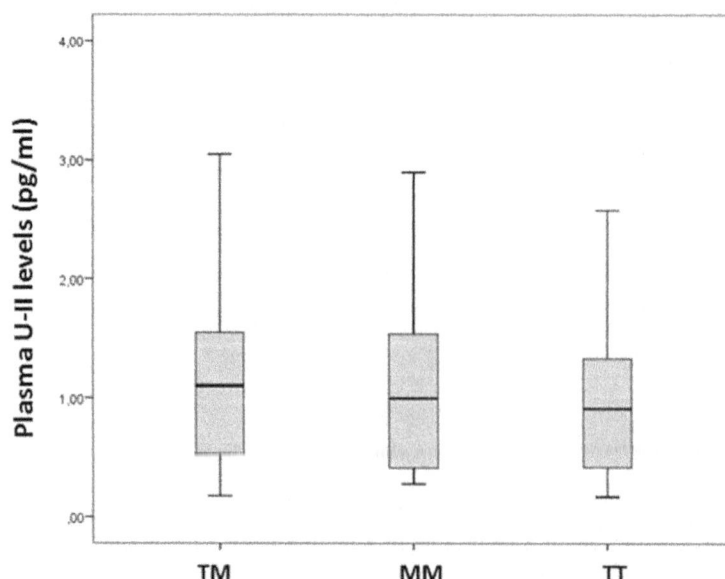

**Fig. 3** The relationship between plasma U-II protein level and Thr21Met polymorphism in patients

Non-familial migraines can be considered as polygenic when the diversity of both the number and severity of attacks and the duration of the attacks are considered. Various genes were supposed to be involved in migraine pathophysiology. Our results indicate that a significant association exists between the T21M polymorphism and migraine. The T21M genotype patients were 1.63 times more likely to become migraine than patients with the T21T genotype in the present study. Amino acid change upon Thr21Met polymorphism may affect protein folding efficiency or structure. By this way, differently folded protein may be exposed to protein degradation processes more or less than natively folded protein. Also, some amino acid sequences form signal for degradation. With this amino acid change, degradation signal may be created and this causes U-II level to decrease. Moreover, newly formed Met codon on mRNA may provide potential translation starting point for ribosome, although it is a low probability. So, this causes a truncated U-II protein product. All these possibilities may explain U-II level changes upon Thr21Met variant presence. Also, we revealed that the plasma U-II levels tended to be higher in cases with Thr21Met polymorphism as shown in Fig. 3. However the difference couldn't reach a statistically significant level.

Several publications have indicated a possible relationship between UTS2 gene polymorphisms and hypertension, diabetes mellitus, Behçet's disease, and systemic sclerosis [17, 36–38]. Recently, genome-wide studies have provided new insights for genes associated with migraine disease (the ion channel gene, TRPM8, FHL5, ASTN2, and LRP1 [39] but UTS2 gene was not one of them. Since, we believe that it is worthy to evaluate this vasoactive peptide in migraine pathophysiology since vascular changes predominantly take place in migraine cases in both attack and attack-free periods.

## Conclusion

Our study suggests that U-II may play a role in migraine pathogenesis, also Thr21Met polymorphism was associated with the risk of migraine disease. Further studies are needed for considering the role of U-II in migraine pathophysiology and for deciding if UTS2 gene may be a novel candidate gene in migraine cases.

## Abbreviations

BMI: body mass index; CGRP: calcitonin gene-related peptide; CI: confidence interval; ET-1: endothelin-1; FHM: familial hemiplegic migraine; GPR14: G-protein coupled receptor; hUT2R: human receptor for U-II; ICHD-3: International Classification of Headache Disorders; MDRD: Modification of Diet in Renal Disease; MIDAS: Migraine Disability Assessment Scale; MWoA: migraine without aura; NPY: neuropeptide Y; NSAID: nonsteroidal anti-inflammatory drug; OR: odds ratio; S89N: Ser89Asn; SD: standard deviation; SP: substance P; T21M: Thr21Met; U-II: urotensin-2; UTR: U-II receptor; VIP: vasoactive intestinal peptide.

## Competing interests
The authors declare that they have no competing interests.

## Authors' contributions
SG and SK conceived and designed the study. SG, FŞ, EA, SE, MK, HD, AA, ET were responsible for data acquisition. SG, SK, S.KUL and AMN were in charge of data analysis and interpretation and drafted the manuscript. SG, AMN were responsible for critical revision of this manuscript. All authors approved the final version of this manuscript.

## Acknowledgements
None.

## Author details
[1]Department of Neurology, Faculty of Medicine, University of Gaziantep, Gaziantep, Turkey. [2]Ulubey Vocational Higher School, Ordu University, Ordu, Turkey. [3]Department of Neurology, Emine-Bahaeddin Nakiboglu Medical Faculty, Zirve University, Gaziantep, Turkey. [4]Neurology Clinics, Medical Park Hospital, Gaziantep, Turkey. [5]Department of Medical Biology, Faculty of Medicine, University of Gaziantep, Gaziantep, Turkey. [6]Division Of Neurology, Turkish Ministry Of Health Siirt State Hospital, Siirt, Turkey. [7]Department of Biostatistics, Faculty of Medicine, University of Gaziantep, Gaziantep, Turkey.

## References
1. Lipton RB, Bigal ME (2005) Migraine: epidemiology, impact, and risk factors for progression. Headache 45(Suppl 1):S3–S13. doi:10.1111/j.1526-4610.2005.4501001.x
2. Demarquay G, Mauguière F (2015) Central nervous system underpinnings of sensory hypersensitivity in migraine: insights from Neuroimaging and electrophysiological studies. Headache. doi:10.1111/head.12651
3. Fang J, An X, Chen S, Yu Z, Ma Q, Qu H (2015) Case-control study of GRIA1 and GRIA3 gene variants in migraine. J Headache Pain 17(1):2. doi:10.1186/s10194-016-0592-2
4. de Vries B, Frants RR, Ferrari MD, van den Maagdenberg AM (2009) Molecular genetics of migraine. Hum Genet 126(1):115–132. doi:10.1007/s00439-009-0684-z
5. Schürks M (2012) Genetics of migraine in the age of genome-wide association studies. J Headache Pain 13(1):1–9. doi:10.1007/s10194-011-0399-0
6. Mulder EJ, Van Baal C, Gaist D, Kallela M, Kaprio J, Svensson DA, Nyholt DR, Martin NG, MacGregor AJ, Cherkas LF, Boomsma DI, Palotie A (2003) Genetic and environmental influences on migraine: a twin study across six countries. Twin Res 6(5):422–431. doi:10.1375/136905203770326420
7. Onan D, Hannan RD, Thomas WG (2004) Urotensin II: The old kid in town. Trends Endocrinol Metab 15(4):175–182. doi:10.1016/j.tem.2004.03.007
8. Lavecchia A, Cosconati S, Novellino E (2005) Architecture of the human urotensin II receptor: comparison of the binding domains of peptide and non-peptide urotensin II agonists. J Med Chem 48(7):2480–2492. doi:10.1021/jm049110x
9. Jégou S, Cartier D, Dubessy C, Gonzalez BJ, Chatenet D, Tostivint H, Scalbert E, LePrince J, Vaudry H, Lihrmann I (2006) Localization of the urotensin II receptor in the rat central nervous system. J Comp Neurol 495(1):21–36. doi:10.1002/cne.20845
10. Clark SD, Nothacker HP, Wang Z, Saito Y, Leslie FM, Civelli O (2001) The urotensin II receptor is expressed in the cholinergic mesopontine tegmentum of the rat. Brain Res 923(1–2):120–127. doi:10.1016/S0006-8993(01)03208-5
11. MacLean MR, Alexander D, Stirrat A, Gallagher M, Douglas SA, Ohlstein EH, Morecroft I, Polland K (2000) Contractile responses to human urotensin-II in rat and human pulmonary arteries: effect of endothelial factors and chronic hypoxia in the rat. Br J Pharmacol 130(2):201–204. doi:10.1038/sj.bjp.0703314
12. Maguire JJ, Kuc RE, Davenport AP (2000) Orphan-receptor ligand human urotensin II: Receptor localization in human tissues and comparison of vasoconstrictor responses with endothelin-1. Br J Pharmacol 131(3):441–446. doi:10.1038/sj.bjp.0703601
13. Ross B, McKendy K, Giaid A (2010) Role of urotensin II in health and disease. Am J Physiol Regul Integr Comp Physiol 298(5):R1156–R1172. doi:10.1152/ajpregu.00706.2009

14. Huitron-Resendiz S, Kristensen MP, Sánchez-Alavez M, Clark SD, Grupke SL, Tyler C, Suzuki C, Nothacker HP, Civelli O, Criado JR, Henriksen SJ, Leonard CS, de Lecea L (2005) Urotensin II modulates rapid eye movement sleep through activation of brainstem cholinergic neurons. J Neurosci 25(23): 5465–5474. doi:10.1523/JNEUROSCI.4501-04.2005

15. Douglas SA, Dhanak D, Johns DG (2004) From 'gills to pills': urotensin-II as a regulator of mammalian cardiorenal function. Trends Pharmacol Sci 25(2):76–85. doi:10.1016/j.tips.2003.12.005

16. Gartlon JE, Ashmeade T, Duxon M, Hagan JJ, Jones DN (2004) Urotensin-II, a neuropeptide ligand for GPR14, induces c-fos in the rat brain. Eur J Pharmacol 493(1–3):95–98. doi:10.1016/j.ejphar.2004.04.009

17. Suzuki S, Wenyi Z, Hirai M, Hinokio Y, Suzuki C, Yamada T, Yoshizumi S, Suzuki M, Tanizawa Y, Matsutani A, Oka Y (2004) Genetic variations at urotensin II and urotensin II receptor genes and risk of type 2 diabetes mellitus in Japanese. Peptides 25(10):1803–1808. doi:10.1016/j.peptides.2004.03.030

18. Olesen J, Steiner TJ (2004) The International classification of headache disorders, 2nd edn (ICDH-II). J Neurol Neurosurg Psychiatry 75(6):808–811

19. Michaels WM, Grootendorst DC, Verduijn M, Elliott EG, Dekker FW (2010) Performance of the Cockcroft-Gault, MDRD, and new CKD-EPI formulas in relation to GFR, age, and body size. Clin J Am Soc Nephrol 5(6):1003–1009. doi:10.2215/CJN.06870909

20. Cauchi M, Robertson NP (2016) CGRP and migraine. J Neurol 263(1):192–194. doi:10.1007/s00415-015-8000-4

21. Karsan N, Goadsby PJ (2015) Calcitonin gene-related peptide and migraine. Curr Opin Neurol 28(3):250–254. doi:10.1097/WCO.0000000000000191

22. Tajti J, Szok D, Majlath Z, Tuka B, Csati A, Vécsei L (2015) Migraine and neuropeptides. Neuropeptides 52:19–30. doi:10.1016/j.npep.2015.03.006

23. Cernuda-Morollon E, Martinez-Camblor P, Ramon C, Larrosa D, Serrano-Pertierra E, Pascual J (2014) CGRP and VIP levels as predictors of efficacy of Onabotulinumtoxin type A in chronic migraine. Headache 54(6):987–995. doi:10.1111/head.12372

24. Vaudry H, Do Rego JC, Le Mevel JC, Chatenet D, Tostivint H, Fournier A, Tonon MC, Pelletier G, Conlon JM, Leprince J (2010) Urotensin II, From fish to human. Ann N Y Acad Sci 1200:53–66. doi:10.1111/j.1749-6632.2010.05514.x

25. do Rego JC, Leprince J, Scalbert E, Vaudry H, Costentin J (2008) Behavioral actions of urotensin-II. Peptides 29(5):838–844. doi:10.1016/j.peptides.2007.12.016

26. de Lecea L, Bourgin P (2008) Neuropeptide interactions and REM sleep: a role for Urotensin II? Peptides 29(5):845–851. doi:10.1016/j.peptides.2008.02.009

27. Ng LL, Loke I, O'Brien RJ, Squire IB, Davies JE (2002) Plasma urotensin in human systolic heart failure. Circulation 106(23):2877–2880. doi:10.1161/01.CIR.0000044388.19119.02

28. Khan SQ, Bhandari SS, Quinn P, Davies JE, Ng LL (2007) Urotensin II is raised in acute myocardial infarction and low levels predict risk of adverse clinical outcome in humans. Int J Cardiol 117(3):323–328. doi:10.1016/j.ijcard.2006.05.016

29. Cheung BM, Leung R, Man YB, Wong LY (2004) Plasma concentration of urotensin II is raised in hypertension. J Hypertens 22(7):1341–1344. doi:10.1097/01.hjh.0000125452.28861.f1

30. Tietjen GE (2009) Migraine as a systemic vasculopathy. Cephalalgia 29(9): 987–96. doi:10.1111/j.1468-2982.2009.01937.x

31. Malik R, Winsvold B, Auffenberg E, Dichgans M, Freilinger T (2015) The migraine-stroke connection: A genetic perspective. Cephalalgia. Dec 9. 0333102415621055. [Epub ahead of print]

32. Tietjen EG (2007) Migraine and ischaemic heart disease and stroke: potential mechanisms and treatment implications. Cephalalgia 27(8):981–987

33. Pezzini A, Del Zotto E, Giossi A, Volonghi I, Grassi M, Padovani A (2009) The migraine-ischemic stroke connection: potential pathogenic mechanisms. Curr Mol Med 9(2):215–26

34. Cutrer FM (2010) Pathophysiology of migraine. Semin Neurol 30(2):120–130. doi:10.1055/s-0030-1249222

35. Goadsby PJ (2009) Pathophysiology of migraine. Neurol Clin 27(2):335–360. doi:10.1016/j.ncl.2008.11.012

36. Wenyi Z, Suzuki S, Hirai M, Hinokio Y, Tanizawa Y, Matsutani A, Satoh J, Oka Y (2003) Role of urotensin II gene in genetic susceptibility to Type 2 diabetes mellitus in Japanese subjects. Diabetologia 46(7):972–976

37. Ong KL, Wong LY, Man YB, Leung RY, Song YQ, Lam KS, Cheung BM (2006) Haplotypes in the urotensin II gene and urotensin II receptor gene are associated with insulin resistance and impaired glucose tolerance. Peptides 27(7):1659–1667

38. Oztuzcu S, Ulasli M, Pehlivan Y, Cevik MO, Cengiz B, Igci YZ, Okumuş S, Arslan A, Onat AM (2013) Thr21Met (T21M) but not Ser89Asn (S89N) polymorphisms of the urotensin-II (UTS-II) gene are associated with Behcet's disease (BD). Peptides 42:97–100. doi:10.1016/j

39. Tobias Freilinger, Verneri Anttila, Boukje de Vries, Rainer Malik, Mikko Kallela, Gisela M Terwindt, Patricia Pozo-Rosich, Bendik Winsvold, Dale R Nyholt, Willebrordus P J van Oosterhout, Ville Artto, Unda Todt, Eija Hämäläinen, Jèssica Fernández-Morales, Mark A Louter, Mari A Kaunisto, Jean Schoenen, Olli Raitakari, Terho Lehtimäki, Marta Vila-Pueyo, Hartmut Göbel, Erich Wichmann, Cèlia Sintas, Andre G Uitterlinden, Albert Hofman, Fernando Rivadeneira, Axel Heinze, Erling Tronvik, Cornelia M van Duijn, Jaakko Kaprio, Bru Cormand, Maija Wessman, Rune R Frants, Thomas eitinger, Bertram Müller-Myhsok, John-Anker Zwart, Markus Färkkilä, Alfons Macaya, Michel Derrari, Christian Kubisch, Aarno Palotie, Martin Dichgans, Arn M J M van den Maagdenberg & International Headache Genetics Consortium (2012) Genome-wide association analysis identifies susceptibility loci for migraine without aura. Nature Genetics 44:777–782. doi:10.1038/ng.2307

# Cost-effectiveness analysis of non-invasive vagus nerve stimulation for the treatment of chronic cluster headache

James Morris[1*], Andreas Straube[2], Hans-Christoph Diener[3], Fayyaz Ahmed[4], Nicholas Silver[5], Simon Walker[1], Eric Liebler[6] and Charly Gaul[3,7]

## Abstract

**Background:** Cluster headache (CH) is a debilitating condition that is generally associated with substantial health care costs. Few therapies are approved for abortive or prophylactic treatment. Results from the prospective, randomised, open-label PREVA study suggested that adjunctive treatment with a novel non-invasive vagus nerve stimulation (nVNS) device led to decreased attack frequency and abortive medication use in patients with chronic CH (cCH). Herein, we evaluate whether nVNS is cost-effective compared with the current standard of care (SoC) for cCH.

**Methods:** A pharmacoeconomic model from the German statutory health insurance perspective was developed to estimate the 1-year cost-effectiveness of nVNS + SoC (versus SoC alone) using data from PREVA. Short-term treatment response data were taken from the clinical trial; longer-term response was modelled under scenarios of response maintenance, constant rate of response loss, and diminishing rate of response loss. Health-related quality of life was estimated by modelling EQ-5D™ data from PREVA; benefits were defined as quality-adjusted life-years (QALY). Abortive medication use data from PREVA, along with costs for the nVNS device and abortive therapies (i.e. intranasal zolmitriptan, subcutaneous sumatriptan, and inhaled oxygen), were used to assess health care costs in the German setting.

**Results:** The analysis resulted in mean expected yearly costs of €7096.69 for nVNS + SoC and €7511.35 for SoC alone and mean QALY of 0.607 for nVNS + SoC and 0.522 for SoC alone, suggesting that nVNS generates greater health benefits for lower overall cost. Abortive medication costs were 23 % lower with nVNS + SoC than with SoC alone. In the alternative scenarios (i.e. constant rate of response loss and diminishing rate of response loss), nVNS + SoC was more effective and cost saving than SoC alone.

**Conclusions:** In all scenarios modelled from a German perspective, nVNS was cost-effective compared with current SoC, which suggests that adjunctive nVNS therapy provides economic benefits in the treatment of cCH. Notably, the current analysis included only costs associated with abortive treatments. Treatment with nVNS will likely promote further economic benefit when other potential sources of cost savings (e.g. reduced frequency of clinic visits) are considered.

**Keywords:** Chronic cluster headache, Vagus nerve stimulation, Non-invasive, Cost-effectiveness, Germany, Pharmacoeconomics, United Kingdom

* Correspondence: james.morris@cogentia.co.uk
[1]Cogentia Healthcare Consulting Ltd., Richmond House, 16-20 Regent Street, Cambridge CB2 1DB, UK
Full list of author information is available at the end of the article

# Background

Cluster headache (CH) is a debilitating condition associated with intense pain and cranial autonomic symptoms, which cause marked disability [1]. The disorder adversely affects quality of life [2] and is associated with substantial health care costs (more than €11,000 per year) [3]. The condition can be chronic or episodic. Both direct costs (e.g. medication, clinic visits) and indirect costs (e.g. reduced work capacity) have been found to be substantially higher for patients with chronic CH (cCH) than for those with episodic CH [3]. Few drugs (e.g. subcutaneous [SC] sumatriptan, intranasal [IN] zolmitriptan, and dihydroergotamine [DHE] injection) are approved by various regulatory agencies for abortive treatment [4, 5]. Lithium is approved for CH prophylaxis in Germany [6] and is used off-label in other areas. Other agents such as verapamil and topiramate are also used off-label despite a lack of rigorous, well-controlled studies to support their use in the prevention of CH attacks [7–9]. Although short-term methylprednisone therapy may be effective in CH prophylaxis, several safety concerns preclude its long-term use [8].

Vagus nerve stimulation (VNS) is a neuromodulatory technique that is well established for epilepsy and depression and has been applied to a variety of other disorders including Alzheimer disease, migraine, and CH [10–12]. It is thought to suppress pain through inhibition of vagal afferents in the trigeminal nucleus caudalis (TNC) [13] and by blocking or reversing increases in TNC glutamate levels [14]; VNS has also been implicated in modulation of the cholinergic anti-inflammatory pathway [15–17].

In an initial open-label study ($N = 19$), non-invasive vagus nerve stimulation (nVNS) was found to be effective in the prevention and treatment of CH [11]. Subsequently, a larger ($N = 97$), prospective, open-label, randomised study (PREVA [18]) evaluated the safety and efficacy of adjunctive treatment with a novel nVNS device (gamma-Core®) in patients with cCH. In the PREVA trial, compared with standard of care (SoC) alone, adjunctive nVNS (nVNS + SoC) was associated with significantly greater decreases from baseline in the number of CH attacks per week and the use of abortive medications. Compared with SoC alone, nVNS + SoC was also associated with a significantly higher response rate (i.e. the proportion of participants with a ≥50 % reduction from baseline in the number of CH attacks per week; 40 % for nVNS + SoC vs 8.3 % for SoC alone, $P < 0.001$) and significantly greater improvements from baseline in quality-of-life measures, with no serious treatment-related adverse events.

The present analysis was undertaken to quantify the economic impact of nVNS therapy in patients with cCH. By developing a pharmacoeconomic model and applying it to data from the PREVA study, we evaluated whether nVNS is a cost-effective treatment option compared with the current standard practice in a European setting. Analysis using German costs is the focus of this paper because Germans represented the largest proportion of PREVA participants. To corroborate our findings and widen their applicability, we conducted a similar analysis using UK costs, which is briefly described in the Discussion section.

# Methods

## Study design

The principal data source for this analysis was the PREVA study (clinicaltrials.gov identifier NCT01701245), which compared the effectiveness of nVNS added to SoC with that of SoC alone as prophylactic therapy for cCH. For each participant, SoC was individualised and typically included prophylactic medications (e.g. verapamil, lithium) and abortive agents (e.g. inhaled oxygen, triptans). The study design (Fig. 1) and methodology of PREVA have been described in detail previously [18]. The PREVA study was conducted in accordance with the principles and requirements of the Declaration of Helsinki, Good

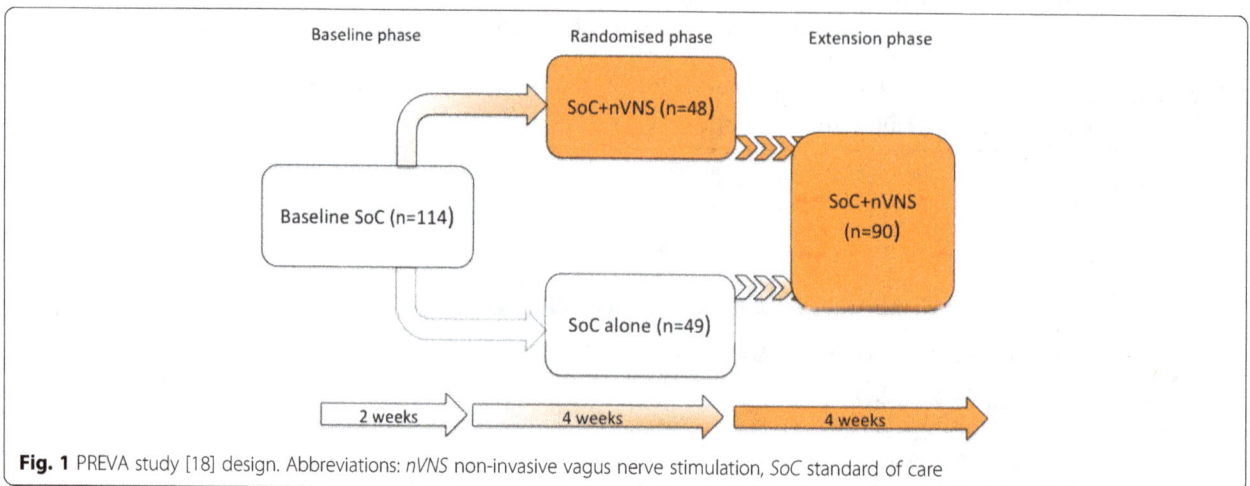

**Fig. 1** PREVA study [18] design. Abbreviations: *nVNS* non-invasive vagus nerve stimulation, *SoC* standard of care

Clinical Practices, and clinical trial registration. All PREVA investigators obtained institutional review board approval, and all PREVA participants provided written informed consent.

### Model structure and parameter estimates

Figure 2 depicts the 1-year model that was used to estimate the cost-effectiveness of adjunctive nVNS therapy from the German statutory health insurance perspective. Model parameter estimates were derived from data on the efficacy of nVNS and the use of abortive medications from the randomised phase of PREVA. *Treatment response* was defined as ≥50 % reduction from baseline in the number of CH attacks per week. Beyond the randomised phase, responders in the SoC group were assumed to be non-responders, and non-responders in the nVNS + SoC group were assumed to discontinue prophylactic treatment with nVNS but continue use of abortive treatments. Four late responders in the nVNS + SoC group (i.e. patients who were not classified as responders during the randomised phase but responded during the extension phase) were included as responders in the base case. An alternative scenario in which the 4 late responders were classified as non-responders was also modelled in a sensitivity analysis.

To estimate the probability of response in the base case analysis, subjects from the nVNS + SoC group who were responders throughout the extension phase were assumed to maintain this response until the end of the model time horizon (1 year). In addition to the base case analysis, 3 alternative scenarios were explored. An exponential survival curve function was fitted to data from

patients in the nVNS + SoC group on the basis of their response statuses at the end of the randomised phase and at the end of the extension phase. In the first alternative scenario, the exponential function was used to predict patient response status beyond 4 weeks (i.e. beyond the randomised phase) assuming a constant monthly rate (~31 %) of response loss throughout the course of the model. The second scenario was modelled assuming a diminishing rate of response loss; that is, the rate at which response was lost beyond 4 weeks (as predicted by the exponential function) was reduced by a fixed percentage (10 %) each month. In the final scenario, no patients in the SoC-alone group were assumed to have responded initially, and all other assumptions were the same as in the base case.

Benefits in this analysis were defined as quality-adjusted life-years (QALY). Health-related quality of life (HRQoL) for responders and non-responders was estimated by modelling EQ-5D™ index data from PREVA in an ordinary least squares regression analysis to control for potential imbalances at baseline between treatment arms. Results from the regression analysis suggested that response was associated with an increase of 0.2366 in EQ-5D index score and that nVNS therapy (regardless of response) was associated with an increase of 0.01246 in EQ-5D index score. Using the German tariff, HRQoL utility scores were estimated for responders and non-responders and applied to the model states (the UK tariff was applied for the UK analysis).

Data on abortive medication use from the last 14 days of the PREVA randomised phase (Table 1) were used to

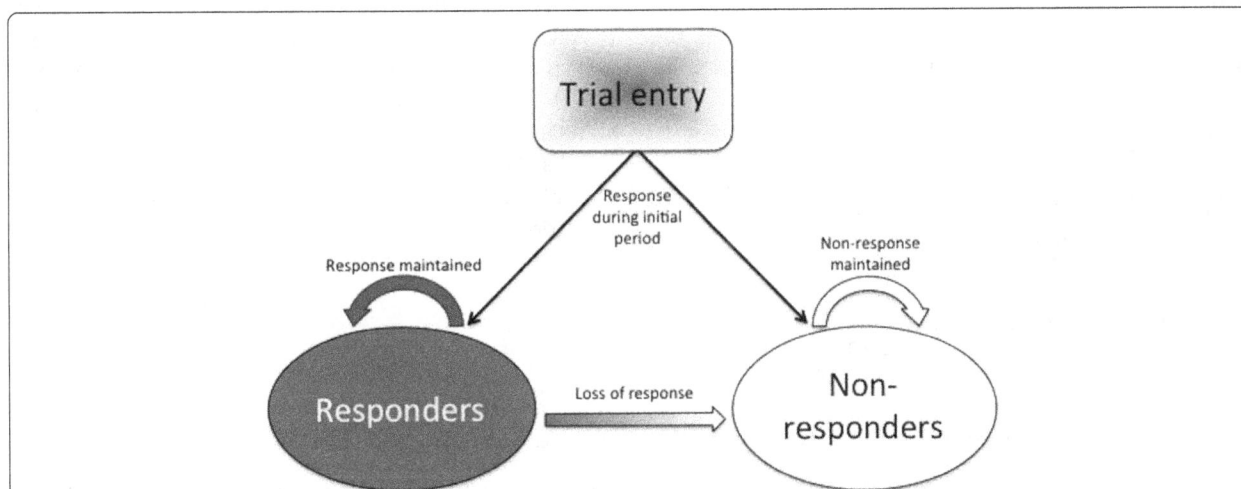

**Fig. 2** Pharmacoeconomic model structure. *Response* was defined as a ≥50 % reduction from baseline in the number of CH attacks during the randomised period (or during month 2 in the case of 4 late responders). Responders in the SoC group were modelled as non-responders beyond the randomised phase. Probability of response was modelled for the base case (response maintained) and for the following alternative scenarios: 1) constant rate of response loss, 2) diminishing rate of response loss, and 3) no initial response in the SoC group. Abbreviations: *CH* cluster headache; *SoC* standard of care

**Table 1** Abortive medication use during the last 14 days of the PREVA randomised phase

| Abortive medication | No. of uses, mean (SD) | |
| --- | --- | --- |
| | nVNS + SoC (n = 45) | SoC alone (n = 48) |
| IN zolmitriptan | 1.6 (5.5) | 1.3 (3.6) |
| SC sumatriptan | 2.8 (4.0) | 7.5 (9.6) |
| Inhaled oxygen | 6.5 (11.1) | 10.8 (15.3) |

Abbreviations: *IN* intranasal, *nVNS* non-invasive vagus nerve stimulation, *SC* subcutaneous, *SD* standard deviation, *SoC* standard of care

assess health care resource utilisation. Patients in the nVNS + SoC group who maintained responder status were assumed to continue using the same amount of resources as those observed in the overall nVNS + SoC group during the randomised phase. Non-responders were assumed to have the same resource use as that observed in the SoC group during the randomised phase. Unit costs for nVNS, triptans, and inhaled oxygen are shown in Table 2. The nVNS use cost was the listed price in Germany, and unit costs for IN zolmitriptan and SC sumatriptan were determined from the Lauer-Taxe® [19]. Costs for inhaled oxygen were derived using the estimated daily cost for oxygen from a previous study [3] and data from the baseline phase of PREVA.

All economic models are associated with uncertainty; we used a conventional method to reflect this in the analysis by developing a probabilistic model using a Markov chain Monte Carlo simulation to quantify how parameter uncertainty affects model results (i.e. the cost-effectiveness estimates for nVNS + SoC) [20, 21] (Table 3). Distributions for each model parameter of interest were estimated in line with best practice. A probabilistic analysis with 1000 simulations for each scenario was conducted, and mean values from this analysis were calculated. Each simulation was plotted on the cost-effectiveness plane to show the spread of results.

**Table 2** Unit cost of treatments

| Treatment | Description | Cost per dose, € |
| --- | --- | --- |
| IN zolmitriptan | AscoTop® Nasal 5 mg/Dosis Nasenspray, Solution €86.22: 6 single-dose nasal sprays, PZN 03107201 | 14.07[a] |
| SC sumatriptan | Sumatriptan-Hormosan Inject 6 mg/0.5-mL Solution €64.40: 2 pre-filled syringes, PZN 04700154 | 31.31[a] |
| Inhaled oxygen | Estimated cost per CH attack | 2.87 |
| nVNS | gammaCore device pre-loaded with 300 stimulations | 0.87 |

Abbreviations: *IN* intranasal, *nVNS* non-invasive vagus nerve stimulation, *SC* subcutaneous
[a]Prices include mandatory pharmacy discount of €1.77 per pack
Published prices for zolmitriptan and sumatriptan were taken from Lauer-Taxe (cheapest available price selected) [19]. Price for oxygen was estimated using daily cost from Gaul et al [3]

**Table 3** Parameters for the probabilistic sensitivity analysis

| Parameter | Mean | SE | Distribution |
| --- | --- | --- | --- |
| Probability of response with nVNS + SoC | 0.489 | 0.074 | Beta |
| Probability of response with SoC alone | 0.083 | 0.039 | Beta |
| Probability of discontinued response | 0.310 | 0.378 | Normal[a] |
| Utility score (nVNS + SoC responder) | 0.772 | NA | Multivariate normal |
| Utility score (nVNS + SoC non-responder) | 0.536 | NA | Multivariate normal |
| Utility score (SoC alone responder) | 0.760 | NA | Multivariate normal |
| Utility score (SoC alone non-responder) | 0.523 | NA | Multivariate normal |
| *Resource use per 14 days* | | | |
| With nVNS + SoC | | | |
| Zolmitriptan | 1.6 | 0.82 | Gamma |
| Sumatriptan | 2.8 | 0.60 | Gamma |
| Oxygen | 6.5 | 1.65 | Gamma |
| With SoC alone | | | |
| Zolmitriptan | 1.3 | 0.52 | Gamma |
| Sumatriptan | 7.5 | 1.38 | Gamma |
| Oxygen | 10.8 | 2.21 | Gamma |

Abbreviations: *NA* not applicable, *nVNS* non-invasive vagus nerve stimulation, *SE* standard error, *SoC* standard of care
[a]Based on exponential survival function

## Results
### Base case
For the German base case, the analysis resulted in mean expected costs of €7096.69 for nVNS + SoC and €7511.35 for SoC alone and mean QALY of 0.607 for nVNS + SoC and 0.522 for SoC alone. Thus, nVNS + SoC appears to generate greater health benefits for lower overall cost (Table 4). Approximately 80 % of the probabilistic simulations resulted in cost savings for nVNS + SoC (versus SoC alone), and the vast majority of the simulations plotted fell below the commonly used €20,000/QALY gained threshold (i.e. the amount that commissioners of health care services are willing to pay per additional unit of health with new technologies)

**Table 4** Base case[a] cost-effectiveness analysis

| Treatment group | Mean cost, € | Mean QALY | ICER[b] |
| --- | --- | --- | --- |
| nVNS + SoC | 7096.96 | 0.607 | nVNS dominant over SoC[c] |
| SoC alone | 7511.35 | 0.522 | |

Abbreviations: *ICER* incremental cost-effectiveness ratio, *nVNS* non-invasive vagus nerve stimulation, *QALY* quality-adjusted life-year, *SoC* standard of care
Probabilistic estimates are based on mean results across all Monte Carlo simulations [21]
[a]In the base case, subjects in the nVNS + SoC group who responded through the extension phase were assumed to maintain response
[b]The expense of gaining an additional QALY with adjunctive nVNS therapy (vs SoC alone)
[c]Indicates that adjunctive nVNS therapy was more effective and cost saving than SoC alone

(Fig. 3) [22–24]. Overall abortive medication costs were 23 % lower in the nVNS + SoC group than in the SoC-alone group (Fig. 4). Compared with the SoC-alone group, the nVNS + SoC group had 29 % lower SC sumatriptan costs, 19 % lower inhaled oxygen costs, and 75 % higher IN zolmitriptan costs.

### Alternative scenarios and sensitivity analysis

Altering the model by varying the likelihood for loss of response in either group had little effect on the relative cost-effectiveness of nVNS (Table 5). In the alternative scenarios explored, the percentages of the probabilistic simulations that resulted in cost savings for nVNS + SoC (versus SoC alone) were ~71 % for *constant rate of response loss* and ~79 % for both *diminishing rate of response loss* and *no response for SoC*. Results from the sensitivity analysis suggest that exclusion of the 4 late responders to nVNS (i.e. designating them as non-responders in the model) had a modest impact on cost-effectiveness. For all scenarios modelled in the sensitivity analysis, nVNS + SoC was more effective and cost saving (Table 6).

### Discussion

The treatment of CH is challenging, and many of the commonly used abortive and preventive medications are associated with serious safety risks, poor tolerability, and/or marginal efficacy. For acute treatment, triptans are contraindicated in patients with cardiovascular disease [25, 26]. Drug costs or restrictions on prescribing and/or coverage may further limit triptan accessibility for many patients [27, 28]. Long-term frequent use of triptans, as may be needed for cCH management, can in turn lead to the development of medication overuse headache [29, 30], which, although rare, has been reported in patients with CH [31, 32]. Oxygen may delay rather than abort CH attacks in some patients and has portability limitations [25, 26], and DHE may be associated with fibrosis (e.g. cardiac, pulmonary, pleural), ergotism, and chest tightness [26, 33]. For prophylactic treatment, verapamil has a high potential for drug interactions, and the large dosages required for CH treatment are associated with adverse cardiac events such as arrhythmias, as well as oedema [26]. Lithium requires progressive titration and frequent drug-level monitoring because of its narrow therapeutic window and the risk

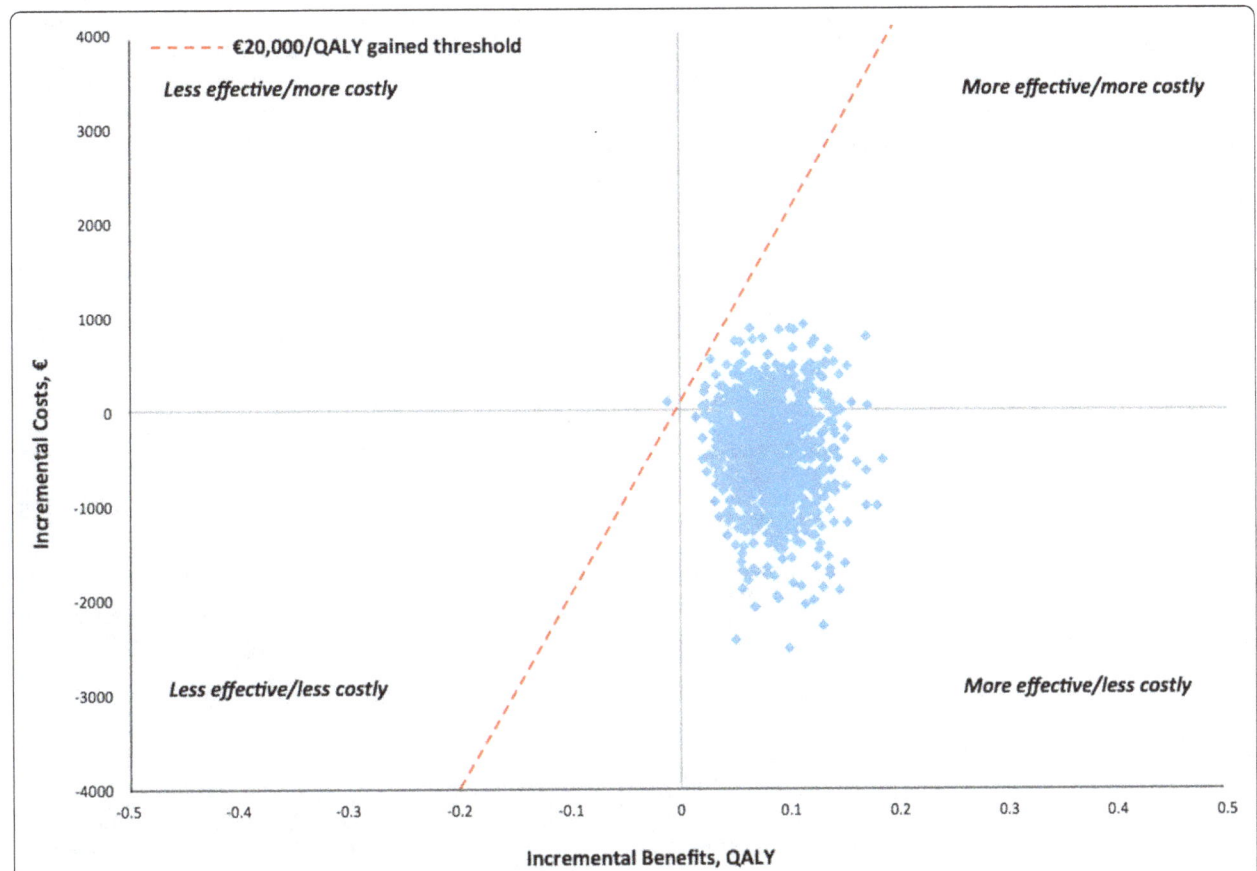

**Fig. 3** Plot of the base case model simulations (cost-effectiveness plane). Abbreviation: *QALY* quality-adjusted life-year

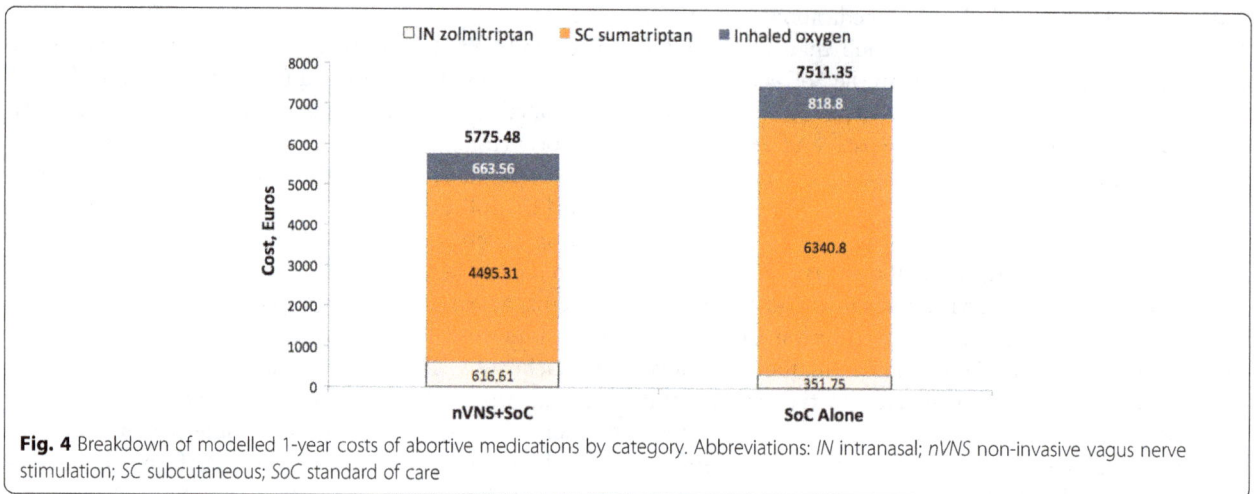

**Fig. 4** Breakdown of modelled 1-year costs of abortive medications by category. Abbreviations: *IN* intranasal; *nVNS* non-invasive vagus nerve stimulation; *SC* subcutaneous; *SoC* standard of care

of toxicity [25, 26, 34], and topiramate is often poorly tolerated owing to its cognitive side effects [26]. Thus, more practical and cost-effective treatment approaches for CH are needed. Results from the PREVA study [18] suggest that in addition to reducing the frequency of CH attacks, adjunctive nVNS therapy may decrease the need for abortive medications and improve quality of life in patients with cCH. The current pharmacoeconomic analysis indicates that adjunctive nVNS is likely to result in cost savings when compared with SoC alone. Notably, the present analysis was conservative in that it included only the costs associated with use of abortive medications without accounting for other potential sources of cost savings (e.g. reduced frequency of clinic visits, fewer hospitalisations, increased productivity).

Currently, there are few good options for acute or prophylactic treatment of CH. Neuromodulation methods such as sphenopalatine ganglion (SPG) stimulation and occipital nerve stimulation (ONS) have shown some promise in CH prevention, but most studies of these techniques have been small and/or have lacked control arms [35, 36]. Furthermore, SPG and ONS are invasive, expensive, and associated with risks inherent with implanted devices (e.g. infection, pain at the site of implantation, electrode migration). The findings that nVNS is effective in cCH prophylaxis [18], is not associated with risks that are inherent in invasive neuromodulation methods, and offers cost savings over the current standard practice suggest that this therapy warrants a prominent place in the management of cCH.

The current analysis is subject to certain limitations. The PREVA study provided data from an 8-week period,

**Table 5** Cost-effectiveness analysis for alternative scenarios

| Scenario Treatment group | Mean cost, € | Mean QALY | ICER[a] |
|---|---|---|---|
| **Constant rate of response loss** | | | |
| nVNS + SoC | 7377.41 | 0.558 | nVNS dominant over SoC[b] |
| SoC alone | 7518.56 | 0.526 | |
| **Diminishing rate of response loss** | | | |
| nVNS + SoC | 7141.30 | 0.599 | nVNS dominant over SoC[b] |
| SoC alone | 7508.98 | 0.525 | |
| **No response for SoC** | | | |
| nVNS + SoC | 7085.34 | 0.610 | nVNS dominant over SoC[b] |
| SoC alone | 7507.94 | 0.524 | |

Abbreviations: *ICER* incremental cost-effectiveness ratio, *nVNS* non-invasive vagus nerve stimulation, *QALY* quality-adjusted life-year, *SoC* standard of care
Probabilistic estimates are based on mean results across all Monte Carlo simulations [21]
[a]The expense of gaining an additional QALY with adjunctive nVNS therapy (vs SoC alone)
[b]Indicates that adjunctive nVNS therapy was more effective and cost saving than SoC alone

**Table 6** Cost-effectiveness sensitivity analysis (4 late responders excluded)

| Scenario Treatment group | Mean cost, € | Mean QALY | ICER[a] |
|---|---|---|---|
| **Response maintained** | | | |
| nVNS + SoC | 7380.93 | 0.566 | nVNS dominant over SoC[b] |
| SoC alone | 7540.28 | 0.536 | |
| **Constant rate of response loss** | | | |
| nVNS + SoC | 7392.09 | 0.550 | nVNS dominant over SoC[b] |
| SoC alone | 7440.13 | 0.539 | |
| **Diminishing rate of response loss** | | | |
| nVNS + SoC | 7279.89 | 0.560 | nVNS dominant over SoC[b] |
| SoC alone | 7385.29 | 0.537 | |

Abbreviations: *ICER* incremental cost-effectiveness ratio, *nVNS* non-invasive vagus nerve stimulation, *QALY* quality-adjusted life-year, *SoC* standard of care
[a]The expense of gaining an additional QALY with adjunctive nVNS therapy (vs SoC alone)
[b]Indicates that adjunctive nVNS therapy was more effective and cost saving than SoC alone

which were extrapolated to assess cost-effectiveness over 1 year. Although there have been few cost-effectiveness evaluations of neuromodulatory techniques for the treatment of primary headache disorders, such studies have generally included time horizons of at least 3 years [37–39]. Considering the time frame of PREVA, a 1-year time horizon was chosen for this analysis to preserve robustness and to avoid introducing unnecessary uncertainty. As in patients with epilepsy [40], evidence suggests that patients with headache may have improved response to VNS with longer-term treatment [41, 42]. Although increases in response rate with long-term VNS have yet to be explored in CH, the current analysis could be viewed as conservative because the duration of PREVA may not have allowed demonstration of the full benefit of nVNS.

Recently, the National Institute for Health and Care Excellence (NICE) Interventional Procedures Advisory Committee noted that the relapsing/remitting nature of CH and migraines as well as the potential for placebo effects should be considered when interpreting evidence of treatment efficacy for these conditions [43]. Indeed, because periods of relapse and remission are common among patients with primary headache disorders, research in this area may be susceptible to regression artefacts [44, 45]. However, the PREVA study included data from patients with cCH only. By *International Classification of Headache Disorders* definition [46], cCH is not associated with extended periods of remission (i.e. ≥1 month), suggesting that the phenomenon of regression to the mean (e.g. aberrantly high attack frequency at baseline followed by a decrease in attack frequency regardless of treatment group) would not be expected. Because the PREVA study lacked a sham treatment group, the degree to which the placebo effect might have contributed to the cost-effectiveness of nVNS is unclear. Nevertheless, the clinically relevant design of the PREVA study was valuable in that it allowed for observation of medication use in a control group that likely reflects real-world use.

As with any probabilistic analysis, some degree of uncertainty is inherent in the current investigation. To address this, a sensitivity analysis and a range of alternative scenarios were included, and results from all of these suggested that nVNS + SoC was more effective and cost saving than SoC alone. Results were relatively insensitive to assumptions about late responders in the nVNS + SoC arm. In the sensitivity analysis, where the 4 late-responding patients were classified as non-responders, nVNS + SoC was dominant over SoC alone in all modelled scenarios.

The current analysis cannot be directly extrapolated across all of Europe because it evaluates cost-effectiveness from a German health insurance perspective. To explore the generalisability of our findings, we conducted the same analysis from a UK perspective and found similar results. For the base case, the probabilistic analysis resulted in mean expected costs of £5409.83 for nVNS + SoC and £5393.31 for SoC alone and mean QALY of 0.538 for nVNS + SoC and 0.438 for SoC alone. The incremental cost-effectiveness ratio of nVNS + SoC was £166.12, and 47 % of the probabilistic simulations resulted in cost savings for nVNS + SoC over SoC alone (J. Morris, unpublished data, 2016). The degree to which these results can be generalised to other countries may vary depending on specific drug prices and the availability of generic medications in those markets.

Lastly, the current cost-effectiveness projections included only the costs associated with the use of abortive treatments. This suggests that our analysis is conservative, as data on additional health care resource use (e.g. clinic visits) would likely lead to a disproportionate cost increase for the SoC-alone group. Likewise, potential health benefits from decreased use of abortive medications (e.g. drug-related side effects) and effects on indirect costs (e.g. increased work capacity), which could further enhance the economic profile of nVNS, were not considered herein. The economic benefits of nVNS could be established with greater certainty by incorporating additional cost components into future studies.

## Conclusions

The current study provides evidence of the efficacy and economic benefits of nVNS therapy for patients with cCH in the context of the German and UK health care systems. In all scenarios modelled, nVNS was more cost-effective than the current standard practice. These findings are especially meaningful given the substantial economic burden associated with CH [3] and considering that new technologies are cited as major drivers of increasing health care expenditures [47, 48]. Our results suggest that new technologies such as nVNS may help decrease overall treatment costs, information that likely will be important to clinicians, patients, and payers when treatment decisions are made.

### Availability of data and materials

Clinical data from the PREVA study are available in the following publication: Gaul C, et al (2015) Non-invasive vagus nerve stimulation for PREVention and Acute treatment of chronic cluster headache (PREVA): a randomised controlled study [Published online September 21]. Cephalalgia. doi:10.1177/0333102415607070.

Economic data supporting the conclusions in this manuscript are on file at Cogentia Healthcare Consulting Ltd. and electroCore, LLC, and are confidential in order to support economic filings in the affected countries.

## Abbreviations

cCH: chronic cluster headache; CH: cluster headache; DHE: dihydroergotamine; HRQoL: health-related quality of life; IN: intranasal; NICE: National Institute for Health and Care Excellence; nVNS: non-invasive vagus nerve stimulation; ONS: occipital nerve stimulation; QALY: quality-adjusted life-year; SC: subcutaneous; SoC: standard of care; SPG: sphenopalatine ganglion; TNC: trigeminal nucleus caudalis; VNS: vagus nerve stimulation.

## Competing interests

James Morris is an employee of Cogentia Healthcare Consulting Ltd. Andreas Straube has received honoraria for educational talks and advisory boards from Allergan Germany; Boehringer Ingelheim; Cerbotech; Desitin Pharma; electroCore, LLC; Hormosan Pharma; MSD Germany; and Teva. Hans-Christoph Diener has received honoraria for participation in clinical trials, contribution to advisory boards, or oral presentations from Addex Pharmaceuticals; Alder Biopharmaceuticals; Allergan, Inc.; Almirall, SA; Amgen, Inc.; AstraZeneca; Autonomic Technologies, Inc.; Bayer Vital; Berlin-Chemie; Boehringer Ingelheim; Bristol-Myers Squibb; Chordate Medical; Coherex Medical; CoLucid Pharmaceuticals, Inc.; electroCore, LLC; GlaxoSmithKline; Grünenthal; Janssen-Cilag; Johnson & Johnson; Labrys Biologics Inc.; La Roche; Lilly; 3 M; Medtronic; Menarini Pharma; Minster Pharmaceuticals; MSD; NeuroScore; Novartis; Pfizer, Inc.; Pharma Medica Research Inc.; Pierre Fabre Laboratories; Sanofi; Schaper & Brümmer; St. Jude Medical; Teva; and Weber & Weber. Financial support for research projects has been provided by Allergan, Inc.; Almirall; AstraZeneca; Bayer; electroCore, LLC; GlaxoSmithKline; Janssen-Cilag; MSD; and Pfizer, Inc. Headache research at the Department of Neurology in Essen is supported by the German Research Council (DFG), the German Ministry of Education and Research (BMBF), and the European Union. Dr. Diener has no ownership interest in and does not own stocks of any pharmaceutical company.
Fayyaz Ahmed has nothing to disclose.
Nicholas Silver has received honoraria from Allergan, Inc., and electroCore, LLC; investigator fees from Amgen Inc. and Eli Lilly and Company; and investigator fees paid to the Walton Centre.
Simon Walker is an employee of Cogentia Healthcare Consulting Ltd.
Eric Liebler is an employee of electroCore, LLC, and receives stock ownership.
Charly Gaul has received honoraria from Allergan, Inc.; Autonomic Technologies, Inc.; Bayer; Berlin-Chemie; Boehringer Ingelheim; Desitin Pharmaceuticals; electroCore, LLC; Grünenthal; Hormosan Pharma; MSD; and St. Jude Medical. Dr. Gaul has no ownership interests and does not own any pharmaceutical company stocks.

## Authors' contributions

JM contributed to the design and construction of the pharmacoeconomic model and data analysis and interpretation, as well as to drafting and revision of the manuscript. AS, H-CD, FA, and NS were principal investigators in the PREVA clinical study and provided clinical expertise in data interpretation and revision of the manuscript. SW contributed to the design and construction of the pharmacoeconomic model, data analysis and interpretation, and revision of the manuscript. EL contributed to the design and construction of the pharmacoeconomic model and data interpretation, as well as to drafting and revision of the manuscript. CG was the primary principal investigator in the PREVA clinical study and provided clinical expertise in data interpretation and revision of the manuscript. All authors read and approved the final manuscript draft.

## Acknowledgements

Technical and editorial support for this manuscript was provided by Elizabeth Barton, MS, of MedLogix Communications, LLC, and funded by electroCore, LLC.

## Author details

[1]Cogentia Healthcare Consulting Ltd., Richmond House, 16-20 Regent Street, Cambridge CB2 1DB, UK. [2]Ludwig Maximilian University of Munich, Marchioninistr 15, Munich D81377, Germany. [3]Department of Neurology and Headache Center, University Hospital Essen, Hufelandstrasse 55, 45122 Essen, Germany. [4]Hull and Yorkshire Hospitals, Hull Royal Infirmary, Anlaby Road, Hull HU3 2JZ, UK. [5]The Walton Centre for Neurology and Neurosurgery, Lower Lane, Liverpool L9 7LJ, UK. [6]electroCore, LLC, 150 Allen Road, Suite 201, Basking Ridge, NJ 07920, USA. [7]Migraine and Headache Clinic Königstein, Ölmühlweg 31, 61462 Königstein im Taunus, Germany.

## References

1. Martelletti P, Mitsikostas DD (2015) Cluster headache: a quasi-rare disorder needing a reappraisal. J Headache Pain 16:59. doi:10.1186/s10194-015-0545-1
2. Jürgens TP, Gaul C, Lindwurm A, Dresler T, Paelecke-Habermann Y, Schmidt-Wilcke T, Lürding R, Henkel K, Leinisch E (2011) Impairment in episodic and chronic cluster headache. Cephalalgia 31(6):671–682. doi:10.1177/0333102410391489
3. Gaul C, Finken J, Biermann J, Mostardt S, Diener HC, Müller O, Wasem J, Neumann A (2011) Treatment costs and indirect costs of cluster headache: a health economics analysis. Cephalalgia 31(16):1664–1672. doi:10.1177/0333102411425866
4. Hedlund C, Rapoport AM, Dodick DW, Goadsby PJ (2009) Zolmitriptan nasal spray in the acute treatment of cluster headache: a meta-analysis of two studies. Headache 49(9):1315–1323. doi:10.1111/j.1526-4610.2009.01518.x
5. D.H.E. 45 [package insert]. Aliso Viejo, CA: Valeant Pharmaceuticals North America; 2014.
6. Holle D, Burmeister J, Scherag A, Ose C, Diener HC, Obermann M, Pred CH Study Group (2013) Study protocol of Prednisone in episodic Cluster Headache (PredCH): a randomized, double-blind, placebo-controlled parallel group trial to evaluate the efficacy and safety of oral prednisone as an add-on therapy in the prophylactic treatment of episodic cluster headache with verapamil. BMC Neurol 13:99. doi:10.1186/1471-2377-13-99
7. Francis GJ, Becker WJ, Pringsheim TM (2010) Acute and preventive pharmacologic treatment of cluster headache. Neurology 75(5):463–473. doi:10.1212/WNL.0b013e3181eb58c8
8. Freitag FG, Schloemer F (2014) Medical management of adult headache. Otolaryngol Clin North Am 47(2):221–237. doi:10.1016/j.otc.2013.11.002
9. May A, Leone M, Afra J, Linde M, Sándor PS, Evers S, Goadsby PJ, Force ET (2006) EFNS guidelines on the treatment of cluster headache and other trigeminal-autonomic cephalalgias. Eur J Neurol 13(10):1066–1077. doi:10.1111/j.1468-1331.2006.01566.x
10. Beekwilder JP, Beems T (2010) Overview of the clinical applications of vagus nerve stimulation. J Clin Neurophysiol 27(2):130–138. doi:10.1097/WNP.0b013e3181d64d8a
11. Nesbitt AD, Marin JC, Tompkins E, Ruttledge MH, Goadsby PJ (2015) Initial use of a novel noninvasive vagus nerve stimulator for cluster headache treatment. Neurology 84(12):1249–1253. doi:10.1212/WNL.0000000000001394
12. Yuan H, Silberstein SD (2016) Vagus nerve and vagus nerve stimulation, a comprehensive review: part I. Headache 56(1):71–78. doi:10.1111/head.12647
13. Bossut DF, Maixner W (1996) Effects of cardiac vagal afferent electrostimulation on the responses of trigeminal and trigeminothalamic neurons to noxious orofacial stimulation. Pain 65(1):101–109
14. Oshinsky ML, Murphy AL, Hekierski H Jr, Cooper M, Simon BJ (2014) Noninvasive vagus nerve stimulation as treatment for trigeminal allodynia. Pain 155(5):1037–1042. doi:10.1016/j.pain.2014.02.009
15. Brock C, Errico JP, Simon B, Imthon AK, Drewes A, Aziz Q, Lerman I, Farmer AD (2015) A report on 2 studies of the effects of non-invasive vagus nerve stimulation (nVNS) on autonomic and inflammatory parameters in healthy humans. http://vnsociety.com/wp-content/uploads/2015/11/Brock-2015-WCI-Poster-A-Report-on-2-Studies-of-the-Effects-of-nVNS-on-Autonomic-and-Inflammatory-Parameters-in-Healthy-Humans.pdf. Accessed 2 December 2015
16. Levine YA, Koopman FA, Faltys M, Caravaca A, Bendele A, Zitnik R, Vervoordeldonk MJ, Tak PP (2014) Neurostimulation of the cholinergic anti-inflammatory pathway ameliorates disease in rat collagen-induced arthritis. PLoS One 9(8):e104530. doi:10.1371/journal.pone.0104530
17. Olofsson PS, Levine YA, Caravaca A, Chavan SS, Pavlov VA, Faltys M, Tracey KJ (2015) Single-pulse and unidirectional electrical activation of the cervical vagus nerve reduces tumor necrosis factor in endotoxemia. Bioelectron Med 2:37–42. doi:10.15424/bioelectronmed.2015.00006
18. Gaul C, Diener HC, Silver N, Magis D, Reuter U, Andersson A, Liebler EJ, Straube A, PREVA Study Group (2015) Non-invasive vagus nerve stimulation for PREVention and Acute treatment of chronic cluster headache (PREVA): a randomised controlled study [Published online September 21]. Cephalalgia. doi:10.1177/0333102415607070

19. Lauer-Taxe online, available by subscription (2015) http://www.lauer-fischer.de/LF. Accessed March 2015

20. Briggs A, Sculpher M, Claxton K (2006) Decision modelling for health economic evaluation. Oxford University Press, Oxford, UK

21. Drummond MF, Sculpher MJ, Claxton K, Stoddart GL, Torrance GW (2015) Methods for the economic evaluation of health care programmes, 4th edn. Oxford University Press, Oxford, UK

22. Boersma C, Broere A, Postma MJ (2010) Quantification of the potential impact of cost-effectiveness thresholds on Dutch drug expenditures using retrospective analysis. Value Health 13(6):853–856. doi:10.1111/j.1524-4733.2010.00736.x

23. Brouwer W, van Exel J, Baker R, Donaldson C (2008) The new myth: the social value of the QALY. Pharmacoeconomics 26(1):1–4

24. Simoens S (2010) How to assess the value of medicines? Front Pharmacol 1:115. doi:10.3389/fphar.2010.00115

25. Martelletti P (2015) Cluster headache management and beyond. Expert Opin Pharmacother 16(10):1411–1415. doi:10.1517/14656566.2015.1052741

26. Pomeroy JL, Marmura MJ (2013) Pharmacotherapy options for the management of cluster headache. Clin Med Insight Ther 5:53–74. doi:10.4137/CMT.S10251

27. Khan S, Mascarenhas A, Moore JE, Knowles S, Gomes T (2015) Access to triptans for acute episodic migraine: a qualitative study. Headache 55(suppl 4):199–211. doi:10.1111/head.12593

28. Amadio A, Lee K, Yao Z, Camacho X, Knowles S, Lay C, Paterson JM, Hunt J, Gomes T, Ontario Drug Policy Research Network (2015) Public drug coverage and its impact on triptan use across Canada: a population-based study. Headache 55(suppl 4):212–220. doi:10.1111/head.12508

29. Saper JR, Da Silva AN (2013) Medication overuse headache: history, features, prevention and management strategies. CNS Drugs 27(11):867–877. doi:10.1007/s40263-013-0081-y

30. Silberstein SD Medication overuse headache. http://www.americanheadachesociety.org/assets/1/7/Stephen_Silberstein_-_Medication_Overuse_Headache.pdf. Accessed 12 January 2016

31. Paemeleire K, Evers S, Goadsby PJ (2008) Medication-overuse headache in patients with cluster headache. Curr Pain Headache Rep 12(2):122–127

32. Goadsby PJ, Cittadini E, Burns B, Cohen AS (2008) Trigeminal autonomic cephalalgias: diagnostic and therapeutic developments. Curr Opin Neurol 21(3):323–330. doi:10.1097/WCO.0b013e3282fa6d76

33. European Medicines Agency (2013) CHMP referral assessment report: ergot derivatives containing medicinal products. http://www.ema.europa.eu/docs/en_GB/document_library/Referrals_document/Ergot_derivatives-containing_products/WC500161303.pdf. Accessed 10 November 2015

34. Lee DC, Gupta A (2015) Lithium toxicity. http://emedicine.medscape.com/article/815523-overview. Accessed 8 February 2016

35. Schoenen J, Jensen RH, Lantéri-Minet M, Láinez MJ, Gaul C, Goodman AM, Caparso A, May A (2013) Stimulation of the sphenopalatine ganglion (SPG) for cluster headache treatment. Pathway CH-1: a randomized, sham-controlled study. Cephalalgia 33(10):816–830. doi:10.1177/0333102412473667

36. Schwedt TJ, Vargas B (2015) Neurostimulation for treatment of migraine and cluster headache. Pain Med 16(9):1827–1834. doi:10.1111/pme.12792

37. Pietzsch JB, Garner A, Gaul C, May A (2015) Cost-effectiveness of stimulation of the sphenopalatine ganglion (SPG) for the treatment of chronic cluster headache: a model-based analysis based on the Pathway CH-1 study. J Headache Pain 16:530. doi:10.1186/s10194-015-0530-8

38. Jenkins B, Tepper SJ (2011) Neurostimulation for primary headache disorders: part 2, review of central neurostimulators for primary headache, overall therapeutic efficacy, safety, cost, patient selection, and future research in headache neuromodulation. Headache 51(9):1408–1418. doi:10.1111/j.1526-4610.2011.01967.x

39. Leone M, Franzini A, Cecchini AP, Mea E, Broggi G, Bussone G (2009) Costs of hypothalamic stimulation in chronic drug-resistant cluster headache: preliminary data. Neurol Sci 30(suppl 1):S43–47. doi:10.1007/s10072-009-0057-3

40. Elliott RE, Morsi A, Tanweer O, Grobelny B, Geller E, Carlson C, Devinsky O, Doyle WK (2011) Efficacy of vagus nerve stimulation over time: review of 65 consecutive patients with treatment-resistant epilepsy treated with VNS > 10 years. Epilepsy Behav 20(3):478–483. doi:10.1016/j.yebeh.2010.12.042

41. Silberstein SD, Da Silva AN, Calhoun AH, Grosberg BM, Lipton RB, Cady RK, Goadsby PJ, Simmons K, Mullin C, Saper JR, Liebler EJ (2014) Chronic migraine prevention with non-invasive vagus nerve stimulation in a prospective pilot study (the EVENT study): report from the open-label phase. Presented at: 56th Annual Scientific Meeting of the American Headache Society. June 26-29, 2014. http://www.ecorelibrary.com/landing/pdf/AHS%20EVENT%20Double-blind%20Poster_PRINT%206-24-14.pdf

42. Yuan H, Silberstein SD (2015) Vagus nerve stimulation and headache. Headache. doi:10.1111/head.12721

43. National Institute for Health and Care Excellence (2015) Transcutaneous stimulation of the cervical branch of the vagus nerve for cluster headache and migraine. http://www.nice.org.uk/guidance/GID-IP1116/documents/interventional-procedure-consultation-document. Published November 2015. Accessed 11 January 2016

44. Houle TT, Turner DP, Houle TA, Smitherman TA, Martin V, Penzien DB, Lipton RB (2013) Rounding behavior in the reporting of headache frequency complicates headache chronification research. Headache 53(6):908–919. doi:10.1111/head.12126

45. Turner DP, Smitherman TA, Penzien DB, Lipton RB, Houle TT (2013) Rethinking headache chronification. Headache 53(6):901–907. doi:10.1111/head.12127

46. Headache Classification Committee of the International Headache Society (2013) The International Classification of Headache Disorders, 3rd edition (beta version). Cephalalgia 33(9):629–808. doi:10.1177/0333102413485658

47. Skinner JS (2013) The costly paradox of health-care technology. MIT Tech Rev http://www.technologyreview.com/news/518876/the-costly-paradox-of-health-care-technology/. Published September 5, 2013. Accessed 8 December 2015

48. Regalado A (2013) We need a Moore's law for medicine. MIT Tech Rev http://www.technologyreview.com/news/518871/we-need-a-moores-law-for-medicine/. Published September 3, 2013. Accessed 8 December 2015

# Onabotulinumtoxin-A treatment in Greek patients with chronic migraine

Michail Vikelis[1,2,3*†], Andreas A. Argyriou[4†], Emmanouil V. Dermitzakis[5], Konstantinos C. Spingos[6] and Dimos D. Mitsikostas[3]

## Abstract

**Background:** Chronic migraine is a disabling condition, with limited treatment options. We conducted an open label, single arm, prospective clinical trial, to assess the efficacy and safety of onabotulinumtoxin-A in Greek patients with chronic migraine. Since recent evidence suggests that a meaningful clinical response may be delayed until after a third onabotulinumtoxin-A administration, we aimed at assessing outcomes at this time point.

**Methods:** A total of 119 patients with CM, scheduled to be treated with Onabotulinumtoxin-A (Botox ®) every 3 months, according to the approved indication and standard clinical practice, were prospectively enrolled. Data documenting changes from baseline (T0—trimester before Onabotulinumtoxin-A first administration) to the period after its third administration (T3) in (i) mean number of monthly headache days (ii) migraine severity as expressed by the mean number of days with peak headache intensity of >4/10 in a 0–10 numerical scale, and (iii) mean number of days with use of any acute headache medication, were collected from patients' headache diaries at each visit.

**Results:** Of the 119 patients, a total of 81 received 3 courses of onabotulinumtoxin-A and were included in the efficacy population. In those 81 patients, there was a significant decrease in mean headache days/month between T0 and T3 ($21.3 \pm 5.4$ vs $7.7 \pm 4.8$; $P < 0.001$); a significant decrease in days with peak headache intensity of >4/10 ($11.9 \pm 5.5$ vs $3.7 \pm 3.3$; $P < 0.001$) and finally, the change in days using acute headache medications per month between was also significant ($16.2 \pm 7.8$ vs $5.2 \pm 4.3$; $P < 0.001$). Adverse events were few and of non- serious nature.

**Conclusion:** Our results strongly support the use of onabotulinumtoxin-A for the prophylaxis of CM, as this intervention proved effective, safe and well tolerated in our cohort of Greek patients.

**Keywords:** Migraine, Chronic migraine, Treatment, Prevention, Prophylaxis, Onabotulinumtoxin-A

## Background

Migraine is the 3rd most prevalent medical disorder and ranks among the leading causes of all disease-associated disability worldwide [1, 2]. Based on its frequency, migraine is subdivided into two forms, i.e., episodic (less than 15 days monthly) and chronic migraine (more than 15 headache days monthly, of which at least 8 are of migrainous type or respond to migraine-specific medication, for more than 3 months) [3]. Compared to episodic migraine, chronic migraine (CM) is associated with increased pain intensity, pain-associated symptoms, such as nausea, photophobia, phonophobia, as well as pain-related comorbidities. Moreover, patients with CM seem to have a longer average duration of headache than those with episodic migraine [4].

CM also causes greater disability in patients with increased missing household work per month, reduced productivity in household work and higher missed family activities, compared to episodic migraineurs [5]. Hence, CM has been demonstrated to significantly downgrade the health-related quality of life (HRQOL) of patients [6]. Psychiatric comorbidities seem to substantially complicate its incidence and severity [7, 8]. CM might affect up to 1 of 5 migraine patients, resulting in an estimated prevalence of about 1.4 to 2.2 % of the general population [9].

To date, the only approved treatment for CM is prophylaxis with onabotulinumtoxin A (Botox*). Its official approval in CM was given after the evaluation of its efficacy

* Correspondence: mvikelis@headaches.gr
[†]Equal contributors
[1]Headache Clinic, Mediterraneo Hospital, Glyfada, Greece
[2]Glyfada Headache Clinic, 8 Lazaraki Str, Glyfada 16675, Greece
Full list of author information is available at the end of the article

and safety in the Phase III randomized placebo-controlled identical clinical trials PREEMPT (Phase III REsearch Evaluating Migraine Prophylaxis Therapy) I and II [10, 11]. Pooled analysis of these studies, showed that onabotulinumtoxinA was effective in significantly reducing the mean frequency of headache days from baseline (week 4) to the primary endpoint at week 24, as well as in other secondary efficacy variables, including frequency of migraine, and cumulative hours of headache. Most adverse events were mild to moderate [12].

Given that recent literature contains publications reporting the outcome after administering Onabotulinumtoxin-A against CM in other South-European populations [13–17], but to our knowledge no such report exists from Greece, the aim of the current study was to explore and share our clinical experience with Onabotulinumtoxin-A in the treatment of CM in a cohort of Greek patients.

## Methods
### Study design
This study was an open-label, single-arm, prospective multicentre, clinical study, conducted in accordance with the principles of the Helsinki Declaration. Eligibility was confirmed by a protocol-specific checklist and written informed consent was obtained from each patient. Participants were enrolled from five headache centres, located in four different nodal geographic parts of Greece, including the major urban areas of Athens, Thessaloniki, Patras and the island of Corfu. The study was approved by the principal investigator's Institutional Review Board (Mediterraneo Hospital, protocol no. 1640).

### Patient selection
The study was conducted between January 2014 and April 2016. To be eligible for enrolment, participants had to be diagnosed with CM with or without medication overuse and be scheduled to receive Onabotulinumtoxin-A, according to the approved indication and the standard clinical practice.

As a national policy and shared guideline in all Greece geographical regions, the medication is approved for chronic migraine and fully reimbursed by the public social security system for patients who inadequately responded or were intolerant to previous treatments. Hence, all of our patients were treated with Onabotulinumtoxin-A if they were diagnosed with CM and, according to current reimbursement policy in Greece, were considered as non-responders to previous preventive medications, due either to lack of efficacy or intolerance. Administration of previous orally administered migraine preventives had to be stopped at least three months prior to study entry.

Enrolled patients were also required to be adult and be able to fully understand the study information provided by the investigators. Exclusion criteria included any contraindication to Onabotulinumtoxin-A, according to the approved summary of Product's Characteristics (SmPc) [18].

### Intervention
The study cohort consisted of patients scheduled to receive therapy with Onabotulinumtoxin-A (Botox® 100UI/fl, Allergan-Hellas), at fixed cranial and cervical sites at a fixed dose of 155 UI every three months, according to the PREEMPT paradigm and the approved Botox® SmPc [10, 18]. Administration of additional 40UI of Botox® was allowed, in line with the PREEMPT modified "follow the pain" paradigm, at the injector's discretion [19]. No deviation from the maximum target dose (195UI) was allowed. Patients who could not tolerate the commenced fixed dose were counted as early withdrawers due to intolerability.

### Efficacy evaluation
The primary objective of our study was to evaluate the efficacy of Onabotulinumtoxin-A as expressed by the change in mean number of monthly headache days from baseline (T0—3 months period before the first Onabotulinumtoxin-A administration) to the period after its third administration (T3). Our secondary objectives included the estimation of the crude percentage of responders to intervention. Patients were classified as responders if at T3 at least 50 % reduction in headache days was achieved and further sub-classified as good responders (at least 75 % reduction in migraine days) and excellent responders (100 % reduction in migraine days—migraine free). The percentage of reduction (50, 75, 100 %) in headache days was calculated by averaging the number of days with headache per month for the three months after each treatment and comparing this with the relative number for the three months before each treatment.

Other secondary objectives included the change in migraine severity as expressed by the change in number of days with peak headache intensity of more than 4 out of 10 in a 0–10 numerical scale (moderate/severe pain), and finally the change in days with any acute headache medications used between T0 and T3. Each patient enrolled was interviewed at baseline (T0), and after each Onabotulinumtoxin-A administration. The same neurologist performed the clinical evaluation and Onabotulinumtoxin-A injections for each individual enrolled. Patients' headache diaries were used as a source to document changes in the efficacy variables during the treatment period.

As mentioned above, our therapeutic plan was to administer at least 3 courses of onabotulinumtoxin-A to each participant before assessing efficacy (efficacy population) and thus no drop-outs were allowed earlier, unless the patients asked for their withdrawal from the intervention for any reason, including perceived lack of efficacy, adverse events, intolerance, or any other. To quantify this, we recorded the reasons for discontinuation of Onabotulinumtoxin-A administration before T3. Patients lost to follow-up for any reason consisted the Intention to Treat population (ITT) and were counted as non-responders per se.

## Safety evaluation

At each visit, patients were encouraged to report any adverse effects occurring throughout the study period either spontaneously or in response to general, non-direct questioning. Each local investigator was responsible for documenting the type and severity of overall adverse events and then categorized them for potential relationship to onabotulinumtoxin-A therapy.

## Statistical analysis

Descriptive statistics were generated for all variables. Changes in mean values of efficacy variables between T0 and T3 were assessed using the Wilcoxon rank test for paired data. All tests were two-sided and significance was set at $P < 0.05$. Statistics were performed using the SPSS for Windows (release 17.0; SPSS Inc., Chicago, IL).

## Results

A total of 119 patients (ITT population) were initially enrolled and 81 (68.1 %) of them achieved treatment with the 3$^{rd}$ course of Onabotulinumtoxin-A, thus being included in the efficacy population analysis. A total of 38 subjects asked their withdrawal from the protocol before T3 for various reasons. Table 1 describes in detail the reasons accounting for early treatment discontinuation in those 38 cases. Noteworthy, and as outlined in Table 1, there were 8 cases that dropped out early due to "perceived good response". Among those 8 patients, 3 returned with a relapse within 1 to 6 months after their withdrawal, 3 were lost to follow up and 2 remained in significant remission.

The 81 patients that attained the 3$^{rd}$ course of treatment were 8 males (9.9 %) and 73 females (90.1 %) with a mean age of $43.5 \pm 9.8$ (range: 21–75) years. Patients

**Table 1** Reasons accounting for early drop-outs ($n = 38$), before the administration of the 3$^{rd}$ Onabotulinumtoxin-A session

| Reasons of early withdrawal | N (%) |
| --- | --- |
| Perceived lack of efficacy by patients at T1 or T2 administration | 19 (50 %) |
| Patients significantly improved at T1 or T2 and perceived that no additional sessions were needed | 8 (21 %) |
| Lost to follow-up | 7 (18.3 %) |
| Financial limitations | 2 (5.3 %) |
| Intolerance to intervention | 2 (5.3 %) |

T1, T2: Trimesters after the 1$^{st}$ and 2$^{nd}$ Onabotulinumtoxin-A session, respectively

had failed of a mean number of $2.9 \pm 1.3$ (range: 1–7) previous medications, including, on a per case basis, flunarizine, valproic acid, topiramate, propranolol and amitriptyline. A total of 39/81 (48.1 %) patients had coexistent medication overuse headache (MOH) at T0, according to ICHD-III beta criteria [3]. Psychiatric comorbidities, diagnosed according to the Diagnostic and Statistical Manual of Mental Disorders, Fifth Edition [20], were common, being evident in 52/81 patients (64.2 %). Of those 52 patients, 19 (23.5 %) had anxiety disorders, 16 (19.8 %) had depression, 14 (17.3 %) and 3 (3.7 %) had bipolar disorder. Treatment, if needed, was at their psychiatrists' discretion, but it was recommended the use of a stable dose during the study's period.

The analysis of response variables in the efficacy population ($n = 81$) showed that there was a significant decrease in mean monthly headache days between T0 and T3 ($21.3 \pm 5.4$—range: 15–30 vs $7.7 \pm 4.8$—range: 2–19; $P < 0.001$). A total of 65/81 (80.2 %) patients were classified as responders, because they achieved response either at 50 % ($n = 20$; 24.7 %) or at 75 % ($n = 45$; 55.6 %). The remaining 16 patients (19.8 %) were considered as non-responders due to lack of efficacy at T3 (response less than 50 %), although 6 of them (37.5 % of non responders) achieved a 30 % reduction in headache days.

On an ITT basis, the analysis of results also favoured the intervention with Onabotulinumtoxin-A, as the majority of patients in total group (65/119; 54.6 %) experienced remission of at least 50 %. The percentage of first time responders after the third Onabotulinumtoxin-A course was 9.2 %, as 6/65 patients had not responded to first two sessions and responded to the third.

In addition, a significant decrease in migraine severity, as expressed by the change in the number of monthly days with peak headache intensity of more that 4 (moderate/severe pain) in a 0–10 numerical scale was noted between T0 and T3 ($11.9 \pm 5.5$—range: 4–30 vs $3.7 \pm 3.3$—range: 0–18; $P < 0.001$). Finally, the change in days using acute headache medications per month between T0 and T3 was also significant ($16.2 \pm 7.8$—range: 5–30 vs $5.2 \pm 4.3$—range: 0–19; $P < 0.001$). Changes in all efficacy variables between T0 and T3 (mean and median values) are summarised in Table 2.

Subgroup analysis of patients with coexistent MOH (39/81) showed that Onabotulinumtoxin-A treatment significantly reduced the mean monthly headache days at T3 compared with T0 ($24.4 \pm 5.4$—range: 16–30 vs $10.7 \pm 4.5$—range: 2–19; $P < 0.001$). Amongst patients with MOH, 29/39 (74.4 %) patients were classified as responders, because they achieved response either at 50 % ($n = 20$; 51.3 %) or at 75 % ($n = 9$; 23.1 %). In those MOH patients, there was a significant reduction in days using acute headache medications per month between T0 and T3 ($23.0 \pm 5.5$ vs $7.9 \pm 4.4$; $P < 0.001$).

**Table 2** Changes in efficacy variables from baseline (T0—trimester before initiation of therapy) to the trimester after a 3rd administration of Onabotulinumtoxin-A (Botox ®) (T3) in 81 patients comprising the efficacy population

| Efficacy variables | T0 Mean ± SD Range Median | T3 Mean ± SD) Range Median | P value |
|---|---|---|---|
| Headache days/month | 21.3 ± 5.4 | 7.7 ± 4.8 | |
| | 15–30 | 2–19 | P < 0.001 |
| | 20 | 6 | |
| Number of days with peak | 11.9 ± 5.5 | 3.7 ± 3.3 | |
| headache intensity of more than 4/10, /month | 4–30 | 0–18 | P < 0.001 |
| | 10 | 3 | |
| Days with any acute headache medication/month | 16.2 ± 7.8 5–30 14 | 5.2 ± 4.3 0–19 4 | P < 0.001 |

There were few reported events of side effects, which were transient and not severe enough to justify treatment discontinuation. We recorded side effects at the following rates: wheals in the injection site ($n = 5$; 6.2 %), mild ptosis ($n = 5$; 6.2 %), lateral eyebrow elevation ($n = 3$; 3.7 %), and shoulder and/or neck pain ($n = 3$; 3.7 %). Overall, onabotulinumtoxin-A treatment was documented to be generally safe and based on just 2 cases of early withdrawal from intervention before T3 due to intolerability (neck pain in both cases), it was also proven to be well tolerated.

## Discussion

The mode of action of Onabotulinumtoxin-A in CM is not yet completely understood. It is perceived to act by interrupting peripheral nociceptor sensitisation and, subsequently, central sensitisation, which are among the central neurophysiological events of individual migraine attacks and, when often repeated, are considered to be key factors in migraine chronification [21, 22].

Since its formal approval by the official authorities, Onabotulinumtoxin-A has reached local market availability in several countries. In Greece, the use of Onabotulinumtoxin-A for CM was approved in late 2013, and as such there is a rather limited use in Greece up to date and subsequent scarcity of data on its clinical practice. To our knowledge, literature does not contain any report on the outcome of Onabotulinumtoxin-A intervention in a population of Greek patients with CM.

In the current setting, we documented a significant improvement in all efficacy variables after 3 sessions or 9 months of Onabotulinumtoxin-A exposure. Patients comprising the efficacy population ($n = 81$) obtained an 80.2 % response rate at ≥ 50 %, whereas a corresponding rate of 54.6 % was noted in the ITT population.

Onabotulinumtoxin-A proved safe and well tolerated. A similar beneficial effect was observed in patients with coexistent MOH. As such, our results, overall, are in agreement with previously published studies applying similar study design in patients with or without MOH [13–17, 23–26].

To fully explore the efficacy of intervention and be able to capture patients who have not responded to initial treatment cycles, we sustained exposure to Onabotulinumtoxin-A for several months (9 months) and assessed response after the administration of its 3rd course. Our decision to assess efficacy at T3 was supported by recent evidence suggesting that a meaningful clinical response to Onabotulinumtoxin-A treatment in CM may take time to occur [27, 28]. In a secondary analysis of PREEMPT, the percentage of first time responders after the third Onabotulinumtoxin-A course was 10.3 % [28]. A comparable rate (9.2 %) was observed in our study, thereby bolstering the argument that a delayed response to Onabotulinumtoxin-A therapy might not be that uncommon.

The main limitation of our study was the relatively high percentage of early drop-outs before T3 ($n = 38$; 32 %) from the initial cohort of 119 patients enrolled. Even so, the sample size of our efficacy population ($n = 81$) was larger compared to other studies with similar design [13–16]. Moreover, ITT analysis also favoured Onabotulinumtoxin-A treatment in the current setting. Other limitations include the open-label, single-arm study design we applied and the non-inclusion in the protocol of specific tools assessing disability, depression and HRQOL changes over the treatment period. In any case, we conducted and herein reported the outcome of the first prospective study that was performed to reflect real-life clinical experience with Onabotulinumtoxin-A in Greek CM patients. The long-term follow-up (12–24 months) of patients included in this study is ongoing.

## Conclusions

Treatment with Onabotulinumtoxin-A proved effective, safe and well tolerated in our setting. Further studies are warranted to explore the predictors of response to Onabotulinumtoxin-A treatment in CM patients with or without MOH. In our opinion, exploring predictors of response in essential, since new treatments for CM, such as monoclonal Abs would be available in the coming years and physicians will have to decide which treatment fits better each patient.

**Abbreviations**
CM: Chronic migraine; HRQOL: Health-related quality of life; MHO: Medication overuse headache

**Funding**
No funding source had a role in the preparation and conduction of this trial or in the preparation of the manuscript and the decision to submit it for publication. Journal's article-processing charge was covered by Allergan.

## Authors' contributions

MV, KS and ED designed the protocol. MV, AA, KS and ED recruited patients and performed the assessments. AA performed the statistical analysis. AA, MV and KS drafted the manuscript. ED and DDM reviewed critically the final draft. All authors read and approved the final manuscript.

## Competing interests

MV has received honoraria and travel grants from Allergan, Greece, Brain Therapeutics, Greece and is an investigator in an Amgen-sponsored clinical trial on migraine prophylaxis. AA has received honoraria and travel grants from Allergan, Greece. EVD has received honoraria and travel grants from Allergan, Greece and is an investigator in an Amgen-sponsored clinical trial on migraine prophylaxis. KS has received honoraria and travel grants from Allergan, Greece. DDM participated in the Advisory Board of Amgen, Novartis, Eli Lilly, Teva, Merck-Serono, Sanofi-Genzyme, and received honoraria and travel grants from Almiral, Menarini, MSD, UCB and Pfizer.

## Disclosures

No author or any immediate family member has financial relationships with commercial organizations that might appear to present a potential conflict of interest with the material presented.

## Author details

[1]Headache Clinic, Mediterraneo Hospital, Glyfada, Greece. [2]Glyfada Headache Clinic, 8 Lazaraki Str, Glyfada 16675, Greece. [3]Headache Outpatient Clinic, 1st Department of Neurology, National and Kapodistrian University of Athens, Athens, Greece. [4]Neurology Department of the Saint Andrew's State General Hospital of Patras, Patras, Greece. [5]Department of Neurology, "Geniki Kliniki" Euromedica, Thessaloniki, Greece. [6]Corfu Headache Clinic, Corfu, Greece.

## References

1.   Murray CJ, Vos T, Lozano R et al (2012) Disability-adjusted life years (DALYs) for 291 diseases and injuries in 21 regions, 1990-2010: a systematic analysis for the Global Burden of Disease Study 2010. Lancet 380:2197–223
2.   No authors listed (2015) The Global Burden of Diseases: living with disability. Lancet 386:2118.
3.   Headache Classification Committee of the International Headache Society (IHS) (2013) The international classification of headache disorders, 3rd edition (beta version). Cephalalgia 33:629–808
4.   Blumenfeld AM, Varon SF, Wilcox TK, Buse DC, Kawata AK, Manack A, Goadsby PJ, Lipton RB (2011) Disability, HRQoL and resource use among chronic and episodic migraineurs: results from the International Burden of Migraine Study (IBMS). Cephalalgia 31:301–15
5.   Bigal ME, Serrano D, Reed M, Lipton RB (2008) Chronic migraine in the population: Burden, diagnosis, and satisfaction with treatment. Neurology 71:559–566
6.   Stewart WF, Wood GC, Manack A, Varon SF, Buse DC, Lipton RB (2010) Employment and work impact of chronic migraine and episodic migraine. J Occup Environ Med 52:8–14
7.   Buse DC, Manack A, Serrano D, Turkel C, Lipton RB (2010) Sociodemographic and comorbidity profiles of chronic migraine and episodic migraine sufferers. J Neurol Neurosurg Psychiatry 81:428–32
8.   Mitsikostas DD, Thomas AM (1999) Comorbidity of headache and depressive disorders. Cephalalgia 19:211–7
9.   Natoli J, Manack A, Dean B, Butler Q, Turkel CC, Stovner L, Lipton RB (2010) Global prevalence of chronic migraine: a systematic review. Cephalalgia 30:599–609
10.  Aurora SK, Dodick DW, Turkel CC, DeGryse RE, Silberstein SD, Lipton RB, Diener HC, Brin MF, PREEMPT 1 Chronic Migraine Study Group (2010) OnabotulinumtoxinA for treatment of chronic migraine: Results from the double-blind, randomized placebo controlled phase of the PREEMPT 1 trial. Cephalalgia 30:793–803
11.  Diener HC, Dodick DW, Aurora SK, Turkel CC, DeGryse RE, Lipton RB, Silberstein SD, Brin MF, PREEMPT 2 Chronic Migraine Study Group (2010) OnabotulinumtoxinA for treatment of chronic migraine: Results from the double-blind, randomized, placebo-controlled phase of the PREEMPT 2 trial. Cephalalgia 30:804–14
12.  Dodick DW, Turkel CC, DeGryse R, Aurora SK, Silberstein SD, Lipton RB, Diener HC, Brin MF, PREEMPT Chronic Migraine Study Group (2010) OnabotulinumtoxinA for treatment of chronic migraine: Pooled results from the double-blind, randomized, placebo-controlled phases of the PREEMPT clinical program. Headache 50:921–36
13.  Grazzi L (2013) Onabotulinum toxin A for treatment of chronic migraine with medication overuse. Neurol Sci 34(Suppl 1):S27–8
14.  Grazzi L, Usai S (2015) Onabotulinum toxin A (Botox) for chronic migraine treatment: an Italian experience. Neurol Sci 36(Suppl 1):33–5
15.  Pedraza MI, de la Cruz C, Ruiz M, López-Mesonero L, Martínez E, de Lera M, Guerrero ÁL (2015) OnabotulinumtoxinA treatment for chronic migraine: experience in 52 patients treated with the PREEMPT paradigm. Springerplus 4:176
16.  Russo M, Manzoni GC, Taga A, Genovese A, Veronesi L, Pasquarella C, Sansebastiano GE, Torelli P (2016) The use of onabotulinum toxin A (Botox®) in the treatment of chronic migraine at the Parma Headache Centre: a prospective observational study. Neurol Sci 37:1127–31
17.  Cernuda-Morollón E, Ramón C, Larrosa D, Alvarez R, Riesco N, Pascual J (2015) Long-term experience with onabotulinumtoxinA in the treatment of chronic migraine: What happens after one year? Cephalalgia 35:864–8
18.  The pharmaceutical catalogue eRx.gr. http://erx.gr/p/z/?type=pl&bcode= 2802480201018. Accessed 13 June 2016.
19.  Blumenfeld A, Silberstein SD, Dodick DW, Aurora SK, Turkel CC, Binder WJ (2010) Method of injection of onabotulinumtoxinA for chronic migraine: a safe, well-tolerated, and effective treatment paradigm based on the PREEMPT clinical program. Headache 50:1406–18
20.  American Psychiatric Association (2013) Diagnostic and statistical manual of mental disorders, Fifthth edn. American Psychiatric Publishing, Arlington, Sections 1.2.3 & 1.2.4 & 1.2.5. ISBN 978-0-89042-555-8
21.  Whitcup SM, Turkel CC, DeGryse RE, Brin MF (2014) Development of onabotulinumtoxinA for chronic migraine. Ann N Y Acad Sci 1329:67–80
22.  Szok D, Csáti A, Vécsei L, Tajti J (2015) Treatment of chronic migraine with OnabotulinumtoxinA: mode of action, efficacy and safety. Toxins 7:2659–73
23.  Negro A, Curto M, Lionetto L, Martelletti P (2015) A two years open-label prospective study of OnabotulinumtoxinA 195 U in medication overuse headache: a real-world experience. J Headache Pain 17:1
24.  Khalil M, Zafar HW, Quarshie V, Ahmed F (2014) Prospective analysis of the use of OnabotulinumtoxinA (BOTOX) in the treatment of chronic migraine; real-life data in 254 patients from Hull, U.K. J Headache Pain 15:54
25.  Negro A, Curto M, Lionetto L, Crialesi D, Martelletti P (2015) OnabotulinumtoxinA 155 U in medication overuse headache: a two years prospective study. Springerplus 4:826
26.  Ahmed F, Zafar HW, Buture A, Khalil M. Does analgesic overuse matter? Response to OnabotulinumtoxinA in patients with chronic. Springerplus. 2015; 9:589.
27.  Burstein R, Zhang X, Levy D, Aoki KR, Brin MF (2014) Selective inhibition of meningeal nociceptors by botulinum neurotoxin type A: therapeutic implications for migraine and other pains. Cephalalgia 34:853–69
28.  Silberstein SD, Dodick DW, Aurora SK, Diener HC, DeGryse RE, Lipton RB, Turkel CC (2015) Per cent of patients with chronic migraine who responded per onabotulinumtoxinA treatment cycle: PREEMPT. J Neurol Neurosurg Psychiatry 86:996–1001

# Risk of medication overuse headache across classes of treatments for acute migraine

Kristian Thorlund[1,2*], Christina Sun-Edelstein[3], Eric Druyts[2,4], Steve Kanters[2,5], Shanil Ebrahim[1], Rahul Bhambri[6], Elodie Ramos[6], Edward J. Mills[1,2], Michel Lanteri-Minet[7,9] and Stewart Tepper[8]

## Abstract

**Background:** The most commonly prescribed medications used to treat migraine acutely are single analgesics, ergots, opioids, and triptans. Due to varying mechanisms of action across drug classes, there is reason to believe that some classes may be less likely than others to elicit Medication Overuse Headache (MOH) than others. We therefore aimed to determine whether certain classes of acute migraine drugs are more likely to elicit MOH than others.

**Methods:** A comprehensive systematic literature was conducted to identify studies of varying designs that reported on MOH within the considered treatment classes. Only studies that reported MOH according to the International Classification of Headache Disorders (ICHD) were considered. Since no causal comparative design studies were identified; data from prevalence studies and surveys were retrieved. Prevalence-based relative risks between treatment classes were calculated by integrating both medication overuse and medication use from published studies. For each pair wise comparison, pooled relative risks were calculated as the inverse variance weighted average.

**Results:** A total of 29 studies informed the relative risk between treatment classes, all of which reported country-specific data. Five studies reported country-specific medication use data. For triptans versus analgesics the study relative risks generally favored triptans. The pooled relative risk was 0.65 (i.e., relative risk reduction of 35 %). For ergots versus analgesics, a similar trend was observed in favor of ergots with a relative risk of 0.41. For triptans versus ergots, the direction of effect was mixed, and the pooled relative risk was 1.07. Both triptans and ergots appeared favorable when compared to opioids, with pooled relative risks of 0.35 and 0.76, respectively. However, the evidence was limited for these comparisons. Analgesics and opioids also appeared to yield similar risk of MOH (pooled relative risk 1.09).

**Conclusion:** Our study suggests that in patients receiving acute migraine treatment, analgesics and opioids are associated with a higher risk of developing MOH compared with other treatments. These findings provide incentive for better monitoring of use of analgesics and opioids for treating acute migraine, and suggest possible clinical preference for use of so-called "migraine-specific" treatments, that is, triptans and ergots.

## Background

Medication-overuse headache (MOH) is caused by overuse of medications for migraines or other pain disorders. According to the International Classification of Headache Disorders, 3rd Edition, Beta (ICHD-3), MOH is defined as headache occurring on 15 or more days per month

* Correspondence: kthorlund@redwoodoutcomes.com
[1]Department of Clinical Epidemiology & Biostatistics, McMaster University, Hamilton, ON, Canada
[2]Redwood Outcomes, 302-1505 2nd Ave. West, Vancouver, BC, Canada
Full list of author information is available at the end of the article

developing as a consequence of regular overuse of acute or symptomatic headache medication (on 10 or more, or 15 or more days per month, depending on the medication) for more than 3 months [1].

MOH manifests as increased frequency and intensity of headaches or migraine attacks and enhanced sensitivity to stimuli that elicit these episodes [2] Although the mechanisms underlying MOH are not fully elucidated, it is hypothesized that repeated medication use could elicit increased headache attacks as a consequence of neuronal plasticity that may increase responsiveness to triggers. The prevalence of MOH is 1–2 % in the general population worldwide, and because of the estimated socio-economic cost, it is likely to be the most costly neurological disorder known [3–6].

Commonly prescribed medications for migraines may include analgesics, ergots, opioids, and triptans. Due to varying mechanisms of action across drug classes, there is reason to believe that some classes may be less likely than others to elicit MOH. Because of the estimated socio-economic burden of MOH, it is therefore important to establish which drug class generally is least likely to elicit MOH.

The aim of this study was therefore to determine whether certain classes of acute migraine drugs are more likely to elicit MOH than others. To achieve this, we performed a comprehensive systematic literature review of available evidence and, to the extent data allowed, extrapolated the comparative risks of MOH associated with available drug classes.

## Methods
### Eligibility criteria
Eligible studies could be either observational or clinical (randomized or non-randomized) in nature. Only studies that included adults 18 years of age and older who were suffering from acute migraine were eligible. Eligible studies must have reported MOH by treatment class (i.e. analgesic, ergot, opioid, or triptan), and according to versions of ICHD-2 [1, 7–9].

### Search strategy
In consultation with an academic medical librarian, we conducted a systematic search of the medical literature using MEDLINE, EMBASE, and the Cochrane Controlled Trials Register (from inception to March 24, 2014). The search strategy was sensitive and broad, consisting of the following: 'medication overuse headache' and 'migraine'. Conference abstracts provided through the EMBASE search were also reviewed to determine if there were relevant studies recently completed. Additionally, hand searches of the bibliographies of published systematic reviews and health technology assessments were performed. All searches were performed independently, in duplicate.

### Data extraction
We extracted data on the total number of patients, the number of patients with MOH by treatment class (i.e. analgesics, ergots, opioids, and triptans), MOH diagnostic criteria, and the country/region of each study. These data were extracted from the baseline characteristics of the studies. Two reviewers independently extracted and recorded all data in a Microsoft Excel spreadsheet. All data extraction were then checked by a third reviewer.

### Materials
Out of 443 abstracts reviewed, a total of 29 studies were eligible [10–39]. Additional file 1: Figure S1 shows the flow chart, and Additional file 1: Table S1 show the list of studies excluded following full-text review with accompanying reason for exclusion. Table 1 presents the characteristics of the included studies. All included studies had been published since the year 2004, when the ICHD-2 was first released. Eleven of the included studies adhered to the definition of MOH in version 1 of the ICHD-2, whereas 9 studies adhered to the revision put forward in 2005, and 9 studies adhered to the appendix put forward in 2006. No studies made use of ICHD-3, released in beta in 2013. All studies took place in Europe (1 in Denmark, 3 in France, 2 in Germany, 19 in Italy, 2 in Norway, 1 in Spain, and 1 in Sweden). Two studies were population based, the remaining were based out of a clinical setting (i.e., investigator headache centers, hospital departments of neurology, of headache and pain clinics).

In general, the included studies reported on use of treatment classes, but did not distinguish which individual agent or agents (e.g., sumatriptan or eletriptan for triptans) had been administered to patients. Thus, analysis by individual agents was not possible. However, since all eligible studies were published between 2006 and 2013, it is reasonable to assume that most patients receiving ergots received dihydroergotamine (DHE) and not the older ergotamine tartrate.

All studies reported MOH as prevalence estimates within included study population; no study reported MOH as an outcome. All included studies were either observational (prospective or retrospective), clinical cohorts, or population surveys.

### Data considerations
As indicated in section 3.4, no trials or observational studies looking at multiple migraine interventions reported development of MOH as an outcome. For this reason, the comparison between interventions had to be based on studies reporting prevalence estimates of MOH. While relatively few available studies were specifically designed to estimate prevalence, several still provided data on the proportion of patients using each of the interventions that had developed MOH. For example, several survey studies reported in their baseline table the number and proportion of enrolled patients with MOH. Other publications described the characteristics of migraine patients in one or more clinics, which included the number and proportion of patients with MOH. To justify inclusion of studies not designed to estimate prevalence, we made the assumption that prevalence estimates were not confounded by the designs of these studies. We verified that the eligibility criteria in these studies did not include criteria related to MOH.

**Table 1** Summary of study characteristics

| Study | Country | Diagnosis classification | Study setting | No. patients | No. medication overuse headache | | | |
|---|---|---|---|---|---|---|---|---|
| | | | | | Analgesics | Ergots | Opioids | Triptans |
| Altieri et al. 2009 [11] | Italy | ICHD-2 [7] | Clinic | 27 | 11 | NR | NR | 4 |
| Ayzenberg et al. 2008 [12] | Germany | ICHD-2 [7] | Clinic | 29 | 14 | NR | NR | 15 |
| Biagianti et al. 2012 [13] | Italy | ICHD-2 Revised [8] | Clinic | 52 | 26 | NR | NR | 20 |
| Boe et al. 2007 [14] | Norway | ICHD-2 Appendix [7] | Clinic | 100 | 20 | 1 | NR | 23 |
| Coppola et al. 2010 [15] | Italy | ICHD-2 Appendix [7] | Clinic | 29 | 10 | NR | NR | 9 |
| Cupini et al. 2009 [16] | Italy | ICHD-2 Appendix [7] | Clinic | 33 | NR | 1 | NR | 4 |
| Di Lorenzo et al. 2009 [17] | Italy | ICHD-2 [7] | Clinic | 107 | 18 | NR | NR | 29 |
| Donnet et al. 2009 [18] | France | ICHD-2 [7] | Population | 320 | 157 | 25 | 29 | 64 |
| Dousset et al. 2013 [19] | France | ICHD-2 Appendix [7] | Clinic | 42 | 8 | 1 | 0 | 9 |
| Galli et al. 2011 [20] | Italy | ICHD-2Appendix [7] | Clinic | 82 | 21 | 2 | 3 | 22 |
| Gambini et al. 2013 [21] | Italy | ICHD-2 Revised [8] | Clinic | 63 | 33 | NR | NR | 21 |
| Gomez-Beldarrain et al. 2011 [22] | Spain | ICHD-2Revised [8] | Clinic | 42 | 25 | NR | NR | 3 |
| Hagen et al. 2009 [23] | Norway | ICHD-2 Appendix [7] | Clinic | 56 | 18 | NR | 14 | 17 |
| Jonsson et al. 2011 [6] | Sweden | ICHD-2 Appendix [7] | Population | 799 | 517 | 7 | 33 | 66 |
| Lorenzo et al. 2012 [24] | Italy | ICHD-2 Appendix [7] | Clinic | 43 | 17 | NR | NR | 8 |
| Pageler et al. 2008 [25] | Germany | ICHD-2 [7] | Clinic | 20 | 1 | 3 | NR | 5 |
| Perrotta et al. 2010 [26] | Italy | ICHD-2 [7] | Clinic | 31 | 11 | NR | NR | 19 |
| Perrotta et al. 2012 [27] | Italy | ICHD-2 [7] | Clinic | 27 | 4 | NR | NR | 6 |
| Radat et al. 2013 [28] | France | ICHD-2 [7] | Clinic | 17 | 2 | NR | 2 | 4 |
| Rainero et al. 2006 [29] | Italy | ICHD-2 [7] | Clinic | 18 | NR | 2 | NR | 3 |
| Relja et al. 2006 [30] | Italy | ICHD-2 [7] | Clinic | 101 | 38 | 9 | 0 | 12 |
| Rossi et al. 2006 [31] | Italy | ICHD-2 Revised [8] | Clinic | 118 | 63 | 3 | NR | 24 |
| Rossi et al. 2011 [32] | Italy | ICHD-2 Revised [8] | Clinic | 100 | 57 | 1 | NR | 23 |
| Sances et al. 2010 [33] | Italy | ICHD2 Revised [8] | Clinic | 172 | 42 | 5 | 5 | 50 |
| Sandrini et al. 2011 [34] | Italy | ICHD-2 Appendix [7] | Clinic | 56 | 23 | 2 | NR | 20 |
| Terrazzino et al. 2010 [35] | Italy | ICHD-2 Revised [8] | Clinic | 227 | 79 | 2 | 1 | 32 |
| Trucco et al. 2010 [36] | Italy | ICHD-2Revised [8] | Clinic | 70 | 18 | 0 | NR | 9 |
| Valguarnera et al. 2010 [37] | Italy | ICHD2 [7] | Clinic | 95 | 20 | 2 | 2 | 30 |
| Zeeberg et al. 2006 [38] | Denmark | ICHD2 Revised [8] | Clinic | 216 | 63 | 8 | 12 | 43 |

Since the prevalence of MOH is highly correlated with the prevalence of drug dispensing, prevalence estimates do not provide a good basis for comparison of risk of MOH associated with the different interventions. For example, triptans are prescribed more frequently than ergots, and so we expect to see higher numbers of triptan-related MOH occurrences than ergot-related MOH occurrences. To form a fair basis for comparisons of the relevant interventions, it is therefore also necessary to know the frequency of treatment use. These were estimated post-hoc by a systematic review of the literature, and were incorporated in the calculations of comparative risk of MOH. To this end, we systematically searched MEDLINE and EMBASE for population-based studies providing estimates of medication use prevalence for the countries/regions represented in the eligible MOH prevalence studies.

The prevalence of medication use for migraine was derived from 5 studies identified in our literature review (See Table 2) [23, 40–43]. Because the data on medication prevalence use was limited, some assumptions needed to be made. For all countries, the prevalence of opioid use among those with migraine was not available. The closest evidence of opioid use prevalence that we identified was a Swedish study including chronic headache patients. This study yielded an opioid use prevalence of 4.1 %. Since use of opioids is known to be low in Europe (which is where all included studies came from) and since we believed it reasonable to assume opioid use among chronic daily headache patients would likely be higher than opioid use among acute migraine patients, we assumed an opioid use prevalence of 2 % for all included studies.

**Table 2** Prevalence of medication use for episodic migraine in Europe (column 2) and the applied adjustment factors in calculating MOH prevalence and risk ratios (columns 3–6)

| Country/Region | Drug class (Prevalence, %) | Analgesics | Ergotamines | Opioids | Triptans |
|---|---|---|---|---|---|
| Denmark [41] | Analgesics (NA) | – | NA | NA | NA |
| | Ergotamines (NA) | NA | – | NA | NA |
| | Opioids (2.0) | NA | NA | – | 1:13 (0.08) |
| | Triptans (26.0) | NA | NA | 13:1 (13.0) | – |
| France [40, 42] | Analgesics (12.0) | – | 4:1 (4.00) | 6:1 (6.0) | 6:10 (0.58) |
| | Ergotamines (3.0) | 1:4 (0.25) | – | 3:2 (1.50) | 1:7 (0.14) |
| | Opioids (2.0) | 1:6 (0.17) | 2:3 (0.67) | – | 1:10 (0.10) |
| | Triptans (20.8) | 10:6 (1.73) | 7:1 (6.93) | 10:1 (10.4) | – |
| Germany [40, 42] | Analgesics (31.0) | – | 9:2 (4.43) | 15:1 (15.0) | 2:1 (2.14) |
| | Ergotamines (7.0) | 2:9 (0.23) | – | 7:2 (3.50) | 1:2 (0.48) |
| | Opioids (2.0) | 1:15 (0.06) | 2:7 (0.29) | – | 1:7 (0.14) |
| | Triptans (14.5) | 1:2 (0.47) | 2:1 (2.07) | 7:1 (7.25) | – |
| Italy [40, 42] | Analgesics (12.0) | – | 12:3 (3.75) | 6:1 (6.00) | 4:5 (0.79) |
| | Ergotamines (3.2) | 3:12 (0.27) | – | 8:5 (1.60) | 1:5 (0.21) |
| | Opioids (2.0) | 1:6 (0.17) | 5:8 (0.63) | – | 1:8 (0.13) |
| | Triptans (15.1) | 5:4 (1.25) | 5:1 (4.72) | 8:1 (7.55) | – |
| Norway [43] | Analgesics (NA) | – | NA | NA | NA |
| | Ergotamines (NA) | NA | – | NA | NA |
| | Opioids (2.0) | NA | NA | – | 1:19 (0.05) |
| | Triptans (37.0) | NA | NA | 19:1 (18.5) | – |
| Spain [40] | Analgesics (16.4) | – | 4:5 (0.82) | 8:1 (8.20) | 1:2 (0.56) |
| | Ergotamines (20.0) | 5:4 (1.22) | – | 10:1 (10.0) | 2:3 (0.69) |
| | Opioids (2.0) | 1:8 (0.12) | 1:10 (0.10) | – | 1:15 (0.07) |
| | Triptans (29.1) | 2:1 (1.77) | 3:2 (1.46) | 15:1 (14.6) | – |
| Sweden [23] | Analgesics (NA) | – | NA | NA | NA |
| | Ergotamines (NA) | NA | – | NA | NA |
| | Opioids (2.0) | NA | NA | – | 3:19 (0.16) |
| | Triptans (26.0) | NA | NA | 19:3 (6.34) | – |

The medication use prevalence estimates presented in parenthesis next to treatment classes in column 2 are taken from included prevalence literature. The ratios (e.g. 3:1) presented in columns 3–6 are approximate ratios of prevalence of use of one medication over another. These ratios are also the adjustments factors multiplied to the unadjusted ratios of MOH for each study to account for the missing information about patients at risk on each medication within each study

## Analysis

For each study we first calculated the proportion of patients with MOH in each treatment class, using the total number of patients as the denominator for both proportions. Subsequently the relative risk was calculated between each pair of treatment classes. As mentioned in the previous section, these relative risks are highly driven by the proportion of patients that received each treatment. For this reason, we applied an adjustment to the relative risk estimates. In particular, we first estimated the ratio with which treatments are being prescribed in clinical practice from prevalence estimates of medication use, and multiplied the inverse of this ratio to the above-obtained relative risks (see Table 2). Further, sensitivity analysis assuming an 8 % medication use prevalence for opioids, was conducted.

The adjusted study relative risks were pooled for each comparison in a fixed-effect meta-analysis. A fixed-effect model was used to provide a fair weighted average of studies. The *meta* function in *R.v.3.0* was used to pool results and produce forest plots. While this function by convention produces 95 % credible intervals, one should only focus on the relative risk estimates and the weighted (pooled) average relative risk, since confidence intervals address sampling error and therefore are not valid under the above adjustments.

## Results

### Triptans versus analgesics

Twenty-five studies informed MOH for both triptans and analgesics in countries where medication use prevalence estimates were also available for both. Adjusted relative risks from these studies are presented in Fig. 1a. Fourteen studies yielded relative risks in favor of triptans, with adjusted relative risks varying from 0.12 to 0.94. In 9 of these 14 studies the relative risk was statistically significant. Eleven studies yielded adjusted relative risks in favor of analgesics, with adjusted relative risk estimates varying from 1.05 to 5.00. The fixed-effect weighted average adjusted relative risk was 0.65, thus suggesting an average 35 % relative risk reduction of MOH associated with triptans compared with analgesics.

### Triptans versus ergots

Fourteen studies informed MOH for both triptans and ergots in countries where medication use prevalence estimates were also available for both. Adjusted relative risks from these studies are presented in Fig.1b. Four studies yielded adjusted relative risk estimates in favor of triptans, two yielded no difference (i.e. relative risk of 1.00), and eight studies yielded adjusted relative risk estimates in favor of ergots. The fixed-effect weighted average relative risk was 1.07.

### Triptans versus opioids

Eleven studies informed MOH for both triptans and opioids in countries where medication use prevalence estimates were also available for both. Adjusted relative risks from these studies are presented in Fig.1c. Five studies yielded adjusted relative risk estimates in favor of triptans, one study suggested no difference, and five studies yielded relative risk estimates in favor of opioids. The fixed-effect weighted average adjusted relative risk was 0.35, suggesting an average 65 % relative risk reduction of MOH with triptans compared with opioids.

### Ergots versus analgesics

Twelve studies informed MOH for both ergots and analgesics in countries where medication use prevalence estimates were also available for both. Adjusted relative risks from these studies are presented in Fig.2a. Eleven of these yielded adjusted relative risk estimates in favor of ergots, and only one small study cell with a zero cell in the analgesics arm yielded a relative risk estimate in favor of analgesics. Among the former 11, adjusted relative risks varied between 0.07 and 0.90. The fixed-effect weighted average adjusted relative risk was 0.41, suggesting an average 59 % relative risk reduction of MOH with ergots compared with analgesics.

### Ergots versus opioids

Seven studies informed MOH for both ergots amines and opioids. Adjusted relative risks from these studies are presented in Fig.2b. Four of these studies yielded adjusted relative risk estimates in favor of ergots (ranging from 0.33 to 0.60), one yielded an adjusted relative risk estimate of 1.00 (i.e., no difference), and two studies, both with zero cells in the opioids arm, yielded relative risk estimates in favor of opioids. The fixed-effect weighted average relative risk was 0.76, suggesting an average 24 % relative risk reduction of MOH with ergots compared with opioids. As noted, this likely reflects mostly DHE use rather than ergotamine tartrate.

### Analgesics versus Opioids

Nine studies informed MOH for both analgesics and opioids. Adjusted relative risks from these studies are presented in Fig.2c. Three studies yielded adjusted relative risk estimates in favor of analgesics, and six studies yielded relative adjusted risk estimates in favor of opioids. The fixed-effect weighted average adjusted relative risk was 1.09, suggesting an average 9 % increased risk of MOH with analgesics compared with opioids.

### Discussion

Our analysis aimed to evaluate rates of MOH depending on the type of medication used. We found a considerably higher rate of MOH associated with analgesics in comparison to triptans and ergots. Our findings also suggest that opioids are either associated with a higher or similar risk of MOH compared to triptans and ergots, but evidence was more limited for these comparisons. These findings should be of interest to patients, clinicians, and policy-makers as many patients may self-medicate, and the magnitude of analgesic use is potentially higher than what has generally been observed in population-based studies.

There are strengths and limitations to our analysis that should be considered. Strengths of this study include our extensive searching to complete the largest and first systematic review of MOH associated with migraine pharmacotherapies. We used an approach that integrated evidence on medication overuse and medication use, the first such effort of which we are aware.

The employed approach further strengthens comparisons between interventions, since all studies provide data on at least two interventions, and so allows for the analysis to retain within-study validity. Studies included had to use the ICHD-2 criteria or later, and thus removed most uncertainty about the appropriateness of the MOH definition, which was particularly variable in older studies. However, this eligibility criterion also came with the limitation that the American Migraine Prevalence and Prevention (AMPP) study was not eligible [35]. In fact, no US studies were eligible under the employed criteria. Therefore, generalizability of our findings to the US population is somewhat limited.

We relied instead on observational studies reporting a mix of pseudo-risk data and medication use data to approximate the relative risk between interventions.

**(A)**

**Risk Ratio**

| Study | RR | W(fixed) |
|---|---|---|
| Altieri et al 2009 | 0.27 | 1.5% |
| Ayzenberg et al 2008 | 1.07 | 1.9% |
| Biagianti et al 2012b | 0.77 | 3.5% |
| Boe et al 2007 | 1.15 | 2.7% |
| Coppola et al 2010 | 0.90 | 1.4% |
| Di Lorenzo et al 2009 | 1.61 | 2.4% |
| Donnet et al 2009 | 0.41 | 21.3% |
| Dousset et al 2013 | 1.12 | 1.1% |
| Galli et al 2011 | 1.05 | 2.9% |
| Gambini et al 2013 | 0.64 | 4.5% |
| Gomez-Beldarrain et al 2011 | 0.12 | 3.4% |
| Hagen et al 2009 | 0.94 | 2.4% |
| Lorenzo et al 2012 | 0.47 | 2.3% |
| Pageler et al 2008 | 5.00 | 0.1% |
| Perrotta et al 2010 | 1.73 | 1.5% |
| Perrotta et al 2012 | 1.50 | 0.5% |
| Radat et al 2013 | 2.00 | 0.3% |
| Relja et al 2006 | 0.32 | 5.2% |
| Rossi et al 2006 | 0.38 | 8.6% |
| Rossi et al 2011 | 0.40 | 7.7% |
| Sances et al 2010b | 1.19 | 5.7% |
| Sandrini et al 2011 | 0.87 | 3.1% |
| Terrazzino et al 2010 | 0.41 | 10.7% |
| Trucco et al 2010 | 0.50 | 2.4% |
| Valguarnera et al 2010 | 1.50 | 2.7% |
| **Fixed effect model** | **0.65** | **100%** |
| Heterogeneity: I-squared=80.4%, | | |

0.1    0.5 1 2    10

**(B)**

| Study | RR | W(fixed) |
|---|---|---|
| Cupini et al 2009 | 1.00 | 1.7% |
| Donnet et al 2009 | 0.36 | 42.7% |
| Dousset et al 2013 | 1.00 | 1.7% |
| Galli et al 2011 | 2.50 | 3.4% |
| Pageler et al 2008 | 0.67 | 5.1% |
| Rainero et al 2006 | 0.50 | 3.4% |
| Relja et al 2006 | 0.33 | 15.4% |
| Rossi et al 2006 | 1.67 | 5.1% |
| Rossi et al 2011 | 5.00 | 1.7% |
| Sances et al 2010b | 2.20 | 8.5% |
| Sandrini et al 2011 | 2.00 | 3.4% |
| Terrazzino et al 2010 | 3.50 | 3.4% |
| Trucco et al 2010 | 5.00 | 0.9% |
| Valguarnera et al 2010 | 3.00 | 3.4% |
| **Fixed effect model** | **1.07** | **100%** |
| Heterogeneity: I-squared=43.1% | | |

0.01    0.1    1    10    100

**(C)**

| Study | RR | W(fixed) |
|---|---|---|
| Donnet et al 2009 | 0.21 | 28.3% |
| Dousset et al 2013 | 3.00 | 0.5% |
| Galli et al 2011 | 1.00 | 2.9% |
| Hagen et al 2009 | 0.07 | 13.7% |
| Jonsson et al 2011 | 0.09 | 32.2% |
| Radat et al 2013 | 0.20 | 2.4% |
| Relja et al 2006 | 5.00 | 0.5% |
| Sances et al 2010b | 1.40 | 4.9% |
| Terrazzino et al 2010 | 4.00 | 1.0% |
| Valguarnera et al 2010 | 2.00 | 2.0% |
| Zeeberg et al 2006 | 0.25 | 11.7% |
| **Fixed effect model** | **0.35** | **100%** |
| Heterogeneity: I-squared=67.3% | | |

0.01    0.1    1    10    100

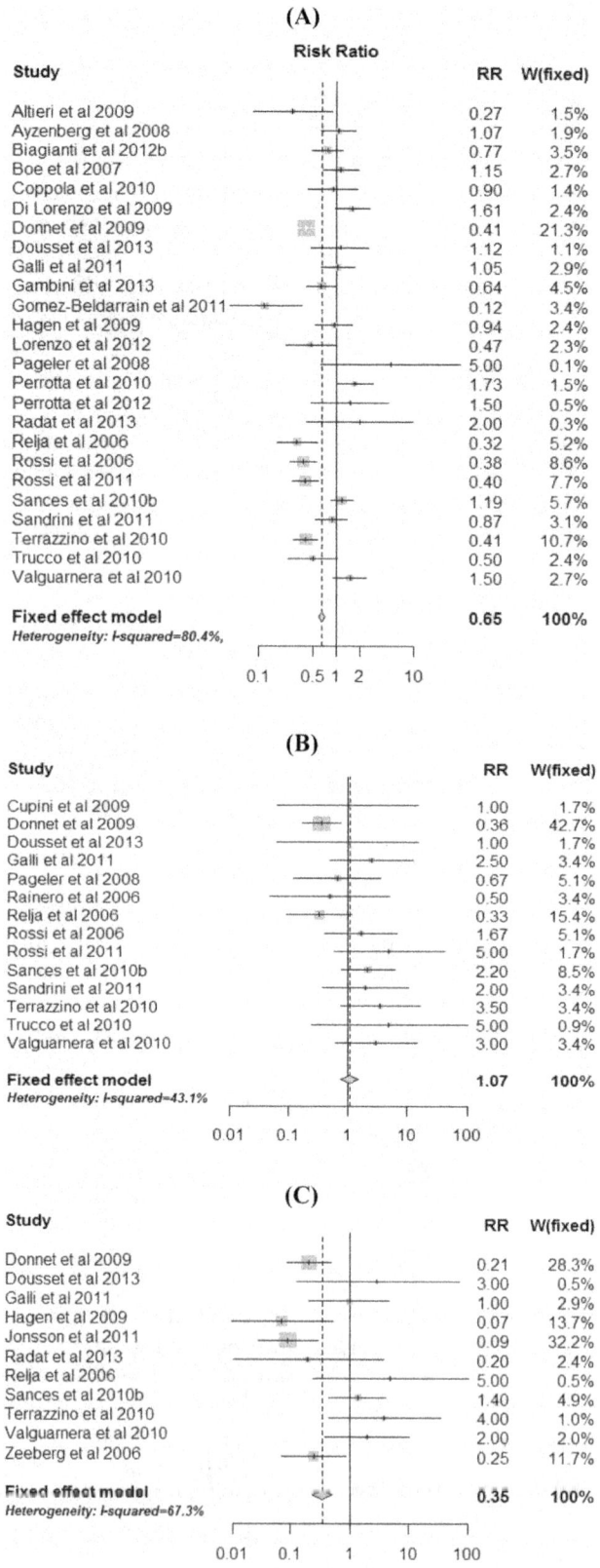

**Fig. 1** Forest plots and weighted average estimate for the relative risk of MOH for the three comparisons: **a** triptans versus analgesics; **b** triptans versus ergots; and **c** triptans versus opioids

**(A)**

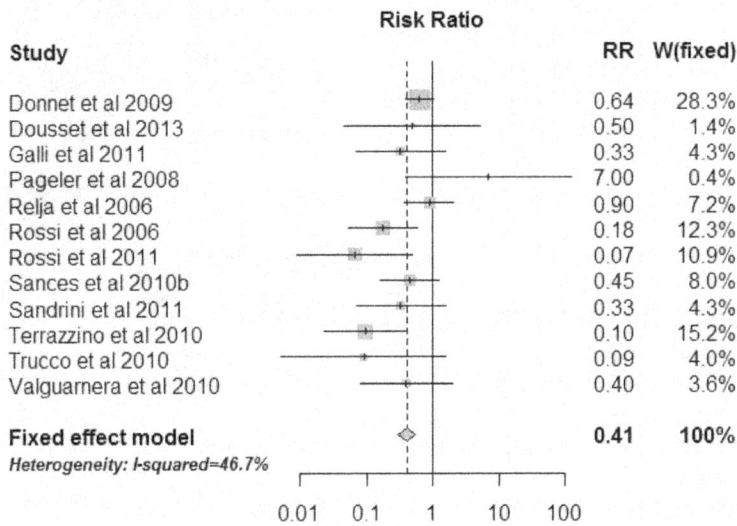

**(B)**

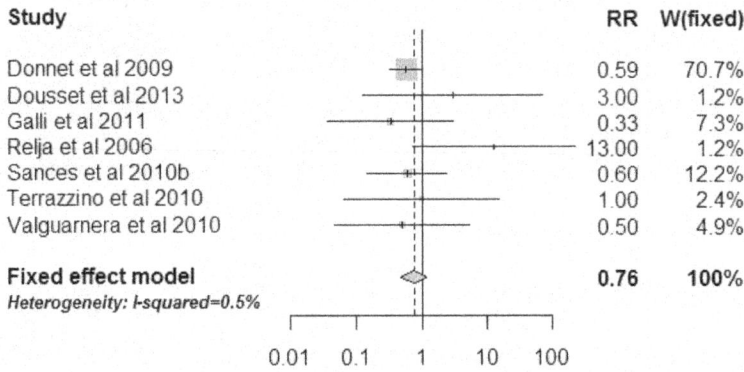

**(C)**

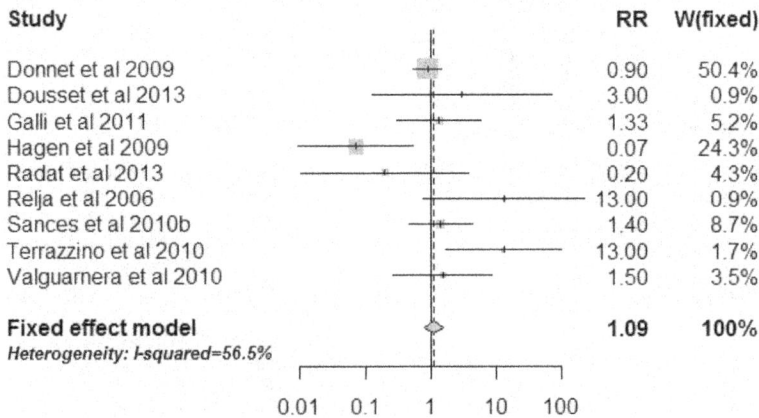

**Fig. 2** Forest plots and weighted average estimate for the relative risk of MOH for the three comparisons: **a** ergots versus analgesics; **b** ergots versus opioids; and **c** analgesics versus opioids

The analytical approached employed to synthesize results from these data relied on assumption that are arguably strong. There may therefore be controversy as to where the evidence fits in the evidence hierarchy. Recognizing the challenges of conducting these evaluations, and given the consistency of our study findings, the investigators believe this systematic review of observational studies provides strong inferences about the causative factors of MOH. The heterogeneity between studies was generally low, in spite of the observational nature of the included studies and the additional uncertainty one might expect from the employed medication use prevalence adjustments. Also, the findings of the individual pair-wise meta-analysis added up 'indirectly'. For example, the direct comparison of triptans and ergots showed similar risk of MOH, and both drug classes had similar relative risk estimates when compared with analgesics (0.65 and 0.41). These consistencies thus add considerable confidence to the findings of the analyses.

There are several possible reasons for our finding increased MOH associated with analgesic and opioid use and less so with triptans and ergots. Analgesics and opioids typically work via targeting pain receptors. On the other hand, both triptans and ergots share serotonergic agonist activity and are vasoconstrictors. Furthermore, analgesics are frequently used in an over-the-counter manner whereby patients self-administer and may do so without the supervision of a clinician. Triptans are, for the most part, prescription medications, and overuse may be better monitored than analgesics. In those countries in which triptans are available without a prescription (e.g. UK, Germany), quantity limits may prevent tendency to overuse.

While our findings are in line with current clinical guidelines and prejudice in favor of targeted migraine-specific pharmacotherapy, they should still only be interpreted as exploratory due to their observational nature. Further, the inclusion of only European studies limits our ability to extrapolate the findings to other global regions.

In summary, our study suggests that in patients with acute episodic migraine, the rate of MOH associated with analgesics and opioids is considerably higher than the rate of MOH associated with triptans and ergots. These findings should be of interest to patients, clinicians, and policymakers, as many patients self-medicate, and the magnitude of analgesic use is potentially higher than what has generally been observed in population-based studies.

## Authors' contributions

KT prepared the first draft of the manuscript and contributed to all revisions, contributed to the concept and study design, contributed to the systematic literature review, contributed to the statistical analyses, and contributed to the interpretation of findings. CSE contributed to the writing of the manuscript, the concept and study design, the systematic literature review, as well as the interpretation of findings. ED and SE contributed to the concept and study design, systematic literature review, and the writing of the manuscript. SK contributed to concept and study design, the statistical analysis and the writing of the manuscript. RB and ER contributed to the concept and study design, the writing of the manuscript and the interpretation of findings. EJM, MLM, and ST, contributed to the concept and study design, the writing of the manuscript, the systematic literature review, and the interpretation of findings. All authors read and approved the final manuscript.

## Competing interests

The study was funded by Pfizer Inc. Redwood Outcomes conducted this study. Drs. Thorlund and Mills are founding partners of Redwood Outcomes and were paid consultants for conducting this study and for the development of this manuscript. Drs. Thorlund and Mills have previously consulted to Boehringer Ingleheim, Merck, Pfizer, Novartis, Janssen, Roche, Novo Nordisk, UCB, Sanofi, BTG, Bayer, Teva, Lundbeck, Lilly, and Gilead on systematic reviews and network meta-analysis. In addition, Drs. Thorlund and Mills have received grant funding from the Canadian Institutes of Health Research (CIHR) Drug Safety & Effectiveness Network to develop methods and educational materials on network meta-analysis. Eric Druyts, and Ping Wu are employees of Redwood Outcomes. Drs Bhambri and Ramos are full-time employees of Pfizer Inc. Dr. Lanteri-Milnet has received compensation from Allergan, Almirall SAS, Amgen, Astellas, AstraZeneca Pharmaceuticals, ATI, BMS, Boehringer, Boston Scientific, CoLucid, Convergence, Glaxo-SmithKline, Grunenthal, Lilly, Johnson & Johnson, Medtronic, Menarini, MSD, Pierre Fabre, Pfizer, ReckittBenckiser, Saint-Jude, Sanofi-Aventis, UCB, Zambon. Dr. Sun-Edelstein has received lecture fees from Pfizer and MSD. Dr. Tepper has received grant funding from Alder, Allergan, Amgen, ATI, ElectroCore, eNeura, GSK, Teva, Pernix, Optinose/Avanir/Otsuka; served as a consultant to Acorda, Allergan, Amgen, ATI, Avanir, Depomed, Impax, Pfizer, Scion Neurostim, Teva, Zosana; participated in speakers bureau activities for Allergan, Depomed, Impax, Pernix, Teva and Advisory activities for Allergan, Amgen, ATI, Avanir, Dr. Reddy's, Merck, Teva, Pfizer. Dr. Tepper further holds stock in ATI. Drs. Ebrahim and Kanters have nothing to disclose.

## Author details

[1]Department of Clinical Epidemiology & Biostatistics, McMaster University, Hamilton, ON, Canada. [2]Redwood Outcomes, 302-1505 2nd Ave. West, Vancouver, BC, Canada. [3]Department of Medicine, St. Vincent's Hospital, The University of Melbourne, Melbourne, Australia. [4]Department of Medicine, Faculty of Medicine, University of British Columbia, Vancouver, BC, Canada. [5]School of Population and Public Health, Faculty of Medicine, University of British Columbia, Vancouver, BC, Canada. [6]Pfizer Ltd, New York, NY, USA. [7]Pain Department, CHU Nice, France - FHU InovPain, Université Nice Côte d'Azur, Nice, France. [8]Geisel School of Medicine at Dartmouth, Hanover, NH, USA. [9]INSERM U1107, Neuo-Dol, Trigeminal Pain and Migraine Université Auvergne, Clermont-Ferrand, France.

## References

1.  Headache Classification Committee of the International Headache Society (IHS). The International Classification of Headache Disorders, 3rd edition (beta version). Cephalalgia. 2013;33:629–808.
2.  De Felice M, Ossipov MH, Porreca F (2011) Update on medication-overuse headache. Curr Pain Headache Rep 15:79–83
3.  Russell MB, Lundqvist C (2012) Prevention and management of medication overuse headache. Curr Opin Neurol 25:290–5
4.  Grande RB, Aaseth K, Gulbrandsen P, Lundqvist C, Russell MB (2008) Prevalence of primary chronic headache in a population-based sample of 30- to 44-year-old persons. The Akershus study of chronic headache. Neuroepidemiology 30:76–83
5.  Aaseth K, Grande RB, Kvaerner KJ, Gulbrandsen P, Lundqvist C, Russell MB (2008) Prevalence of secondary chronic headaches in a population-based

sample of 30-44-year-old persons. The Akershus study of chronic headache. Cephalalgia 28:705–13

6. Jensen R, Stovner LJ (2008) Epidemiology and comorbidity of headache. Lancet Neurol 7:354–61

7. Headache Classification Committee of The International Headache Society (2004) The International Classification of Headache Disorders, 2nd edition. Cephalalgia 24:1–160

8. Silberstein S, Olesen J, Bousser M (2005) The International Classification of Headache Disorders, 2nd edition (ICHD-II)-revision of criteria for 8.2 Medication-overuse headache. Cephalagia 25:460–465

9. Olesen J, Bousser M, Diener H (2006) New appendix criteria open for a broader concept of chronic migraine. Cephalagia 26:742–746

10. Altieri M, Di Giambattista R, Di Clemente L, Fagiolo D, Tarolla E, Mercurio A, Vicenzini E, Tarsitani L, Lenzi GL, Biondi M, Di Piero V (2009) Combined pharmacological and short-term psychodynamic psychotherapy for probable medication overuse headache: a pilot study. Cephalalgia 29:293–9

11. Ayzenberg I, Oberman M, Leineweber K, Franke L, Yoon MS, Diener HC, Katsarava Z (2008) Increased activity of serotonin uptake in platelets in medication overuse headache following regular intake of analgesics and triptans. J Headache Pain 9:109–112

12. Biagianti B, Grazzi L, Gambini O, Usai S, Muffatti R, Scarone S, Bussone G (2012) Decision-making deficit in chronic migraine patients with medication overuse. Neurol Sci 33(Suppl 1):S151–5

13. Boe MG, Mygland A, Salvesen R (2007) Prednisolone does not reduce withdrawal headache: a randomized, double-blind study. Neurology 69:26–31

14. Coppola G, Curra A, Di Lorenzo C, Parisi V, Gorini M, Sava SL, Schoenen J, Pierelli F (2010) Abnormal cortical responses to somatosensory stimulation in medication-overuse headache. BMC Neurol 10:126

15. Cupini LM, De Murtas M, Costa C, Mancini M, Eusebi P, Sarchielli P, Calabresi P (2009) Obsessive-compulsive disorder and migraine with medication-overuse headache. Headache 49:1005–13

16. Di Lorenzo C, Di Lorenzo G, Sances G, Ghiotto N, Guaschino E, Grieco GS, Santorelli FM, Casali C, Troisi A, Siracusano A, Pierelli F (2009) Drug consumption in medication overuse headache is influenced by brain-derived neurotrophic factor Val66Met polymorphism. J Headache Pain 10:349–55

17. Donnet A, Lanteri-Minet M, Aucoin F, Allaf B (2009) Use and overuse of antimigraine drugs by pharmacy personnel in France: COTA survey: Research submission. Headache 49:1014–1021

18. Dousset V, Maud M, Legoff M, Radat F, Brochet B, Dartigues JF, Kurth T (2013) Probable medications overuse headaches: validation of a brief easy-to-use screening tool in a headache centre. J Headache Pain 14:81

19. Galli F, Pozzi G, Frustaci A, Allena M, Anastasi S, Chirumbolo A, Ghiotto N, Guidetti V, Matarrese A, Nappi G, Pazzi S, Quartesan R, Sances G, Tassorelli C (2011) Differences in the personality profile of medication-overuse headache sufferers and drug addict patients: a comparative study using MMPI-2. Headache 51:1212–27

20. Gambini O, Biagianti B, Grazzi L, Usai S, Scarone S, Bussone G (2013) Psychiatric screening for migraine patients. Neurol Sci 34(Suppl 1):S61–6

21. Gomez-Beldarrain M, Carrasco M, Bilbao A, Garcia-Monco JC (2011) Orbitofrontal dysfunction predicts poor prognosis in chronic migraine with medication overuse. J Headache Pain 12:459–66

22. Hagen K, Albretsen C, Vilming ST, Salvesen R, Gronning M, Helde G, Gravdahl G, Zwart JA, Stovner LJ (2009) Management of medication overuse headache: 1-year randomized multicentre open-label trial. Cephalalgia 29:221–32

23. Jonsson P, Hedenrud T, Linde M (2011) Epidemiology of medication overuse headache in the general Swedish population. Cephalalgia 31:1015–22

24. Lorenzo CD, Coppola G, Curra A, Grieco G, Santorelli FM, Lepre C, Porretta E, Pascale E, Pierelli F (2012) Cortical response to somatosensory stimulation in medication overuse headache patients is influenced by angiotensin converting enzyme (ACE) I/D genetic polymorphism. Cephalalgia 32:1189–97

25. Pageler L, Katsarava Z, Diener HC, Limmroth V (2008) Prednisone vs. placebo in withdrawal therapy following medication overuse headache. Cephalalgia 28:152–6

26. Perrotta A, Arce-Leal N, Tassorelli C, Gasperi V, Sances G, Blandini F, Serrao M, Bolla M, Pierelli F, Nappi G, Maccarrone M, Sandrini G (2012) Acute reduction of anandamide-hydrolase (FAAH) activity is coupled with a reduction of nociceptive pathways facilitation in medication-overuse headache subjects after withdrawal treatment. Headache 52:1350–61

27. Perrotta A, Serrao M, Sandrini G, Burstein R, Sances G, Rossi P, Bartolo M, Pierelli F, Nappi G (2010) Sensitisation of spinal cord pain processing in medication overuse headache involves supraspinal pain control. Cephalalgia 30:272–84

28. Radat F, Chanraud S, Di Scala G, Dousset V, Allard M (2013) Psychological and neuropsychological correlates of dependence-related behaviour in Medication Overuse Headaches: a one year follow-up study. J Headache Pain 14:59

29. Rainero I, Ferrero M, Rubino E, Valfre W, Pellegrino M, Arvat E, Giordano R, Ghigo E, Limone P, Pinessi L (2006) Endocrine function is altered in chronic migraine patients with medication-overuse. Headache 46:597–603

30. Relja G, Granato A, Bratina A, Antonello RM, Zorzon M (2006) Outcome of medication overuse headache after abrupt in-patient withdrawal. Cephalalgia 26:589–95

31. Rossi P, Di Lorenzo C, Faroni J, Cesarino F, Nappi G (2006) Advice alone vs. structured detoxification programmes for medication overuse headache: a prospective, randomized, open-label trial in transformed migraine patients with low medical needs. Cephalalgia 26:1097–105

32. Rossi P, Faroni JV, Nappi G (2011) Short-term effectiveness of simple advice as a withdrawal strategy in simple and complicated medication overuse headache. Eur J Neurol 18:396–401

33. Sances G, Ghiotto N, Galli F, Guaschino E, Rezzani C, Guidetti V, Nappi G (2010) Risk factors in medication-overuse headache: a 1-year follow-up study (care II protocol). Cephalalgia 30:329–36

34. Sandrini G, Perrotta A, Tassorelli C, Torelli P, Brighina F, Sances G, Nappi G (2011) Botulinum toxin type-A in the prophylactic treatment of medication-overuse headache: a multicenter, double-blind, randomized, placebo-controlled, parallel group study. J Headache Pain 12:427–33

35. Silberstein S, Loder E, Diamond S, Reed ML, Bigal ME, Lipton RB, Group AA (2007) Probable migraine in the United States: results of the American Migraine Prevalence and Prevention (AMPP) study. Cephalalgia 27:220–9

36. Terrazzino S, Sances G, Balsamo F, Viana M, Monaco F, Bellomo G, Martignoni E, Tassorelli C, Nappi G, Canonico PL, Genazzani AA (2010) Role of 2 common variants of 5HT2A gene in medication overuse headache. Headache 50:1587–96

37. Trucco M, Meineri P, Ruiz L, Gionco M (2010) Medication overuse headache: withdrawal and prophylactic therapeutic regimen. Headache 50:989–97

38. Valguarnera F, Tanganelli P (2010) The efficacy of withdrawal therapy in subjects with chronic daily headache and medication overuse following prophylaxis with topiramate and amitriptyline. Neurol Sci 31(Suppl 1):S175–7

39. Zeeberg P, Olesen J, Jensen R (2006) Probable medication-overuse headache: the effect of a 2-month drug-free period. Neurology 66:1894–8

40. Bloudek LM, Stokes M, Buse DC, Wilcox TK, Lipton RB, Goadsby PJ, Varon SF, Blumenfeld AM, Katsarava Z, Pascual J, Lanteri-Minet M, Cortelli P, Martelletti P (2012) Cost of healthcare for patients with migraine in five European countries: results from the International Burden of Migraine Study (IBMS). J Headache Pain 13:361–78

41. Lyngberg AC, Rasmussen BK, Jorgensen T, Jensen R (2005) Secular changes in health care utilization and work absence for migraine and tension-type headache: a population based study. Eur J Epidemiol 20:1007–14

42. MacGregor EA, Brandes J, Eikermann A (2003) Migraine prevalence and treatment patterns: the global Migraine and Zolmitriptan Evaluation survey. Headache 43:19–26

43. Zwart JA, Dyb G, Hagen K, Svebak S, Holmen J (2003) Analgesic use: a predictor of chronic pain and medication overuse headache: the Head-HUNT Study. Neurology 61:160–4

# Real-life data in 115 chronic migraine patients treated with Onabotulinumtoxin A during more than one year

I. Aicua-Rapun[1], E. Martínez-Velasco[2], A. Rojo[3], A. Hernando[1], M. Ruiz[2], A. Carreres[3], E. Porqueres[1], S. Herrero[3], F. Iglesias[1] and A. L. Guerrero[2*]

## Abstract

**Background:** OnabotulinumtoxinA (OnabotA) is effective in Chronic Migraine (CM) during first year of treatment and longer. In real clinical setting, CM patients with acute Medication Overuse (MO) or concurrently receiving oral preventatives are treated with OnabotA. We aim to assess evolution of CM patients beyond first year on OnabotA.

**Methods:** Data were retrospectively collected in three headache units. We analyzed cases who had received at least five sessions of OnabotA according to PREEMPT protocol. We continued OnabotA therapy when a reduction of number of headache days of at least 30% was achieved.

**Results:** We included 115 patients (98 females, 17 males) who completed $7.6 \pm 2.3$ (5–13) OnabotA procedures. Previously they had not responded to topiramate and, at least, one other preventative. Age at inclusion was $45.3 \pm 12$ (14–74) years, and latency between CM onset and OnabotA therapy was $43.1 \pm 38.2$ (6–166) months. At first OnabotA session 92 patients (80%) fulfilled MO criteria and 107 (93%) received a concurrent oral preventative. In 42 cases (36.5%) OnabotA dose was increased over 155 units. After first year in 57 out of 92 patients (61.9%) MO was discontinued. Among those receiving preventatives, in 52 out of 107 they were retired (48.6%). In 22 cases (19.1%) OnabotA administration was delayed to the fourth or fifth month and in 12 (10.4%) it was temporally stopped. Finally, in 18 patients (15.7%) OnabotA was discontinued due to lack of efficacy beyond first year of treatment.

**Conclusion:** Our results suggest that discontinuation of acute medication overuse and oral preventive therapies are achievable objectives in long-term using of OnabotA in CM patients.

**Keywords:** Chronic Migraine, Medication overuse, OnabotulinumtoxinA, Preventatives, Real-life data

## Background

Chronic migraine (CM) is an evolution of migraine, defined as headache occurring on 15 or more days per month during more than 3 months, which has the features of migraine headache on at least 8 days per month [1]. CM is estimated to affect 2% of the population [2]. Most of these patients (50–80%) fulfilled criteria of symptomatic medication overuse with all its somatic and psychological implications [2]. Besides, CM patients

need preventive therapy but, excepting with topiramate, there are no controlled trials evaluating the oral preventatives commonly used in chronic migraine patients [3, 4].

After publication of the PREEMPT clinical program [5–7], in January 2012 OnabotulinumtoxinA (OnabotA) was licensed in Spain for prophylactic treatment of CM "for patients who have not adequately responded or are intolerant to prophylactic drugs for migraine".

In a real-life setting, OnabotA can effectively reduce headache days and migraine days by at least 50%, and increase headache free days from baseline in chronic migraine sufferers [8–10]. Also in a real clinical practice, around 80% of CM patients respond to pericranial

* Correspondence: gueneurol@gmail.com
Partially presented as a Poster at the II Meeting of the European Academy of Neurology, Copenhagen, May 2016.
[2]Neurology Department, Hospital Clínico Universitario de Valladolid, Avda. Ramón y Cajal 3, 47005 Valladolid, Spain

injections of OnabotA during and after the first year of therapy [11].

Our aim is to analyse real-life experience with the use of OnabotA in the treatment of patients with CM refractory or intolerant to oral preventives in three Headache Units beyond first year. We focused on symptomatic medication overuse and concurrent prophylaxis therapy.

## Methods

Cases were selected from prospective registers of patients with CM treated with OnabotA in three headache units located in three tertiary hospitals in Castilla-Leon (Spain). During the inclusion period (January 2012–January 2016), we included adult patients fulfilling criteria for CM [1]. Patients with comorbidities such as anxiety, depression or fibromyalgia and those with common vascular risk factors were also included.

OnabotA was initiated in patients who had not responded positively to at least topiramate (or another neuromodulator if topiramate was not tolerated) and a beta-blocker. We ensured that these drugs were administered at adequate doses and enough time to be effective.

Using a headache diary, patients recorded headache days, migraine days (defined as high intensity, lateralized pain with a significant impairment on daily activities) and the number of days on which they used symptomatic medication, particularly triptans, as well as the number of monthly visits to emergency department as a consequence of headache.

Exclusion criteria for the use of OnabotA were pregnant or breast-feeding women, or excessive use of alcohol. We did not exclude patients who fulfilled criteria for medication overuse, and they were allowed to continue with previous preventive oral medications with no dose increasing.

OnabotA therapy was continued when at least 30% of reduction in headache days was achieved, according to the headache diary. Patients without improvement of at least 30% reduction of headache days after three procedures were considered as no responders and OnabotA was stopped.

We retrospectively analyzed cases who had received at least five sessions of OnabotA. Statistical analysis was performed with the SPSS 20.0 statistical package.

## Results

### Demographic and baseline headache characteristics

A total of 115 patients were included, 98 females (85.2%) and 17 males. Mean age at first procedure was 45.3 ± 12 years (range 14–74 years). The latency between CM diagnosis and OnabotA therapy was 43.1 ± 38.2 months (6–166). They had received 7.6 ± 2.3 oral preventatives (range 5–13) previously to inclusion.

Among the 115 patients, 107 (93%) were receiving a concurrent oral preventive therapy when OnabotA was initiated. Besides, 92 patients (80%) fulfilled medication overuse criteria according to ICHD-3beta, including 47 (40.8%) patients overusing triptans.

In our three centers, 26 additional patients were treated with OnabotA due to a CM during the inclusion period. Among these patients, 21 did not respond after one to three procedures, one dropped out due to adverse effects, and in four cases follow-up was lost.

### Outcome

Our 115 patients completed 7.6 ± 2.3 [5–13] OnabotA procedures (Fig. 1). Follow the pain protocol with additional OnabotA injections to reach up to 195 OnabotA units was used in 42 cases (36.5%), mainly when response time was shorter than 3 months.

In 79 patients (68.7%) the CM remitted to episodic migraine. When considering the concurrent prophylactic treatments, in 52 out of 115 (45.2%) cases, oral drugs were retired and in 16 (13.9%) their dose was reduced.

In 57 out of 92 (61.9%), MO was discontinued. The consumption of any kind of analgesics decreased from an average of 19.1 days per month before the first OnabotA procedure to 8.6 days per month. When considering triptans overuse, its consumption decreased from 18 to 4 days per month.

Due to a good clinical response after third procedure, we were able to delay the OnabotA session to a fourth or fifth month in 22 patients (19.1%), whilst in 12 (10.4%), it was temporally stopped.

Finally, in 18 cases (15.7%) OnabotA therapy was interrupted beyond first year due to a lack of efficacy. Most of these patients had improved between 30 and 50% during first year of treatment.

## Discussion

In our study, baseline characteristics of patients were comparable to those described in the PREEMPT trial

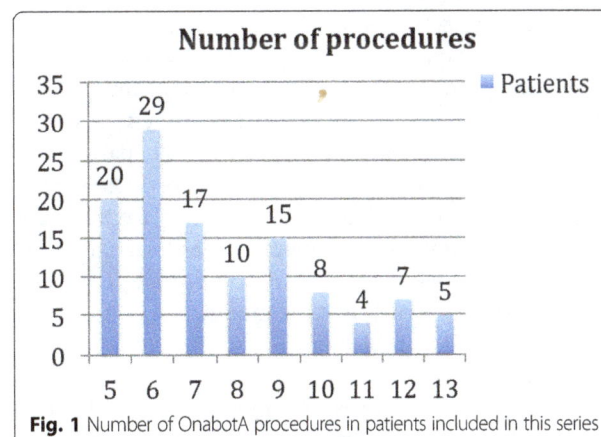

**Fig. 1** Number of OnabotA procedures in patients included in this series

[5–7]. Efficacy of OnabotA in our series was also similar as it was described in studies in a real-life setting [8–15].

In order to properly reflect a real-life setting, we did not exclude patients with symptomatic medication overuse. Within the PREEMPT patient population two-thirds overused acute pain medication during the 28-day baseline period [5, 6] and OnabotA was also effective in CM patients with MO [14]. Other real-life studies considered patients with medication overuse [8, 10] and OnabotA efficacy did not differ between patients with or without MO [16]. In our series, percentage of patients fulfilling medication overuse criteria was similar than observed in PREEMPT program. As additional data not previously offered in real-life studies, we achieved the discontinuation of MO in two thirds of patients.

We also included in our analysis CM patients with concurrent preventive oral therapies; in the same way that Cernuda-Morollon et al. series, percentage of patients receiving a preventative when OnabotA therapy was initiated was high [10]. One of our objectives during OnabotA treatment was to retire concurrent oral therapy and we began to decrease its use after third procedure. We were able (and this is again a point not previously considered in these kind of studies) to retire oral preventatives in almost half of our patients.

The need to modify the OnabotA injection paradigm with the "follow the pain" increasing with up to 40 additional Units remains open, and is commonly left to physician's discretion. Negro et al. [11] showed an increased efficacy of 195 UI compared with 155 UI in a group of patients with chronic migraine with medication overuse, with no increasing in related side effects. Our study was not designed to evaluate the differences between both doses.

During last years, studies considering long-term experience with Onabot A in a real-life setting have been published [10, 17, 18]. OnabotA efficacy showed consistency after first year; percentage of patients in which OnabotA response was not maintained after first year were among 10 and 15% comparing our results with a quite similar series as that by Cernuda-Morollon et al. [10]. Another question still open to discussion is the possibility of ending OnabotA therapy after first year in patients with a good response; it has been shown that when treatment is stopped quality of life parameters worsen [17]. In the same way that previous studies [10, 18], we found that it is not easy to interrupt OnabotA therapy, even temporally. However, in nearly 20% of cases we were able to postpone OnabotA procedures to a fourth of fifth month.

## Conclusion

According to our series, OnabotA efficacy in CM patients is consistent beyond first year of treatment.

Though prolonged interruption of OnabotA is difficult to achieve, we consider that discontinuation of acute medication overuse and oral preventive therapy as well as reduction of frequency of procedures are realistic goals in real-life long-term using of OnabotA in CM patients.

**Funding**

Allergan Inc. funded the article-processing charges. Neither honoraria nor payments were made for authorship. All authors met the ICMJE authorship criteria.

**Competing interest**

The authors declare that they have no competing interest.

**Author details**

[1]Neurology Department, Hospital Universitario de Burgos, Burgos, Spain. [2]Neurology Department, Hospital Clínico Universitario de Valladolid, Avda. Ramón y Cajal 3, 47005 Valladolid, Spain. [3]Neurology Department, Hospital Clínico Universitario, Valladolid, Spain.

**References**

1.  Headache Classification Committee of the International Headache Society (IHS) (2013) The international classification of headache disorders, 3rd edition (beta version). Cephalalgia 33:629–808
2.  Natoli JL, Manack A, Dean B, Butler Q, Turkel CC, Stovner L et al (2010) Global prevalence of chronic migraine: A systematic review. Cephalalgia 30:599–609
3.  Diener HC, Bussone G, Van Oene JC, Lahaye M, Schwalen S, Goadsby P (2007) Topiramate reduces headache days in chronic migraine: A randomized, double blind, placebo-controlled study. Cephalalgia 27:814–823
4.  Silberstein SD, Lipton RB, Dodick DW, Freitag FG, Ramadan N, Matthew N et al (2007) Efficacy and safety of topiramate for the treatment of chronic migraine: A randomized, double-blind, placebo -controlled trial. Headache 47:170–180
5.  Aurora SK, Dodick DW, Turkel CC et al (2010) Onabotulinumtoxin A for treatment of chronic migraine: Results from the double-blind, randomized, placebo-controlled phase of the PREEMPT 1 trial. Cephalalgia 30:793–803
6.  Diener HC, Dodick DW, Aurora SK, Turkel CC, Re DG, Rb L et al (2010) Onabotulinumtoxin A for treatment of chronic migraine: Results from the double blind, randomized, placebo-controlled phase of the PREEMPT 2 trial. Cephalalgia 30:804–814
7.  Aurora SK, Winner P, Freeman MC, Turkel CC, Re DG, Silberstein SD et al (2011) Onabotulinumtoxin A form treatment of chronic migraine: Pooled analyses of the 56-week PREEMPT clinical program. Headache 51:1358–1373
8.  Khalil M, Zafar H, Quarshie V, Fayyaz A (2014) Prospective analysis of the use of Onabotulinumtoxin A (BOTOX) in the treatment of chronic migraine; real life data in 254 patients from Hull. UK J Headache Pain 15:54
9.  Pedraza MI, De la Cruz C, Ruiz M, López-Mesonero L, Martínez E, de Lera M et al (2015) Onabotulinumtoxin A treatment for chronic migraine: experience in 52 patients treated with the PREEMPT paradigm. Springer Plus 4:176
10. Cernuda-Morollón E, Ramón C, Larrosa D, Alvarez R, Riesco N, Pascual J (2015) Long-term experience with onabotulinumtoxin A in the treatment of chronic migraine: What happens after one year? Cephalalgia 35:864–68
11. Negro A, Curto M, Lionetto L, Martelletti P (2016) A two years open-label prospective study of Onabotulinumtoxin A 195 U in medication overuse headache: a real-world experience. J Headache Pain 17:1
12. Russo M, Manzoni GC, Taga A, Genovese A, Veronesi L, Pasquarella C et al (2016) The use of onabotulinum toxin A (Botox) in the treatment of chronic migraine at the Parma Headache Centre: a prospective observational study. Neurol Sci 37:1127–31

13. Grazzi L, Usai S (2015) Onabotulinum toxin A (Botox) for chronic migraine treatment: an Italian experience. Neurol Sci 36(Suppl 1):S33–S35
14. Silberstein SD, Blumenfeld AM, Cady RK, Turner IM, Lipton RB, Diener HC et al (2013) Onabotulinumtoxin A for treatment of chronic migraine: PREEMPT 24-week pooled subgroup analysis of patients who had acute headache medication overuse at baseline. J Neurol Sci 331(1–2):48–56
15. Negro A, Curto M, Luana L, Giamberardino MA, Martelletti P (2016) Chronic migraine treatment: from Onabotulinumtoxin A onwards. Expert Rev Neurother 16:1217–1227
16. Ahmed F, Zafar HW, Buture A, Khalil M (2015) Does analgesic overuse matter? Response to Onabotulinumtoxin A in patients with chronic migraine with or without medication overuse. Springer Plus 4:589
17. Guerzoni S, Pellesi L, Baraldi C, Pini LA (2016) Increased efficacy of regularly repeated cycles with Onabotulinumtoxin A in MOH patients beyond the first year of treatment. J Headache Pain 17:48
18. Kollewe K, Escher CM, Wulff DU, Fathi D, Paracka L, Mohammadi B et al (2016) Long-term treatment of chronic migraine with Onabotulinumtoxin A: efficacy, quality of life and tolerability in a real-life setting. J Neural Transm (Vienna) 123:533–40

# Texture features of periaqueductal gray in the patients with medication-overuse headache

Zhiye Chen[1,2,3], Xiaoyan Chen[2], Mengqi Liu[1,3], Shuangfeng Liu[1], Lin Ma[1*] and Shengyuan Yu[2*]

## Abstract

**Background:** Periaqueductal gray (PAG) is the descending pain modulatory center, and PAG dysfunction had been recognized in migraine. Here we propose to investigate altered PAG texture features (quantitative approach for extracting texture descriptors for images) in the patients with medication-overuse headache (MOH) based on high resolution brain structural image to understand the MOH pathogenesis.

**Methods:** The brain structural images were obtained from 32 normal controls (NC) and 44 MOH patients on 3.0 T MR system. PAG template was created based on the ICBM152 gray matter template, and the individual PAG segment was performed by applying the deformation field to the PAG template after structural image segment. Grey-level co-occurrence matrix (GLCM) was performed to measure the texture parameters including angular second moment (ASM), Contrast, Correlation, inverse difference moment (IDM) and Entropy.

**Results:** Contrast was increased in MOH patients ($9.28 \pm 3.11$) compared with that in NC ($7.94 \pm 0.65$) ($P < 0.05$), and other texture features showed no significant difference between MOH and NC ($P > 0.05$). The area under the ROC curve was 0.697 for Contrast in the distinction of MOH from NC, and the cut-off value of Contrast was 8.11 with sensitivity 70. 5% and specificity 62.5%. The contrast was negatively with the sleep scores ($r = -0.434$, $P = 0.003$).

**Conclusion:** Texture Contrast could be used to identify the altered MR imaging characteristics in MOH in understanding the MOH pathogenesis, and it could also be considered as imaging biomarker in for MOH diagnosis.

**Keywords:** Brain, Magnetic resonance imaging, Medication-overuse headache, Migraine, Periaqueductal gray, Texture analysis

## Background

Periaqueductal gray (PAG) is a center with powerful descending pain modulatory center in the midbrain, which include various layered neurons around the aquaeductus mesencephali [1, 2], and whose dysfunction had been recognized in migraine [3]. PAG, as a substantial descending pain modulatory center, exerts inhibition and facilitation control on nociceptive transmission in the dorsal horn and trigeminal nucleus [4], and the modulatory mechanism was exerted by descending PAG-RVM (rostral ventromedial medulla) pathway contributing to central sensitization and development of secondary hyperalgesia [4, 5]. PAG included multiple types of neurons (eg. L-glutamate,γ-aminobutyric acid (GABA), opioids (particularly enkephalin), substance P), and had distinct connections with the forebrain, brainstem, and nociceptive neurons of lamina I of the spinal cord and trigeminal nucleus [6–9]. Therefore, PAG was confirmed as a critical component of a network responding to pain and receiving functionally input from nociceptive pathways [10–12].

In the previous studies, the specific PAG lesions had been identified in multiple sclerosis [13–17] and infarction [18], and nonspecific PAG lesions was also revealed in episodic migraine (EM) patients in our previous study [19]. The specific lesions was the direct evidence for migraine, and the nonspecific lesions was indirectly used to explain

---
* Correspondence: cjr.malin@vip.163.com; yusy1963@126.com
[1]Department of Radiology, Chinese PLA General Hospital, Beijing 100853, China
[2]Department of Neurology, Chinese PLA General Hospital, Beijing 100853, China
Full list of author information is available at the end of the article

the migraine pathogenesis, which may be associated with iron deposition and may be considered as a possible "generator" of migraine attacks [1, 20, 21]. However, the neuromechinism for nonspecific PAG lesions in migraine was still not elucidated up to now.

Medication-overuse headache (MOH) is a secondary form of chronic headache deriving from episodic migraine (EM) related to the overuse of triptans, analgesics and other acute headache medications [22–24]. Resting-state functional MRI (rs-fMRI) demonstrated altered functional connectivity was revealed in MOH, and suggested that MOH is associated with intrinsic brain network changes rather with macrostructural changes [23]. Voxel-based morphometry (VBM) recognized that increased gray matter in the midbrain presented in MOH [25]. Recently, some studies also confirmed an altered nucleus accumbens functional connectivity of motivational circuits [22] and abnormal connectivity between the PAG and other pain modulatory (frontal) regions in MOH, which were consistent with dysfunctional central pain control [26]. Although the functional and structural MRI recognized the PAG dysfunction in MOH patients, these methods did not presented the detailed changes of the intrinsic natures of PAG in MOH patients.

Texture features are the intrinsic properties of image and provide an efficient image classification to detect subtle alterations in the gray level distribution of an image [27]. Texture feature analysis had been widely applied in the brain tumor [28, 29], epilepsy [30, 31], muscular dystrophy [32], Attention-Deficit/Hyperactivity Disorder classification [33], and mild cognitive impairment [34]. However, MR imaging texture feature analysis was not applied in medication-overuse headache (MOH) so far.

In this study, we hypothesize MOH patients without T2-visible lesions may present altered texture features changes in MR structural images. To address this hypothesis, we prospectively obtained high resolution structural images from 44 MOH patients and 32 NCs without T2-visible lesions on the brain. Gray level co-occurrence matrix(GLCM) [35, 36] was used to calculate the texture parameters of PAG including angular second moment (ASM), Contrast, Correlation, inverse difference moment (IDM) and Entropy in the subjects, which would be used to detect the texture features change for PAG to elucidate the neuromechnism of PAG dysfunction in MOH pathogenesis.

## Methods
### Subjects
Written informed consent was obtained from all participants according to the approval of the ethics committee of the local institutional review board. Forty-four MOH patients and 32 normal controls were recruited from the International Headache Center, Department of Neurology, Chinese PLA General Hospital. All the following inclusion criteria should be fulfilled: 1) MOH refers to ICHD-III beta 8.2, and the definition of migraine refers to ICHD-III beta 1.1 and 1.2 [37]; 2) no migraine preventive medication used in the past 3 months; 3) age between 20 and 60 years; 4) right-handed; 5) absence of any chronic disorders, including hypertension, hypercholesterolemia, diabetes mellitus, cardiovascular diseases, cerebrovascular disorders, neoplastic diseases, infectious diseases, connective tissue diseases, other subtypes of headache, chronic pain other than headache, severe anxiety or depression preceding the onset of headache, psychiatric diseases, etc.; 6) absence of alcohol, nicotine, or other substance abuse; and 7) patient's willingness to engage in the study. Thirty-two normal controls (NCs) were recruited from the hospital's staff and their relatives. Inclusion criteria were similar to those of patients, except for the first two items, and NCs should never have had any primary headache disorders or other types of headache in the past year. The exclusion criteria for NC and MOH were the following: cranium trauma, illness interfering with central nervous system function, psychotic disorder, and regular use of a psychoactive or hormone medication. General demographic and headache information were registered and evaluated in our headache database. Additionally, we evaluated anxiety, depression, and cognitive function of all the participants by using the Hamilton Anxiety Scale (HAMA) [38], the Hamilton Depression Scale (HAMD) [39], and the Montreal Cognitive Assessment (MoCA) Beijing Version (www.mocatest.org). All the patients were given with the Visual Analogue Scale (VAS), migraine disability assessment (MIDSA), and a standard categorical four-grade sleep disturbance scale (SDS)(0, normal; 1, mild sleep disturbance; 2, moderate sleep disturbance; 3, serious sleep disturbance). MRI scans were taken in the interictal stage at least three days after a migraine attack for MOH patients. All the subjects were right-handed and underwent conventional MRI examination to exclude the subjects with cerebral infarction, malacia, or occupying lesions. Alcohol, nicotine, caffeine, and other substances were avoided for at least 12 h before MRI examination.

### MRI acquisition
Images were acquired on a GE 3.0 T MR system (DISCOVERY MR750, GE Healthcare, Milwaukee, WI, USA) and a conventional eight-channel quadrature head coil was used. All subjects were instructed to lie in a supine position, and formed padding was used to limit head movement. A three-dimensional T1-weighted fast spoiled gradient recalled echo (3D T1-FSPGR) sequence generating 180 contiguous axial slices [TR (repetition time) = 6.3 ms, TE (echo time) = 2.8 ms, flip angle = 15°, FOV (field of view) = 25.6 cm × 25.6 cm, Matrix = 256 × 256, NEX (number of acquisition) = 1] was used to perform

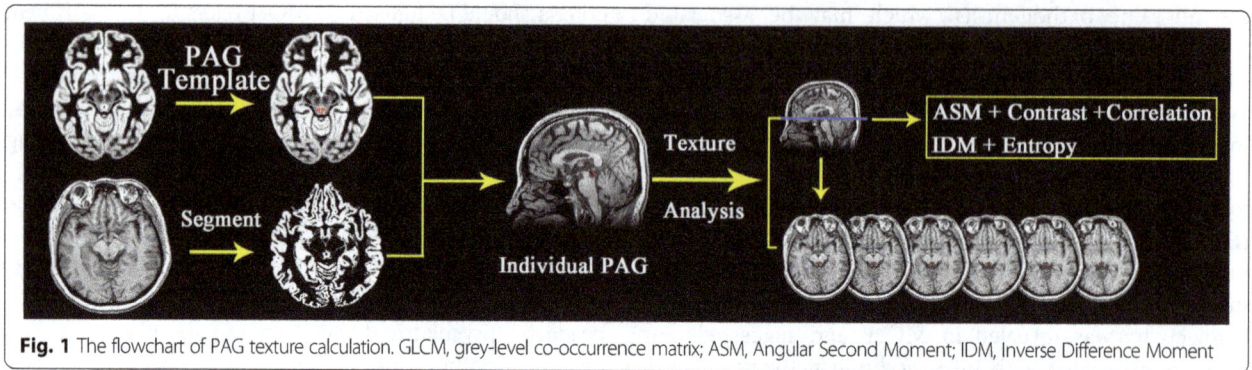

**Fig. 1** The flowchart of PAG texture calculation. GLCM, grey-level co-occurrence matrix; ASM, Angular Second Moment; IDM, Inverse Difference Moment

the new segment and the individual PAG creation. Conventional T2-weighted imaging (T2WI), T1 fluid-attenuated inversion recovery (T1-FLAIR) and diffusion weighted imaging (DWI) were also acquired. All imaging protocols were identical for all subjects. No obvious structural damage and T2-visible lesion were observed on the conventional MR images.

### MR image processing

All MR structural image data were processed using Statistical Parametric Mapping 12 (SPM12) (http://www.fil.ion.ucl.ac.uk/spm/) running under MATLAB 7.6 (The Mathworks, Natick, MA, USA) to perform segment [40]. The image processing included following steps: (1) Create PAG template based on mni_icbm152_gm_-tal_nlin_asym_09a template using MRIcron software (http://people.cas.sc.edu/rorden/mricron/index.html); (2) The structural images segment were performed with the new segment tool of SPM12 software, and the deformation field(iy_subjectid.nii) was generated. (3) Individual PAG mask (wPAG.nii) was generated by apply the deformation field (generated by new segment) to the PAG template using deformations tool of SPM12 software; (4) The individual PAG(wPAG_AddMask.nii) were segmented by an in-house script written on MATLAB (the Math Works, Inc., Natick, MA, USA) platform. The in-house script was provided in the in Additional file 1. (5) The PAG texture parameters were calculated over the whole PAG using gray-level co-occurrence matrix(GLCM) with the GLCM plugins on ImagJ(1.50i)(https://imagej.nih.gov/ij). The texture parameters included ASM, Contrast, Correlation, IDM and Entropy [35, 41] (Fig. 1). These texture parameters were measured on each slice, and the mean texture parameters values over all the slices were regarded as the final texture parameter value.

### Statistical analysis

The statistical analysis was performed by using PASW Statistics 18.0. Independent sample $T$ test was applied to age, HAMA, HAMD, MoCA scores and all the texture parameters. Chi-Square test was applied to sex. Pearson correlation analysis was applied between Contrast and the clinical variables. Significant difference was set at a $P$ value of < 0.05. Receiver operating characteristics (ROC) curve analysis was applied to evaluate the diagnostic efficacy of Contrast.

### Results

#### Demography and neuropsychological test

There was no significant difference for age and sex between MOH and NC, a significant difference for HAMA between MOH($18.25 \pm 8.74$) and NC ($10.19 \pm 2.98$), HAMD between MOH ($19.80 \pm 11.85$) and NC ($8.03 \pm 4.34$), MoCA among MOH ($23.43 \pm 3.72$) and NC ($27.16 \pm 2.32$) (Table 1).

#### Comparison of PAG texture parameters between MOH and NC

Table 2 demonstrated that there was a significant increased Contrast in MOH ($9.28 \pm 3.11$) compared with that in NC ($7.94 \pm 0.65$)($P < 0.05$). The ASM, Correlation,

**Table 1** The clinical characteristics of normal controls and MOH patients

|  | NC | MOH | T value | P value |
|---|---|---|---|---|
| Sex(M/F) | 32(12/20) | 44(9/35) | 2.692[a] | 0.101 |
| Age(year) | 41.34 ± 10.89 | 42.30 ± 9.62 | 0.403 | 0.688 |
| HAMA | 10.19 ± 2.98 | 18.25 ± 8.74 | 5.002 | 0.000 |
| HAMD | 8.03 ± 4.34 | 19.80 ± 11.85 | 5.354 | 0.000 |
| MoCA | 27.16 ± 2.32 | 23.43 ± 3.72 | 4.999 | 0.000 |
| DD(year) | 11.25 ± 9.30 |  |  |  |
| VAS | 7.88 ± 1.45 |  |  |  |
| MIDSA | 101.81 ± 53.95 |  |  |  |
| Frequence(month) | 24.81 ± 6.32 |  |  |  |
| SDS | 2.23 ± 1.36 |  |  |  |

[a]Chi-Square test; *NC* normal control, *MOH* medication-overuse headache, *DD* disease duration, *VAS* visual analogue scale; *HAMA* Hamilton Anxiety Scale, *HAMD* Hamilton Depression Scale, *MoCA* Montreal Cognitive Assessment, *NA* not available, *SDS* standard categorical four-grade sleep disturbance scale (0, normal; 1, mild sleep disturbance; 2, moderate sleep disturbance; 3, serious sleep disturbance)

**Table 2** Comparison of PAG texture parameters among NC and MOH

|  | NC | MOH | T value | P value |
| --- | --- | --- | --- | --- |
| ASM($\times10^{-3}$) | 0.998768 ± 0.000124 | 0.998709 ± 0.000175 | 1.656 | 0.102 |
| Contrast | 7.943417 ± 0.645233 | 9.282469 ± 3.109250992 | 2.395 | 0.019 |
| Correlation | 0.06879277 ± 0.01808873 | 0.062252806 ± 0.030849871 | 1.072 | 0.287 |
| IDM($\times10^{-3}$) | 0.999345 ± 0.000051 | 0.999331992 ± 0.0000595448 | 1.007 | 0.317 |
| Entropy($\times10^{-5}$) | 0.008454 ± 0.000705 | 0.008718528 ± 0.00096365 | 1.317 | 0.192 |

*ASM* Angular Second Moment, *IDM* Inverse Difference Moment

IDM and Entropy showed no significant difference between MOH and NC. Figure 2 presented the distribution of increased Contrast in MOH patients, and the other texture parameters showed no significant change in MOH patients compared with NC patients.

### ROC curve analysis and correlation analysis for Contrast

ROC analysis demonstrated that area under curve (AUC) of Contrast was 0.697 in NC vs. MOH, and the cut-off value was 8.11 with sensitivity 70.5% and specificity 62.5% (Fig. 3). The contrast was negatively with the SDS scores ($r = -0.434$, $P = 0.003$), and presented no significant correlation with other clinical variables.

### Discussion

GLCM has proved to be a popular statistical method of extracting textural feature from MR images. In this study, five texture features were extracted, and previous study recognized that ASM represented the image energy, IDM represented the local homogeneity, Entropy represented the amount of information of the image that is needed for the image compression, and Correlation represented the linear dependency of grey levels of neighboring pixels [42]. In the current study, these four texture features did not showed significant difference between MOH patients and NCs, which suggested these four texture features could not elucidate the MOH pathogenesis, and they were not considered as diagnostic variables.

Contrast represents the amount of local gray level variation in an image, and a high value high value of this parameter may indicate the presence of noise or "wrinkled" textures in the image [30]. In this study, the increased Contrast texture parameter was identified in MOH

patients, which suggested that PAG present increased local gray level variation in MR T1 images. The increased noise in PAG image may be associated with local heterogeneous intensity, which may be influenced by the iron deposition [20, 21] or other factors, and the neuromechanism should be further investigated.

Further ROC analysis revealed that AUC was 0.697 for Contrast, and the cut-off value (8.11) presented with sensitivity 70.5% and specificity 62.5%, which indicated that Contrast might be consider as an imaging biomarker for the diagnosis of MOH. Correlation analysis demonstrated that Contrast was negatively related to SDS scores, which indicated that decreased sleep quality was associated with the MOH pathogenesis. And other clinical variables showed no any correlation with Contrast, and these findings demonstrated that neuropsychological factors and pain intensity may be not associated with the PAG dysfunction in MOH pathogenesis.

In this study, GLCM method was used to calculate the MR image texture features on MOH patients, and texture Contrast was screened from the five texture parameters to explain the PAG dysfunction in MOH patients. However, there were several limitations in our study. Firstly, this study was based on GLCM method to calculate the texture features of PAG, and the other novel texture analysis methods such as histogram analysis and first order texture analysis should be considered in the future. Secondly, only five texture features were calculated in this study, and more texture features should be measured to screen the significant texture features for MOH patients. Lastly, 3D high resolution structural image was used to calculate the PAG texture features because of its high contrast for PAG, and the other MR images such as T2 weighted image and susceptibility

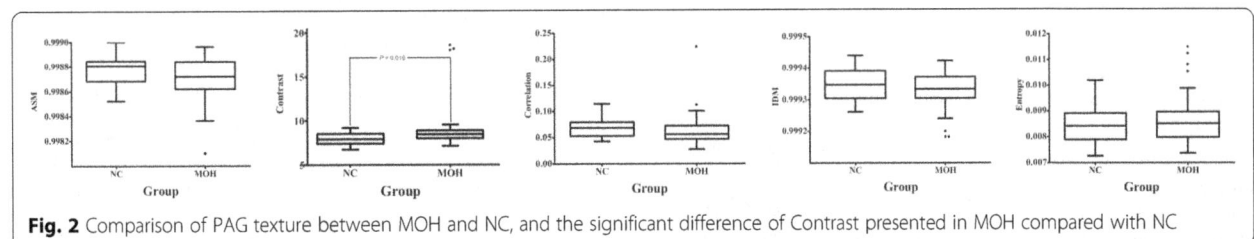

**Fig. 2** Comparison of PAG texture between MOH and NC, and the significant difference of Contrast presented in MOH compared with NC

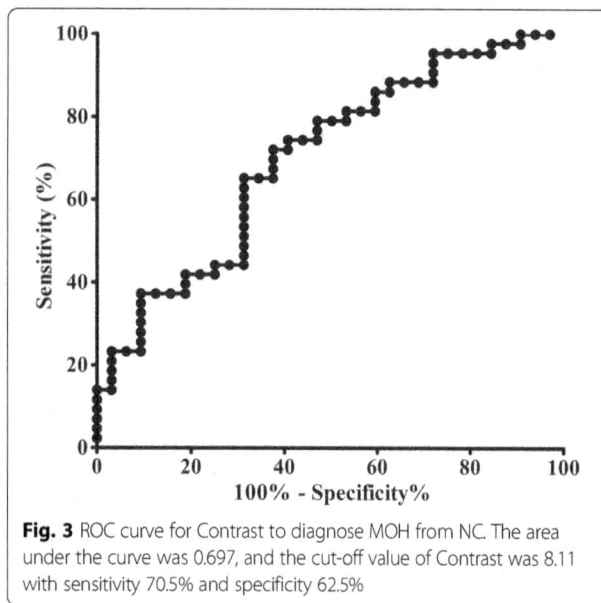

**Fig. 3** ROC curve for Contrast to diagnose MOH from NC. The area under the curve was 0.697, and the cut-off value of Contrast was 8.11 with sensitivity 70.5% and specificity 62.5%

weighted image should also be considered for the texture analysis in the future.

## Conclusion

In conclusion, this study revealed that altered PAG texture Contrast presented in MOH patients undetected by visual assessment, and it may be associated with PAG dysfunction and may be considered as a auxiliary diagnostic and evaluated imaging biomarker in MOH patients.

### Abbreviations
ASM: angular second moment; GLCM: grey-level co-occurrence matrix; IDM: inverse difference moment; MOH: medication-overuse headache; NC: normal controls; PAG: periaqueductal gray

### Acknowledgments
This work was supported by the National Natural Sciences Foundation of China (81371514), the Special Financial Grant from the China Postdoctoral Science Foundation (2014 T70960) and the Foundation for Medical and health Sci & Tech innovation Project of Sanya (2016YW37).

### Authors' contributions
Category 1: (a) Conception and Design: L. M; SY. Y. (b) Acquisition of Data: ZY. C; MQ. L; SF. L; XY. C. (c) Analysis and Interpretation of Data: ZY. C. Category 2: (a) Drafting the Article: ZY. C. (b) Revising It for Intellectual Content: L. M; SY. Y. All authors read and approved the final manuscript.

### Competing interests
The authors declare that they have no competing interests.

### Author details
[1]Department of Radiology, Chinese PLA General Hospital, Beijing 100853, China. [2]Department of Neurology, Chinese PLA General Hospital, Beijing 100853, China. [3]Department of Radiology, Hainan Branch of Chinese PLA General Hospital, Beijing 100853, China.

### References
1. Welch KM, Nagesh V, Aurora SK, Gelman N (2001) Periaqueductal gray matter dysfunction in migraine: cause or the burden of illness? Headache 41:629–37
2. Smith GS, Savery D, Marden C, Lopez Costa JJ, Averill S, Priestley JV, Rattray M (1994) Distribution of messenger RNAs encoding enkephalin, substance P, somatostatin, galanin, vasoactive intestinal polypeptide, neuropeptide Y, and calcitonin gene-related peptide in the midbrain periaqueductal grey in the rat. J Comp Neurol 350:23–40
3. Raskin NH, Yoshio H, Sharon L (1987) Headache may arise from perturbation of brain. Headache 27:416–20
4. Heinricher MM, Tavares I, Leith JL, Lumb BM (2009) Descending control of nociception: specificity, recruitment and plasticity. Brain Res Rev 60:214–25
5. Fields H (2004) State-dependent opioid control of pain. Nat Rev Neurosci 5: 565–75
6. Benarroch EE (2012) Periaqueductal gray: an interface for behavioral control. Neurology 78:210–7
7. An X, Bandler R, Ongür D, Price JL (1998) Prefrontal cortical projections to longitudinal columns in the midbrain periaqueductal gray in Macaque monkeys. J Comp Neurol 401:455–79
8. Herbert H, Saper CB (1992) Organization of medullary adrenergic and noradrenergic projections to the periaqueductal gray matter in the rat. J Comp Neurol 315:34–52
9. Yezierski RP (1988) Spinomesencephalic tract: projections from the lumbosacral spinal cord of the rat, cat, and monkey. J Comp Neurol 267:131–46
10. Keay KA, Bandler R (2002) Distinct central representations of inescapable and escapable pain: observations and speculation. Exp Physiol 87:275–9
11. Parry DM, Macmillan FM, Koutsikou S, Mcmullan S, Lumb BM (2008) Separation of A- versus C-nociceptive inputs into spinal-brainstem circuits. Neuroscience 152:1076–85
12. Lumb BM (2004) Hypothalamic and midbrain circuitry that distinguishes between escapable and inescapable pain. News Physiol Sci 19:22–6
13. Gee JR, Chang J, Dublin AB, Vijayan N (2005) The association of brainstem lesions with migraine-like headache: an imaging study of multiple sclerosis. Headache 45:670–7
14. Haas DC, Kent PF, Friedman DI (1993) Headache caused by a single lesion of multiple sclerosis in the periaqueductal gray area. Headache 33:452–5
15. Lin GY, Wang CW, Chiang TT, Peng GS, Yang FC (2013) Multiple sclerosis presenting initially with a worsening of migraine symptoms. J Headache Pain 14:70
16. Tortorella P, Rocca MA, Colombo B, Annovazzi P, Comi G, Filippi M (2006) Assessment of MRI abnormalities of the brainstem from patients with migraine and multiple sclerosis. J Neurol Sci 244:137–41
17. Fragoso YD, Brooks JB (2007) Two cases of lesions in brainstem in multiple sclerosis and refractory migraine. Headache 47:852–4
18. Wang Y, Wang XS (2013) Migraine-like headache from an infarction in the periaqueductal gray area of the midbrain. Pain Med 14:948–9
19. Chen Z, Chen X, Liu M, Liu S, Ma L, Yu S (2016) Nonspecific periaqueductal gray lesions on T2WI in episodic migraine. J Headache Pain 17:101
20. Kruit MC, Launer LJ, Overbosch J, van Buchem MA, Ferrari MD (2009) Iron accumulation in deep brain nuclei in migraine: a population-based magnetic resonance imaging study. Cephalalgia 29:351–9
21. Tepper SJ, Lowe MJ, Beall E, Phillips MD, Liu K, Stillman MJ et al (2012) Iron deposition in pain-regulatory nuclei in episodic migraine and chronic daily headache by MRI. Headache 52:236–43
22. Torta DM, Costa T, Luda E, Barisone MG, Palmisano P, Duca S et al (2016) Nucleus accumbens functional connectivity discriminates medication-overuse headache. Neuroimage Clin 11:686–93
23. Chanraud S, Di Scala G, Dilharreguy B, Schoenen J, Allard M, Radat F (2014) Brain functional connectivity and morphology changes in medication-overuse headache: Clue for dependence-related processes? Cephalalgia 34:605–15
24. Tepper SJ (2012) Medication-overuse headache. Continuum (Minneap Minn) 18:807–22
25. Riederer F, Gantenbein AR, Marti M, Luechinger R, Kollias S, Sandor PS (2013) Decrease of gray matter volume in the midbrain is associated with treatment response in medication-overuse headache: possible influence of orbitofrontal cortex. J Neurosci 33:15343–9
26. Michels L, Christidi F, Steiger VR, Sandor PS, Gantenbein AR, Landmann G, et

al (2016) Pain modulation is affected differently in medication-overuse headache and chronic myofascial pain - A multimodal MRI study. Cephalalgia. doi:10.1177/0333102416652625

27. Herlidoumême S, Constans JM, Carsin B, Olivie D, Eliat PA, Nadaldesbarats L et al (2003) MRI texture analysis on texture test objects, normal brain and intracranial tumors. Magn Reson Imaging 21:989–93

28. Nachimuthu DS, Baladhandapani A (2014) Multidimensional texture characterization: on analysis for brain tumor tissues using MRS and MRI. J Digit Imaging 27:73–81(9)

29. Mahmoud-Ghoneim D, Toussaint G, Constans JM, de Certaines JD (2003) Three dimensional texture analysis in MRI: a preliminary evaluation in gliomas. Magn Reson Imaging 21:983–7

30. Oliveira MSD, Betting LE, Mory SB, Cendes F, Castellano G (2013) Texture analysis of magnetic resonance images of patients with juvenile myoclonic epilepsy. Epilepsy Behav 27:22–8

31. Caselato GR, Kobayashi E, Bonilha L, Castellano G, Rigas AH, Li LM et al (2003) Hippocampal texture analysis in patients with familial mesial temporal lobe epilepsy. Arq Neuropsiquiatr 61(Suppl 1):83–7

32. Certaines JDD, Larcher T, Duda D, Azzabou N, Eliat PA, Escudero LM et al (2015) Application of texture analysis to muscle MRI: 1-What kind of information should be expected from texture analysis? EPJ Nonlinear Biomed Phys 3:1–14

33. Chang CW, Ho CC, Chen JH (2012) ADHD classification by a texture analysis of anatomical brain MRI data. Front Syst Neurosci 6:66

34. de Oliveira MS, Balthazar ML, D'Abreu A, Yasuda CL, Damasceno BP, Cendes F, Castellano G (2011) MR imaging texture analysis of the corpus callosum and thalamus in amnestic mild cognitive impairment and mild Alzheimer disease. AJNR Am J Neuroradiol 32:60–6

35. Haralick RM, Shanmugam K, Dinstein IH (1973) Textural Features for Image Classification. IEEE Trans Syst Man Cybern smc-3:610–21

36. Rajkovic N, Kolarevic D, Kanjer K, Milosevic NT, Nikolic-Vukosavljevic D, Radulovic M (2016) Comparison of Monofractal, Multifractal and gray level Co-occurrence matrix algorithms in analysis of Breast tumor microscopic images for prognosis of distant metastasis risk. Biomed Microdevices 18:83

37. Headache Classification Committee of the International Headache Society (IHS) (2013) The International Classification of Headache Disorders, 3rd edition (beta version). Cephalalgia 33:629–808.

38. Maier W, Buller R, Philipp M, Heuser I (1988) The Hamilton Anxiety Scale: reliability, validity and sensitivity to change in anxiety and depressive disorders. J Affect Disord 14:61–8

39. Hamilton M (1967) Development of a rating scale for primary depressive illness. Br J Soc Clin Psychol 6:278–96

40. Ashburner J, Friston KJ (2000) Voxel-based morphometry–the methods. Neuroimage 11:805–21

41. Walker RF, Jackway P, Longstaff ID (1995) Improving Co-occurrence Matrix Feature Discrimination. DICTA 3rd Conference on Digital Image Computing: Techniques and Application. Brisbane: University of Queensland, 643–648

42. Mohanaiah P, Sathyanarayana P, Gurukumar L (2014) Image texture feature extraction using GLCM approach. Int J Sci Res Publ 3:1–5

# Increased levels of intramuscular cytokines in patients with jaw muscle pain

S. Louca Jounger[1,2*], N. Christidis[1,2], P. Svensson[1,2,3], T. List[2,4] and M. Ernberg[1,2]

## Abstract

**Background:** The aim of this study was to investigate cytokine levels in the masseter muscle, their response to experimental tooth-clenching and their relation to pain, fatigue and psychological distress in patients with temporomandibular disorders (TMD) myalgia.

**Methods:** Forty women, 20 with TMD myalgia (Diagnostic Criteria for TMD) and 20 age-matched healthy controls participated. Intramuscular microdialysis was performed to sample masseter muscle cytokines. After 140 min (baseline), a 20-minute tooth-clenching task was performed (50% of maximal voluntary contraction force). Pain (Numeric rating scale 0–10) and fatigue (Borg's Ratings of Perceived Exertion 6–20) were assessed throughout microdialysis, while pressure-pain thresholds (PPT) were assessed before and after microdialysis. Perceived stress (PSS-10) and Trait Anxiety (STAI) were assessed before microdialysis.

**Results:** The levels of IL-6, IL-7, IL-8 and IL-13 were higher in patients than controls (Mann Whitney $U$-test; $P$'s < 0.05) during the entire microdialysis. IL-6, IL-8 and IL-13 changed during microdialysis in both groups (Friedman; $P$'s < 0.05), while IL-1β, IL-7 and GM-CSF changed only in patients ($P$'s < 0.01). IL-6 and IL-8 increased in response to tooth-clenching in both groups (Wilcoxon test; $P$'s < 0.05), while IL-7, IL-13 and TNF increased only in patients ($P$'s < 0.05). Patients had higher pain and fatigue than controls before and after tooth-clenching ($P$ < 0.001), and lower PPTs before and after microdialysis ($P$ < 0.05). There were no correlations between cytokine levels, pain or fatigue. Also, there were no differences in stress or anxiety levels between groups.

**Conclusions:** In conclusion, the masseter levels of IL-6, IL-7, IL-8 and IL-13 were elevated in patients with TMD myalgia and increased in response to tooth-clenching. Tooth-clenching increased jaw muscle pain and fatigue, but without correlations to cytokine levels. This implies that subclinical muscle inflammation may be involved in TMD myalgia pathophysiology, but that there is no direct cause-relation between inflammation and pain.

**Keywords:** Cytokines, Bruxism, Masseter muscle, Myalgia, Temporomandibular disorders (TMD)

## Background

Temporomandibular disorders (TMD) are the most common chronic pain conditions in the orofacial region, affecting approximately 10–15% of the adult population [1] and twice as many women as men [2]. The most common subtype is TMD myalgia with jaw muscle pain that is increased by function, pain on palpation, pain referral, restricted mouth opening, and headache [3, 4]. The etiology of TMD and the higher prevalence among women is not well understood.

One hypothesis is that excessive tooth-clenching/grinding might contribute by disturbing the local blood flow in overloaded muscles, leading to ischemia [5]. Epidemiological studies show greater odds of having TMD myalgia when self-reported tooth-clenching is present [6–8]. Ischemia releases neuroactive and inflammatory biomarkers, such as neuropeptides, bradykinin, protons, serotonin (5-HT), glutamate and cytokines that may activate and sensitize nociceptors on peripheral sensory afferents to induce muscle pain and allodynia [9, 10]. Repeated muscle activity may then maintain chronic muscle pain by temporal summation [11]. Previous studies have shown that intense chewing induced pain and fatigue in pain-free healthy participants with similar, but

* Correspondence: sofia.louca@ki.se
[1]Section for Orofacial Pain and Jaw Function, Department of Dental Medicine, Karolinska Institutet, SE 14104, Huddinge, Sweden
[2]Scandinavian Center for Orofacial Neurosciences (SCON), Huddinge, Sweden

transient symptoms as in TMD myalgia patients [12–14]. This observation may suggest that, at least a subset of M-TMD pain patients could be more alike an exercise-induced muscle pain probably caused by ischemia and an accumulation of metabolic biomarkers in the masticatory muscles [12–14]. In another study, experimental tooth-clenching increased jaw muscle pain in patients with M-TMD and caused low levels of pain in controls. Patients with M-TMD had higher levels of 5-HT during the entire experiment, but did not increase in response to tooth-clenching, suggesting that other algesic substances might be released and activate nociceptors that are most likely already sensitized by 5-HT [15].

Studies have shown that several cytokines play a role in acute inflammatory muscle pain and in some chronic muscle pain conditions. There are both pro- and anti-inflammatory cytokines interacting with each other in a balanced matter in order to fight an infection and promote wound healing, and they are often released in a cascade in response to tissue damage. The pro-inflammatory cytokines can initiate an inflammatory response by recruiting other cytokines, macrophages, t-cells and b-cells, initiating the inflammatory response, while anti-inflammatory cytokines can reduce and promote healing by controlling the cytokine response [16].

For example, patients with various chronic pain conditions (neuropathic, nociceptive and mixed pain) had higher serum level of interleukin (IL)-6, IL-1β, IL-2, tumor necrosis factor (TNF), and interferon gamma (IFN-γ) than healthy controls, which correlated with pain intensity [17], and increased cerebrospinal fluid (CSF) and plasma level of IL-8 were reported in patients with widespread pain [18, 19]. In patients with TMD pain increased levels of IL-1β, IL-6, IL-10, TNF, IL-1ra, and monocyte attractant protein-1 (MCP-1) have been reported [19, 20].

Also, muscle levels of TNF and IL-1β were increased in trapezius trigger points in patients with myofascial pain [21, 22], and IL-6 increased in the painful trapezius muscle of patients with whiplash-associated disorders (WAD) [23]. Muscle and plasma levels of IL-6 and IL-8 increase in response to exercise [24, 25]. However, serum IL-10 showed a blunted response to exercise in fibromyalgia [26].

Regardless of their potential role in the development and maintenance of some chronic pain conditions, little is known about the peripheral involvement of cytokines in TMD myalgia. The aim of this study was therefore to compare the levels of the pro- and anti-inflammatory cytokines IL-1β, IL-2, IL-4, IL-5, IL-6, IL-7, IL-8, IL-10, IL-12, IL-13, TNF, IFN-γ, and GM-CSF in the masseter muscle between TMD myalgia patients and healthy controls and the effects of a repetitive tooth-clenching task on their release and relation to masseter pain intensity,

fatigue, and pressure-pain thresholds (PPT). Furthermore, perceived stress and anxiety may also be involved in the pathophysiology of TMD pain [27]. Therefore, questionnaires were used to estimate the potential correlation between biomarkers and psychological variables.

We hypothesized that muscle level of the cytokines would be higher in patients than controls, increase in response to a repetitive tooth-clenching task in a similar manner in both groups, and correlate to pain intensity, fatigue and level of stress and anxiety.

## Methods
### Participants
Twenty women with TMD myalgia and twenty age-matched healthy women were included. Participants were recruited by advertisements and among colleagues and students at the Department of Dental Medicine at the Karolinska Institutet, Huddinge, Sweden where the study was performed. Inclusion criteria for the patients were age over 18, a diagnosis of myalgia according to the Diagnostic Criteria for TMD (DC/TMD) [1] and pain lasting for over 3 months. Inclusion criteria for the controls were age over 18, good general health and no history of/or current pain from the orofacial region. Exclusion criteria for both groups were systemic muscular or joint diseases, WAD, neuropathic pain or neurological disorders, pain of dental origin, and use of analgesics of non-steroidal anti-inflammatory drugs during 48 h before microdialysis.

Based on a previous study [15, 28] the power calculation showed that inclusion of 20 participants in each group would be sufficient to detect a significant difference of 20% (SD 30%) in biomarker levels with 80% power and a significance level of 5%.

The study followed the guidelines of the Declaration of Helsinki and was approved by the Regional Ethical Review Board in Stockholm (2009/2047-32), Sweden. All participants were given written and verbal information before participating and gave their written consent. The participants were compensated upon completion of their participation.

### Experimental protocol
The study used a case–control design with one session lasting for 220 min. After inclusion, psychological distress was assessed; thereafter the maximal voluntary clenching force (MVCF), and PPT were recorded. Participants were reclined in a conventional dental chair and instructed to lie as still as possible during the experiment and to avoid talking. After baseline registrations and local anesthesia, microdialysis was performed in one of the masseter muscles. After 120-minutes (trauma phase), baseline assessments of pain intensity and fatigue were made (120–140 min), followed by a 20-minute

clenching task (exercise). Pain intensity and fatigue were assessed after tooth-clenching. After an additional hour (recovery) the microdialysis catheter was removed and the PPTs were again assessed (Fig. 1).

### Experimental tooth-clenching

MVCF (kg) was assessed with a bite-force transducer (Aalborg University, Denmark) placed between the molars on the most suitable side, from a dental point of view. The same side was used for the clenching task and microdialysis. Participants were instructed to bite as hard as possible on the bite-force transducer for 2–3 s. The mean of three MVCF registrations was calculated. During the experimental tooth-clenching, participants were instructed to repeatedly bite 50% of their mean MVCF for 30-seconds followed by 30-seconds of rest during 20-minutes [15]. Visual feedback was used to maintain the clenching level.

### Assessments of pain intensity, fatigue and pressure-pain threshold

A 0–10 numerical rating scale (NRS) was used to assess pain intensity in the masseter muscle every 20th minute during microdialysis. The Borg Rating of Perceived Exertion Scale (6–20; RPE) was used to measure fatigue [29].

PPT was assessed with an electronic pressure algometer (Somedic Sales AB, Höör, Sweden) with a standardized pressure rate of 50 kPa/s. The tip of the device was 1 cm$^2$, covered with a 1-mm thick rubber-pad. PPT was recorded by applying pressure on the most prominent point of the masseter muscle during contraction, and on the right index finger, which was used as an extra-cranial reference point. Participants pressed a signal-button when the sensation of pressure turned into pain [30]. The mean of three registrations was used in statistical analyzes.

### Psychological distress

The Swedish version of the State-Trait Anxiety Inventory (STAI) was used to assess trait-anxiety. It contains twenty questions measuring the levels of anxiety as a personal characteristic. Scores ranges from 20 to 80, where high scores (>30) indicate higher levels of anxiety [31, 32].

Stress levels were measured with the Swedish version of the Perceived Stress Scale-14 (PSS-14) consisting of 14 stress-related questions of a general nature, including feelings and thoughts during the last month, situations in life that are perceived as stressful, and the current level of experienced stress. The total scoring is 56, and scores below 23.67 are considered normal in healthy participants [33, 34].

### Microdialysis

The most prominent point of the masseter muscle, verified by palpation during contraction, was chosen for microdialysis. The skin overlying the muscle was anaesthetized with a local injection (0.5 ml) of Lidocaine (Xylocaine 20 mg /ml), carefully avoiding anaesthetizing the underlying muscle.

A sterile split able introducer (CMA Microdialysis AB, Solna, Sweden) was inserted intramuscularly in parallel to the muscle fibers at a 45-degree angle to a depth of approximately 40 mm from the skin surface [15, 35].

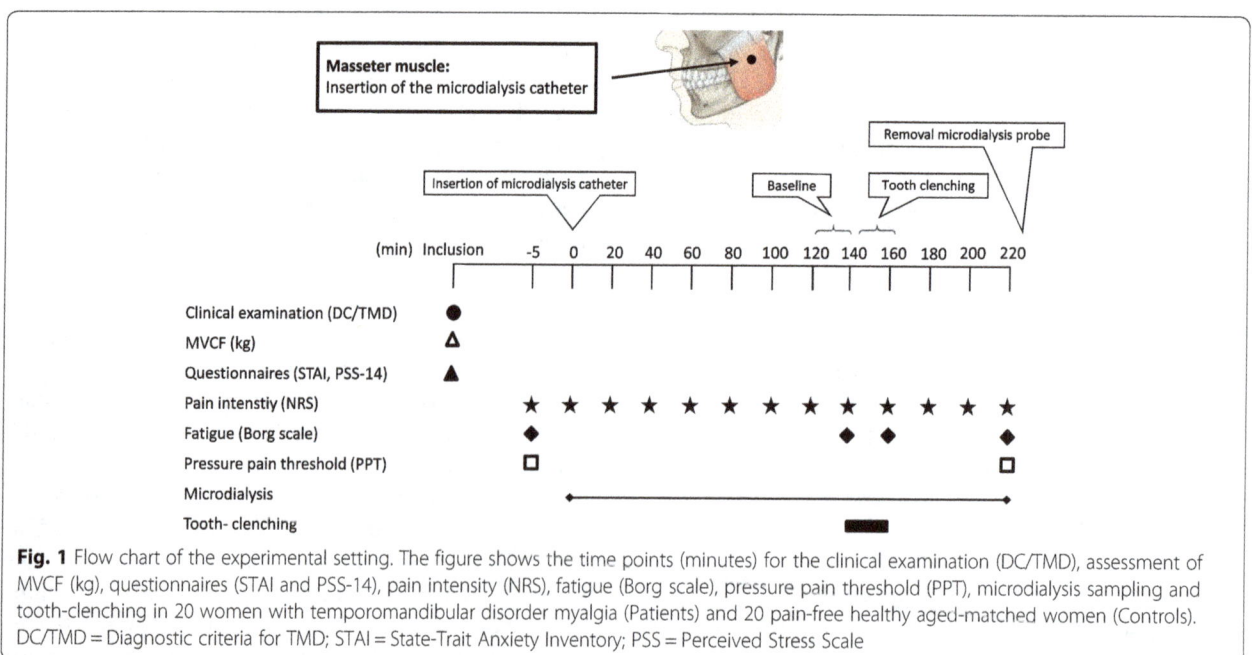

**Fig. 1** Flow chart of the experimental setting. The figure shows the time points (minutes) for the clinical examination (DC/TMD), assessment of MVCF (kg), questionnaires (STAI and PSS-14), pain intensity (NRS), fatigue (Borg scale), pressure pain threshold (PPT), microdialysis sampling and tooth-clenching in 20 women with temporomandibular disorder myalgia (Patients) and 20 pain-free healthy aged-matched women (Controls). DC/TMD = Diagnostic criteria for TMD; STAI = State-Trait Anxiety Inventory; PSS = Perceived Stress Scale

After approximately 20 mm, a slight resistance occurred, typically felt upon penetration of the muscle fascia, and the introducer was additionally inserted 20 mm. A sterile 100 kDa 60 mm long microdialysis catheter with 20 mm membrane length (CMA71 Microdialysis AB, Solna, Sweden) was inserted to the full length, thereafter the introducer was removed by splitting the plastic tube. The catheter was perfused (5 μL/ min) with a Ringer-Acetate solution (Pharmacia & Upjohn, Copenhagen, Denmark) containing 3 mmol glucose and 0.5 mmol lactate from a 2-ml syringe connected to a micro-infusion pump (CMA107, Microdialysis AB, Solna, Sweden). Samples (100 μL) were collected every 20-minutes in capped microvials and immediately frozen (–80 °C). After microdialysis, the catheter was removed and the membrane was checked to ensure that no damaged had occurred.

### Analyzes of dialysate

The cytokines were analyzed with Luminex technology using multiplex immunoassay panels (Milliplex®map kit, Human High sensitivity, T-cell magnetic bead panel, 96-well plate assay, Merck Millipore Darmstadt, Germany) in accordance to the manufacturer's manual.

The limit of detection (LOD) for each cytokine respectively were for IL-1β, IL-2, IL-5, and IL-12: 0.49 pg./mL; IL-4: 1.83 pg./mL; IL-6: 0.18 pg./mL; IL-7: 0.37 pg./mL; IL-8: 0.31 pg./mL, IL-10: 1.46 pg./mL; IL-13: 0.24 pg./mL; GM-CSF: 1.22 pg./mL; IFN-γ: 0.61 pg./mL and for TNF: 0.43 pg./mL.

For each cytokine the number of samples with levels below LOD were calculated. As a quality control, cytokines with >50% of samples below LOD were excluded from further analysis. This was based on findings from our group that some cytokines are undetectable in many individuals, making the results difficult to interpret (Ernberg et al, personal communication). Others have used similar approaches, although with less strict criteria [36].

### Statistics

Data were analyzed with SigmaPlot for Windows, version 11 (Systat Software Inc. Chicago, IL, USA) and STATISTICA, StatSoft Dell Software version 12.0 (Round Rock, Texas USA). For descriptive statistics

mean and standard deviation (SD) or median and inter-quartile range (IQR) were used. Non-parametric statistics were used since most cytokines were not normally distributed and attempts to transform data did not change this. To analyze differences in cytokine levels between groups, the average of all 11 dialysate samples (0–220 min) was calculated and compared with Mann-Whitney $U$-test. Friedman-test was used to analyze changes in cytokine levels over time. Wilcoxon-test compared the time points 140 min (BL) and 160–220 min within groups. Cytokine, pain and fatigue levels after clenching (160 min) were compared between groups with Mann-Whitney $U$-test. Spearman correlations-test with Bonferroni correction for multiple testing was used to analyze correlations between cytokine levels, pain, fatigue and psychological distress. Differences in STAI-trait and PSS-14 scores between groups and differences in PPTs between sides before and after microdialysis were analyzed with unpaired $t$-test. The level of significance was $P < 0.05$.

## Results

### Cytokine levels

IL-2, IL-4, IL-5, IL-10 and IFN-γ were excluded from further statistical analysis since more than 50% of the samples were below LOD (Table 1).

The dialysate levels of the cytokines are shown in Table 2 and Fig. 2. The dialysate levels of IL-6, IL-7, IL-8, and IL-13 were higher in patients than controls during the entire microdialysis. IL-6, IL-8 and IL-13 changed during microdialysis in both groups, while IL-1β, IL-7 and GM-CSF changed only in patients. IL-6 and IL-8 increased in response to tooth-clenching in both groups, while IL-7, IL-13 and TNF only increased in the patients. There were no significant differences in cytokine levels between patients and controls after tooth-clenching (160 min).

### Pain intensity and levels of fatigue

Patients had higher baseline pain intensity and fatigue than controls. Tooth-clenching increased pain intensity in patients and evoked mild pain in controls. It also increased fatigue in both groups (Table 3).

There were no significant correlations between cytokines levels and other variables ($P > 0.102$; $r_s < 0.384$).

**Table 1** Dialysate samples with cytokines levels below LOD

| | IL-1β | IL-2 | IL-4 | IL-5 | IL-6 | IL-7 | IL-8 | IL-10 | IL-12 | IL-13 | TNF | IFN-γ | GM-CSF |
|---|---|---|---|---|---|---|---|---|---|---|---|---|---|
| All | 75 (19.1) | 268 **(68.4)** | 291 **(74.2)** | 264 **(67.3)** | 68 (17.3) | 133 (33.9) | 45 (11.5) | 210 **(53.6)** | 180 (45.9) | 140 (35.7) | 169 (43.1) | 319 **(81.4)** | 178 (45.4) |
| Patients | 54 (24.3) | 133 (59.9) | 188 (84.7) | 144 (64.9) | 38 (17.1) | 82 (36.9) | 18 (8.1) | 118 (53.1) | 127 (57.2) | 64 (28.8) | 100 (45.0) | 165 (74.3) | 118 (53.2) |
| Controls | 21 (12.4) | 135 (79.4) | 103 (60.6) | 120 (70.6) | 30 (17.6) | 51 (30.0) | 27 (15.9) | 92 (53.6) | 53 (31.2) | 76 (44.7) | 69 (40.6) | 154 (90.6) | 60 (35.3) |

Table show the dialysate samples with cytokines levels below LOD in 20 women with Temporomandibular Disorders myalgia (Patients) and 20 pain-free healthy aged-matched women (Controls). Data are presented as n = number of undetectable dialysate samples (%)

*LOD* Limits of detection, *IL* Interleukin, *TNF* Tumor necrosis factor, *IFN* Interferon, *GM-CSF* Granulocyte macrophage colony-stimulating factor. Bold figures denote cytokines with 50% of the samples below LOD (excluded from further analyses)

**Table 2** The average cytokine levels for all samples combined

|                  | IL-1β      | IL-6        | IL-7        | IL-8        | TNF       | GM-CSF      | IL-12      | IL-13       |
|------------------|-----------|-------------|-------------|-------------|-----------|-------------|------------|-------------|
| Dialysate levels |           |             |             |             |           |             |            |             |
| Patients         | 2.3 (7.0) | 25.8 (42.3) | 11.4 (21.5) | 36.2 (51.4) | 4.4 (8.8) | 10.1 (11.2) | 5.5 (11.8) | 4.1 (5.9)   |
| Controls         | 1.6 (2.3) | 11.0 (12.6) | 6.4 (3.2)   | 10.1 (14.7) | 3.5 (1.5) | 14.8 (23.3) | 7.4 (3.0)  | 9.7 (13.4)  |
| *P-values*       | *0.208*   | ***0.015*** | ***0.041*** | ***0.002*** | *0.291*   | *0.199*     | *0.507*    | ***0.002*** |

The average cytokine levels for all samples combined (0–220 min) in 20 women with Temporomandibular Disorders myalgia (Patients) and 20 pain-free healthy age-matched women (Controls). Data are presented as median (IQR)

*IQR* Interquartile range (75 percentile minus 25 percentile), *IL* Interleukin, *TNF* Tumor necrosis factor, *GM-CSF* Granulocyte macrophage colony-stimulating factor. Bold italic figures denote significant group differences ($P < 0.05$)

### Baseline characteristics and PPT

Baseline characteristics of the participants and PPT before and after microdialysis are shown in Table 4. There were no differences between groups in PSS-14 or STAI-trait levels, but the MVCF was lower in patients than controls. PPT over the masseter muscles were lower in patients than controls, in contrast to the reference point, but had not changed after microdialysis in any group (Table 4).

### Discussion

The main findings were that the masseter levels of IL-6, IL-7, IL-8 and IL-13 were higher in TMD myalgia patients than controls and that repetitive tooth-clenching increased the levels of IL-6 and IL-8 in both groups, while IL-7, IL-13 and TNF increased only in patients. Also, tooth-clenching evoked higher pain intensity and fatigue in TMD myalgia patients than controls. Finally, there were no correlations between pain, fatigue and cytokine levels.

Overall, the results from this study supports the hypotheses that 1) the muscle levels of pro- and anti-inflammatory cytokines appear to be elevated in TMD myalgia and 2) severally pro- and anti-inflammatory cytokines increased after repetitive tooth-clenching in both groups. However, there were no significant differences between TMD myalgia patients and controls. This

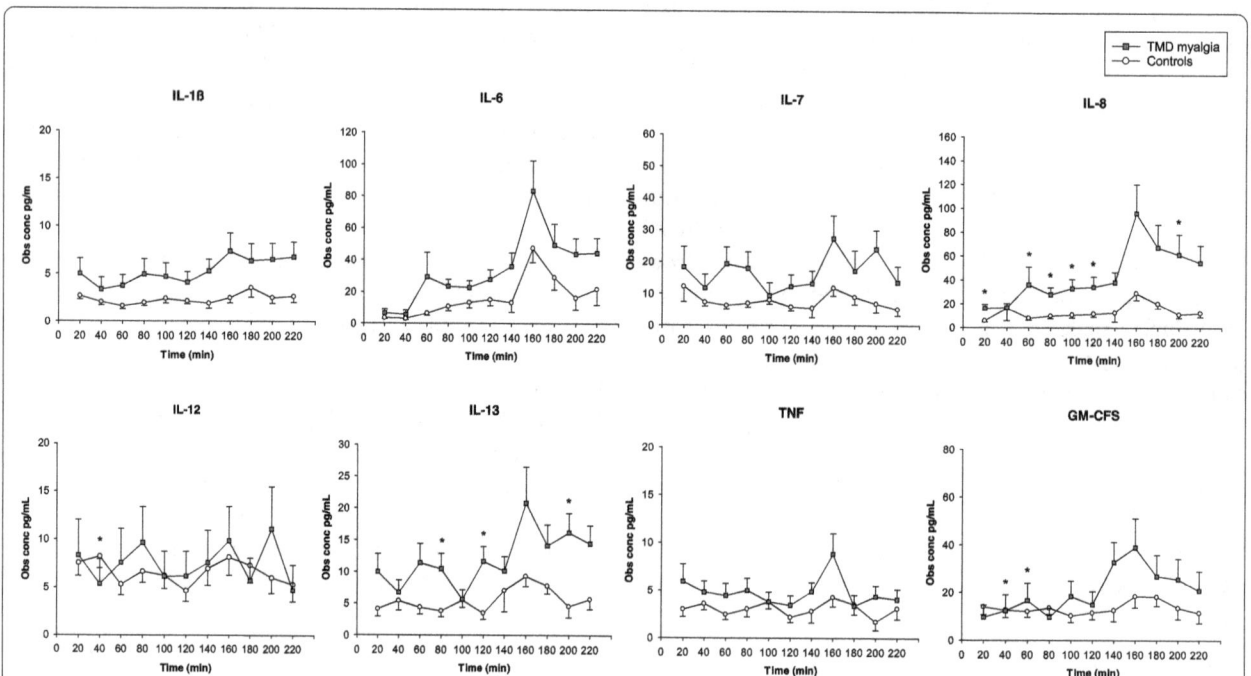

**Fig. 2** The levels of cytokines during microdialysis. Graph showing the levels of cytokines (mean and SEM) during microdialysis in 20 women with temporomandibular disorder myalgia (Patients) and 20 pain-free healthy aged-matched women (Controls). After 140 min (baseline), a 20-minute repetitive tooth-clenching task (140–160 min) was performed followed by one-hour rest (160–220 min). IL-1β ($P = 0.0007$), IL-6 ($P < 0.001$), IL-7 ($P = 0.012$), IL-8 ($P < 0.001$), IL-13 ($P < 0.001$), and GM-CSF ($P = 0.008$) increased with time in the patients, whereas IL-6 ($P < 0.001$), IL-8 ($P < 0.001$), and IL-13 ($P = 0.042$) increased with time in the controls (Friedman test). IL-6 ($P < 0.001$), IL-8 ($P = 0.001$), IL-13 ($P = 0.035$), and TNF ($P = 0.042$) had increased after clenching (160 min) compared to baseline (140 min) in the patients, and IL-6 ($P = 0.004$) and IL-8 ($P = 0.032$) had increased in the controls (Wilcoxon test). There were no significant differences in cytokine levels between patients and controls after clenching (160 min), although there was a trend for IL-8 (Mann-Whitney *U*-test, $P = 0.074$). *= significant difference between the groups ($P < 0.05$)

**Table 3** The median (IQR) pain intensity (NRS) and fatigue (Borg RPE) in the masseter muscle

|  | Before | After | P-values |
|---|---|---|---|
| Pain |  |  |  |
| Patients | 3 (3) | 7 (3) | **<0.001** |
| Controls | 0 (0) | 0 (2) | **0.016** |
| *P-values between groups* | **<0.001** | **<0.001** |  |
| Fatigue |  |  |  |
| Patients | 13 (4) | 19 (1) | **<0.001** |
| Controls | 6 (0) | 14 (3) | **<0.001** |
| *P-values between groups* | **<0.001** | **<0.001** |  |

Table show the median pain intensity and fatigue before and after a 20-minute tooth-clenching task in 20 women with Temporomandibular Disorders myalgia (Patients) and 20 pain-free healthy age-matched women (Controls). *IQR* interquartile range (75 percentile minus 25 percentile), *NRS* Numeric rating scale (0–10), *Borgs's RPE* Borg's ratings of perceived exertion scale (6–20). Bold italic figures denote significant differences (P < 0.05)

lends support for a role of peripheral inflammation to drive chronic muscle pain. However, 3) no correlations with pain, fatigue or PPT levels were found, so in future studies the balance and interaction between pro- and anti-inflammatory cytokines as well as other inflammatory mediators need to be considered.

This is the first study to show elevated muscle levels of the pro-inflammatory cytokines IL-6 and IL-8 and the

**Table 4** Baseline characteristics in 20 women with Temporomandibular Disorders myalgia and 20 healthy pain-free age-matched women

|  | Patients | Controls | P-values |
|---|---|---|---|
| Age (yr) | 31 (10) | 29 (11) |  |
| MVCF (kg) | 356 (205) | 469 (113) | **0.018** |
| STAI-trait (20–80) | 42 (19) | 36 (10) | 0.321 |
| PSS-14 (0–56) | 23 (15) | 20 (9) | 0.392 |
| PPT (kPa) |  |  |  |
| Before |  |  |  |
| Experimental side | 160 (±70) | 239 (±62) | **0.003** |
| Control side | 163 (±46) | 230 (±30) | **<0.001** |
| *P-values between sides* | 0.876 | 0.570 |  |
| Reference point | 412 (±131) | 384 (±115) | 0.573 |
| After |  |  |  |
| Experimental side | 124 (±71) | 232 (±52) | **<0.001** |
| Control side | 147 (±66) | 234 (±48) | **<0.001** |
| *P-values between sides* | 0.298 | 0.919 |  |
| Reference point | 454 (±273) | 425 (±94) | 0.741 |

The baseline characteristics as well as pressure pain thresholds (PPT) before and after microdialysis are shown

Data are presented as median (IQR) or mean (±SD). *IQR* interquartile range (75 percentile minus 25 percentile), *SD* Standard deviation, *MVCF* Maximum voluntary contraction force, *STAI* State- and trait anxiety inventory, *PSS* Perceived stress scale. Bold italic figures denote significant differences (P < 0.05)

anti-inflammatory cytokines IL-7 and IL-13 in painful jaw muscles of patients with TMD myalgia which supports the hypothesis that patients with TMD myalgia have higher levels of cytokines. The results are partly consistent with previous results in other localized myalgias showing increased IL-6 in the painful trapezius muscle of WAD patients [23] and IL-1β and TNF in myofascial trapezius trigger points [21, 22], although one early study did not find any difference in trapezius levels of IL-6 between patients with chronic trapezius myalgia and controls [37]. They are also consistent with very recent results showing that lipopolysaccharide (LPS) stimulated monocytes from patients with TMD show an enhanced production of IL-1β, TNF and IL-6 [38]. Proinflammatory cytokines may act directly on nociceptor terminals to induce pain [39]. Increased muscle levels of other inflammatory markers, such as serotonin and glutamate have also been reported in chronic localized myalgia [15, 23, 35]. These results combined gives support for the involvement of peripheral mechanisms in localized chronic myalgia, and may implicate that patients with chronic pain constantly have their immune system switched on with higher levels of inflammatory mediators leading to peripheral sensitization, which may drive central sensitization processes and pain [40]. The increased muscle levels of IL-7 and IL-13 in the patients in this study imply that anti-inflammatory cytokines are locally produced to counteract this effect, although this may not be sufficient as LPS-stimulated monocytes from TMD-patients showed a blunted response of IL-10 [38].

In patients with TMD elevated plasma levels of both pro- (IL-1β, IL-6, TNF) and anti-inflammatory (IL-10) cytokines were recently reported [20]. Contrary, in TMD patients with widespread pain and in fibromyalgia plasma levels of pro-inflammatory IL-8 were higher [18, 19, 41] and IL-10 lower than controls [18]. This suggests that the balance between pro- and anti-inflammatory cytokines may differ between TMD with and without widespread pain [19] and supports a shift to a more pronounced central pro-inflammatory state in widespread myalgia compared to localized myalgia. Thus, peripheral sensitization may be of greater importance in the pathophysiology of localized myalgias than in widespread pain.

Tooth-clenching increased IL-6, IL-7, IL-8, TNF and IL-13 in TMD myalgia patients and IL-6 and IL-8 in controls, in line with previous studies [25, 37]. IL-6 and IL-8 are regarded as myokines, i.e. cytokines that are produced in the muscle [24], while TNF probably is produced in other tissue [42]. Although plasma cytokines were not analyzed in this study, muscle levels of IL-6 and IL-8 (but not IL-1β or TNF) were reported higher than plasma levels in patients with fibromyalgia, supporting that they are produced in the muscle [25]. It is well described that plasma levels of IL-6 increase in response to exercise. Also, plasma levels of the anti-inflammatory cytokines IL-4, IL-7, IL-10, and IL-13 seem to increase after exercise in healthy subjects [43] and IL-10 also in patients with knee-osteoarthritis [44]. On the contrary, in patients with fibromyalgia, plasma IL-10 showed a blunted response and IL-8 seem to decrease [26, 45]. Thus, patients with localized pain may be able to recruit an anti-inflammatory response after exercise in contrast to patients with generalized pain.

The repetitive tooth-clenching task evoked pain in the controls and increased fatigue in both groups, with higher intensities in TMD myalgia patients in accordance to previous studies using the same methodology [15, 30]. However, other mechanisms than release of cytokines are most probably responsible for this as there were no correlations between the release of cytokines on one hand, and pain or fatigue on the other. This indicates that there is no direct cause-effect relation between pain and cytokine levels. Indeed, the increased pain level may be an effect of the release of other biomarkers [35, 46] or interactions between several other mechanisms [47].

Pain on palpation, reflecting muscle allodynia, is one of the key symptoms of chronic muscle pain why it was not surprising that PPT were lower in patients than controls. Allodynia is generally regarded a sign of central sensitization [48], but peripheral sensitization may participate to the lowered PPT, as there were no differences between TMD myalgia patients and controls in PPT over the reference point. However, masseter PPT did not change in response to tooth-clenching and did not correlate with cytokine levels. This could be the reason why the influence of muscle cytokines on muscle allodynia in TMD myalgia is probably minor, if any at all.

### Limitations and strengths
This is, to our knowledge, the first study investigating the interstitial jaw-muscle release of cytokines in TMD myalgia. Another strength is that a panel with 13 pro- and anti-inflammatory cytokines was used for the analysis in the same dialysate samples so that differences in their pattern after tooth-clenching could be analyzed.

One limitation was that some cytokines were under LOD and had to be excluded. Yet, the most common cytokines reported in previous microdialysis studies could be detected. There are several factors that can affect the dialysate levels, such as the flow-rate, the diffusion-rate through the tissue, the area and weight cut-off of the dialysis membrane, and the composition of the perfusate [49]. Perhaps by adding a colloid to the ringer-solution, the cytokines under LOD could have been detected [50]. Another limitation was that the relative recovery was not analyzed, which could have provided a true value of the extracellular concentrations. Furthermore, the

patients with TMD myalgia were quite young and had a low average pain intensity at baseline, and may therefore not fully represent the general TMD myalgia population. However, the variability in pain intensity and age differs in experimental studies of TMD patients with myalgia. The data in our study is in accordance with findings of a previous study [51]. Finally, the sample was limited only to women that were psychologically healthy why it is unclear if the results can be generalized to male patients and patients with more severe psychological co-morbidities.

### Conclusion
This study showed that the muscle levels of IL-6, IL-7, IL-8 and IL-13 were increased in patients with TMD myalgia and increased further in response to experimental tooth-clenching, as did jaw-muscle pain and fatigue. This give further support that muscle inflammation may drive chronic myalgia, but that patients with TMD myalgia have a normal anti-inflammatory response to exercise. However, the lack of correlation between pain and cytokine levels, indicates that there is no direct cause-relation effect between increased pain and cytokine release and that other peripheral mediators and mechanisms, such as central sensitization are important for pain mediation.

### Abbreviations
5-HT: 5-hydroxytryptamine; serotonin; DC/TMD: Diagnostic Criteria for temporomandibular disorders; IFN-γ: Interferon gamma; IL: Interleukin; NRS: Numeric rating scale; PPT: Pressure pain threshold; PSS: Perceived Stress Scale; STAI-trait: State-Trait Anxiety Inventory; TMD: Temporomandibular disorders; TNF: Tumor necrosis factor; WAD: Whiplash-associated disorders

### Acknowledgements
Jonas Goerlash is gratefully acknowledged for assisting with microdialysis in healthy controls.
This study was supported by grants from the Swedish Research Council (K2009-52P-20943-03-2), the Stockholm County Council (ALF project and SOF-project), the Swedish Rheumatism Association, the Swedish Dental Association, the Department of Dental Medicine at Karolinska Institutet, and the American Dental Association in Sweden (ADSS).

### Authors' contributions
SLJ contributed to conception, study design, data acquisition, analysis, and interpretation, drafted the manuscript; NC, contributed to data analysis and interpretation, drafted the manuscript; PS, and TL contributed to conception, study design, data interpretation, critically reviewed the manuscript; ME contributed to conception, study design, analysis, and interpretation, drafted the manuscript. All authors gave final approval and agree to be accountable for all aspects of the work.

### Competing interests
The authors declare that they have no competing interests.

### Author details
[1]Section for Orofacial Pain and Jaw Function, Department of Dental Medicine, Karolinska Institutet, SE 14104, Huddinge, Sweden. [2]Scandinavian Center for Orofacial Neurosciences (SCON), Huddinge, Sweden. [3]Section of Orofacial Pain and Jaw Function, School of Dentistry and Oral Health, Aarhus University, Vennelyst Boulevard 9, DK-8000 Aarhus C, Denmark. [4]Faculty of Odontology, Malmö University, Malmö, Sweden.

## References

1. Schiffman E, Ohrbach R, Truelove E, Look J, Anderson G, Goulet JP, List T, Svensson P, Gonzalez Y, Lobbezoo F, Michelotti A, Brooks SL, Ceusters W, Drangsholt M, Ettlin D, Gaul C, Goldberg LJ, Haythornthwaite JA, Hollender L, Jensen R, John MT, De Laat A, de Leeuw R, Maixner W, van der Meulen M, Murray GM, Nixdorf DR, Palla S, Petersson A, Pionchon P, Smith B, Visscher CM, Zakrzewska J, Dworkin SF, International Rdc/Tmd Consortium Network IafDR, Orofacial Pain Special Interest Group IAftSoP (2014) Diagnostic Criteria for Temporomandibular Disorders (DC/TMD) for Clinical and Research Applications: recommendations of the International RDC/TMD Consortium Network* and Orofacial Pain Special Interest Groupdagger. J Oral Facial Pain Headache 28(1):6–27. doi:10.11607/jop.1151

2. Dao TT, LeResche L (2000) Gender differences in pain. J Orofac Pain 14(3): 169–184, discussion 184-195

3. Lund JP, Lavigne GJ, Dubner R, Sessle BJ (2001) Orofacial pain - from basic science to clinical management, vol first. vol book, edited. Quintessence Publishing Co, Inc, Illinois

4. Gil-Martinez A, Grande-Alonso M, Lopez-de-Uralde-Villanueva I, Lopez-Lopez A, Fernandez-Carnero J, La Touche R (2016) Chronic temporomandibular disorders: disability, pain intensity and fear of movement. J Headache Pain 17(1):103. doi:10.1186/s10194-016-0690-1

5. Monteiro AA, Kopp S (1989) The sufficiency of blood flow in human masseter muscle during endurance of biting in the intercuspal position and on a force transducer. Proc Finn Dent Soc 85(4-5):261–272

6. Huang GJ, LeResche L, Critchlow CW, Martin MD, Drangsholt MT (2002) Risk factors for diagnostic subgroups of painful temporomandibular disorders (TMD). J Dent Res 81(4):284–288

7. Velly AM, Gornitsky M, Philippe P (2003) Contributing factors to chronic myofascial pain: a case-control study. Pain 104(3):491–499

8. Al-Khotani A, Naimi-Akbar A, Albadawi E, Ernberg M, Hedenberg-Magnusson B, Christidis N (2016) Prevalence of diagnosed temporomandibular disorders among Saudi Arabian children and adolescents. J Headache Pain 17:41. doi:10.1186/s10194-016-0642-9

9. Stauber WT (2004) Factors involved in strain-induced injury in skeletal muscles and outcomes of prolonged exposures. J Electromyogr Kinesiol 14(1):61–70. doi:10.1016/j.jelekin.2003.09.010

10. Slade GD, Ohrbach R, Greenspan JD, Fillingim RB, Bair E, Sanders AE, Dubner R, Diatchenko L, Meloto CB, Smith S, Maixner W (2016) Painful temporomandibular disorder: decade of discovery from OPPERA studies. J Dent Res 95(10):1084–1092. doi:10.1177/0022034516653743

11. Bennett GJ (2012) What is spontaneous pain and who has it? J Pain 13(10): 921–929. doi:10.1016/j.jpain.2012.05.008

12. Koutris M, Lobbezoo F, Naeije M, Wang K, Svensson P, Arendt-Nielsen L, Farina D (2009) Effects of intense chewing exercises on the masticatory sensory-motor system. J Dent Res 88(7):658–662. doi:10.1177/0022034509338573

13. Staahl C, Drewes AM (2004) Experimental human pain models: a review of standardised methods for preclinical testing of analgesics. Basic Clin Pharmacol Toxicol 95(3):97–111. doi:10.1111/J.1742-7843.2004.950301.x

14. Stohler CS (1999) Craniofacial pain and motor function: pathogenesis, clinical correlates, and implications. Crit Rev Oral Biol Med 10(4):504–518

15. Dawson A, Ghafouri B, Gerdle B, List T, Svensson P, Ernberg M (2015) Effects of experimental tooth clenching on pain and intramuscular release of 5-HT and glutamate in patients with myofascial TMD. Clin J Pain 31(8):740–749. doi:10.1097/AJP.0000000000000154

16. Zhang JM, An J (2007) Cytokines, inflammation, and pain. Int Anesthesiol Clin 45(2):27–37. doi:10.1097/AIA.0b013e318034194e

17. Koch A, Zacharowski K, Boehm O, Stevens M, Lipfert P, von Giesen HJ, Wolf A, Freynhagen R (2007) Nitric oxide and pro-inflammatory cytokines correlate with pain intensity in chronic pain patients. Inflamm Res 56(1):32–37. doi:10.1007/s00011-007-6088-4

18. Kadetoff D, Lampa J, Westman M, Andersson M, Kosek E (2012) Evidence of central inflammation in fibromyalgia-increased cerebrospinal fluid interleukin-8 levels. J Neuroimmunol 242(1-2):33–38. doi:10.1016/j.jneuroim.2011.10.013

19. Slade GD, Conrad MS, Diatchenko L, Rashid NU, Zhong S, Smith S, Rhodes J, Medvedev A, Makarov S, Maixner W, Nackley AG (2011) Cytokine biomarkers and chronic pain: association of genes, transcription, and circulating proteins with temporomandibular disorders and widespread palpation tenderness. Pain 152(12):2802–2812. doi:10.1016/j.jpain.2011.09.005

20. Park JW, Chung JW (2016) Inflammatory cytokines and sleep disturbance in patients with temporomandibular disorders. J Oral Facial Pain Headache 30(1):27–33. doi:10.11607/ofph.1367

21. Shah JP, Phillips TM, Danoff JV, Gerber LH (2005) An in vivo microanalytical technique for measuring the local biochemical milieu of human skeletal muscle. J Appl Physiol 99(5):1977–1984

22. Shah JP, Danoff JV, Desai MJ, Parikh S, Nakamura LY, Phillips TM, Gerber LH (2008) Biochemicals associated with pain and inflammation are elevated in sites near to and remote from active myofascial trigger points. Arch Phys Med Rehabil 89(1):16–23. doi:10.1016/j.apmr.2007.10.018

23. Gerdle B, Lemming D, Kristiansen J, Larsson B, Peolsson M, Rosendal L (2007) Biochemical alterations in the trapezius muscle of patients with chronic whiplash associated disorders (WAD) - A microdialysis study. Eur J Pain(London, England). doi:10.1016/j.ejpain.2007.03.009

24. Fischer CP (2006) Interleukin-6 in acute exercise and training: what is the biological relevance? Exerc Immunol Rev 12:6–33

25. Christidis N, Ghafouri B, Larsson A, Palstam A, Mannerkorpi K, Bileviciute-Ljungar I, Lofgren M, Bjersing J, Kosek E, Gerdle B, Ernberg M (2015) Comparison of the levels of Pro-inflammatory cytokines released in the vastus lateralis muscle of patients with fibromyalgia and healthy controls during contractions of the quadriceps muscle–a microdialysis study. PLoS One 10(12):e0143856. doi:10.1371/journal.pone.0143856

26. Torgrimson-Ojerio B, Ross RL, Dieckmann NF, Avery S, Bennett RM, Jones KD, Guarino AJ, Wood LJ (2014) Preliminary evidence of a blunted anti-inflammatory response to exhaustive exercise in fibromyalgia. J Neuroimmunol 277(1-2):160–167. doi:10.1016/j.jneuroim.2014.10.003

27. van Selms MK, Lobbezoo F, Visscher CM, Naeije M (2008) Myofascial temporomandibular disorder pain, parafunctions and psychological stress. J Oral Rehabil 35(1):45–52. doi:10.1111/j.1365-2842.2007.01795.x

28. Larsson B, Rosendal L, Kristiansen J, Sjogaard G, Sogaard K, Ghafouri B, Abdiu A, Kjaer M, Gerdle B (2008) Responses of algesic and metabolic substances to 8 h of repetitive manual work in myalgic human trapezius muscle. Pain 140(3):479–490. doi:10.1016/j.pain.2008.10.001

29. Borg GA (1974) Perceived exertion. Exerc Sport Sci Rev 2:131–153

30. Louca S, Christidis N, Ghafouri B, Gerdle B, Svensson P, List T, Ernberg M (2014) Serotonin, glutamate and glycerol are released after the injection of hypertonic saline into human masseter muscles - a microdialysis study. J Headache Pain 15:89. doi:10.1186/1129-2377-15-89

31. Spielberger CD (1975) The measurement of state and trait anxiety: conceptual and methodological issues. In: Levi L (ed) Emotions-their parameters and measurement. Raven, New York, pp 713–725

32. Forsberg C, Bjorvell H (1993) Swedish population norms for the GHRI, HI and STAI-state. Qual Life Res 2(5):349–356

33. Cohen S, Kamarck T, Mermelstein R (1983) A global measure of perceived stress. J Health Soc Behav 24(4):385

34. Nordin M, Nordin S (2013) Psychometric evaluation and normative data of the Swedish version of the 10-item perceived stress scale. Scand J Psychol 54(6):502–507. doi:10.1111/sjop.12071

35. Ernberg M, Hedenberg-Magnusson B, Alstergren P, Kopp S (1999) The level of serotonin in the superficial masseter muscle in relation to local pain and allodynia. Life Sci 65(3):313–325

36. Chaturvedi AK, Kemp TJ, Pfeiffer RM, Biancotto A, Williams M, Munuo S, Purdue MP, Hsing AW, Pinto L, McCoy JP, Hildesheim A (2011) Evaluation of multiplexed cytokine and inflammation marker measurements: a methodologic study. Cancer Epidemiol Biomarkers Prev 20(9):1902–1911. doi:10.1158/1055-9965.EPI-11-0221

37. Rosendal L, Kristiansen J, Gerdle B, Søgaard K, Peolsson M, Kjaer M, Sörensen J, Larsson B (2005) Increased levels of interstitial potassium but normal levels of muscle IL-6 and LDH in patients with trapezius myalgia. Pain 119(1-3):201–209

38. King C R-DM, Wallet S, Fillingim R. (2016) Altered in vitro production of cytokines in temporomandibular disorder (TMD). Abstract PTH 232 presented at: IASP 2016 International Association for the Study of Pain (IASP): 16th World Congress of Pain; Yokohama, Japan

39. Marchand F, Perretti M, McMahon SB (2005) Role of the immune system in chronic pain. Nat Rev Neurosci 6(7):521–532. doi:10.1038/nrn1700

40. Kidd BL, Urban LA (2001) Mechanisms of inflammatory pain. Br J Anaesth 87(1):3–11

41. Kosek E, Altawil R, Kadetoff D, Finn A, Westman M, Le Maitre E, Andersson M, Jensen-Urstad M, Lampa J (2015) Evidence of different mediators of central inflammation in dysfunctional and inflammatory pain–interleukin-8 in fibromyalgia and interleukin-1 beta in rheumatoid arthritis. J Neuroimmunol 280:49–55. doi:10.1016/j.jneuroim.2015.02.002

42. Pedersen BK, Fischer CP (2007) Beneficial health effects of exercise-the role of IL-6 as a myokine. Trends Pharmacol Sci 28(4):152–156. doi:10.1016/j.tips.2007.02.002

43. Andersson H, Bohn SK, Raastad T, Paulsen G, Blomhoff R, Kadi F (2010) Differences in the inflammatory plasma cytokine response following two elite female soccer games separated by a 72-h recovery. Scand J Med Sci Sports 20(5):740–747. doi:10.1111/j.1600-0838.2009.00989.x

44. Helmark IC, Mikkelsen UR, Borglum J, Rothe A, Petersen MC, Andersen O, Langberg H, Kjaer M (2010) Exercise increases interleukin-10 levels both intraarticularly and peri-synovially in patients with knee osteoarthritis: a randomized controlled trial. Arthritis Res Ther 12(4):R126. doi:10.1186/ar3064

45. Bote ME, Garcia JJ, Hinchado MD, Ortega E (2013) Fibromyalgia: anti-inflammatory and stress responses after acute moderate exercise. PLoS One 8(9):e74524. doi:10.1371/journal.pone.0074524

46. Rosendal L, Larsson B, Kristiansen J, Peolsson M, Sogaard K, Kjaer M, Sorensen J, Gerdle B (2004) Increase in muscle nociceptive substances and anaerobic metabolism in patients with trapezius myalgia: microdialysis in rest and during exercise. Pain 112(3):324–334. doi:10.1016/j.pain.2004.09.017

47. Svensson P, Kumar A (2016) Assessment of risk factors for oro-facial pain and recent developments in classification: implications for management. J Oral Rehabil. doi:10.1111/joor.12447

48. Woolf CJ (2011) Central sensitization: implications for the diagnosis and treatment of pain. Pain 152(3 Suppl):S2–15. doi:10.1016/j.pain.2010.09.030

49. Gerdle B, Ghafouri B, Ernberg M, Larsson B (2014) Chronic musculoskeletal pain: review of mechanisms and biochemical biomarkers as assessed by the microdialysis technique. J Pain Res 7:313–326. doi:10.2147/JPR.S59144

50. Helmy A, Carpenter KL, Skepper JN, Kirkpatrick PJ, Pickard JD, Hutchinson PJ (2009) Microdialysis of cytokines: methodological considerations, scanning electron microscopy, and determination of relative recovery. J Neurotrauma 26(4):549–561. doi:10.1089/neu.2008.0719

51. Shimada A, Castrillon EE, Baad-Hansen L, Ghafouri B, Gerdle B, Wahlen K, Ernberg M, Cairns BE, Svensson P (2016) Increased pain and muscle glutamate concentration after single ingestion of monosodium glutamate by myofascial temporomandibular disorders patients. Eur J Pain 20(9):1502–1512. doi:10.1002/ejp.874

# A multicenter, open-label, long-term safety and tolerability study of DFN-02, an intranasal spray of sumatriptan 10 mg plus permeation enhancer DDM, for the acute treatment of episodic migraine

Sagar Munjal[1]*, Elimor Brand-Schieber[1], Kent Allenby[1], Egilius L.H. Spierings[2], Roger K. Cady[3] and Alan M. Rapoport[4]

## Abstract

**Background:** DFN-02 is a novel intranasal spray formulation composed of sumatriptan 10 mg and a permeation-enhancing excipient comprised of 0.2% 1-O-n-Dodecyl-β-D-Maltopyranoside (DDM). This composition of DFN-02 allows sumatriptan to be rapidly absorbed into the systemic circulation and exhibit pharmacokinetics comparable to subcutaneously administered sumatriptan. Rapid rate of absorption is suggested to be important for optimal efficacy. The objective of this study was to evaluate the safety and tolerability of DFN-02 (10 mg) in the acute treatment of episodic migraine with and without aura over a 6-month period based on the incidence of treatment-emergent adverse events and the evaluation of results of clinical laboratory tests, vital signs, physical examination, and electrocardiograms.

**Methods:** This was a multi-center, open-label, repeat-dose safety study in adults with episodic migraine with and without aura. Subjects diagnosed with migraine with or without aura according to the criteria set forth in the International Classification of Headache Disorders, 2nd edition, who experienced 2 to 6 attacks per month with fewer than 15 headache days per month and at least 48 headache-free hours between attacks, used DFN-02 to treat their migraine attacks acutely over the course of 6 months.

**Results:** A total of 173 subjects was enrolled, 167 (96.5%) subjects used at least 1 dose of study medication and were evaluable for safety, and 134 (77.5%) subjects completed the 6-month study. A total of 2211 migraine attacks was reported, and 3292 doses of DFN-02 were administered; mean per subject monthly use of DFN-02 was 3.6 doses. Adverse events were those expected for triptans, as well as for nasally administered compounds. No new safety signals emerged. Dysgeusia and application site pain were the most commonly reported treatment-emergent adverse events over 6 months (21% and 30.5%, respectively). Most of the treatment-emergent adverse events were mild. There were 5 serious adverse events, all considered unrelated to the study medication; the early discontinuation rate was 22.5% over the 6-month treatment period.

**Conclusion:** DFN-02 was shown to be well tolerated when used over 6 months to treat episodic migraine acutely.

**Keywords:** Episodic migraine, Acute treatment, Intranasal sumatriptan, DDM, Sumatriptan, Long-term safety

* Correspondence: smunjal@drreddys.com
[1]Dr. Reddy's Laboratories Ltd., 107 College Road East Princeton, Princeton, NJ 08540, USA
Full list of author information is available at the end of the article

## Background

In the acute treatment of episodic migraine (ie, patients with fewer than 15 headache days per month [1]), 5-$HT_{1B1D}$ agonists (triptans) are recommended as first-line therapy for moderate and severe attacks and for mild attacks that have been unresponsive to analgesics or nonsteroidal anti-inflammatory drugs in the past [2]. Oral sumatriptan, the most widely used drug in the triptan class [3–5], is effective and safe [6], but it may not be an optimal choice for many attacks. Its poor bioavailability (15%) and slow absorption ($T_{max} \geq 2$ h) lead to a slow onset of action (45–60 min) [7], an issue exacerbated in many patients by migraine-associated gastric stasis [8–10]. To varying degrees, poor absorption and relatively delayed onset of action limit the clinical utility of all oral triptans [4, 6].

For attacks associated with nausea or vomiting, as well as in patients who cannot tolerate or experience dysphagia with oral triptans, evidence-based guidelines recommend the use of non-oral migraine-specific formulations [2]. Currently available alternatives, however, are of limited clinical utility in many patients. Subcutaneous (SC) sumatriptan 6 mg has good efficacy (60% pain-free at 2 h) and a fast onset of action (10 min post-dose) [11], but most SC sumatriptan-treated patients (59%) have injection site reactions, nearly half (42%) experience atypical sensations (eg, tingling, warm/hot, tightness/pressure) [12], and many migraineurs are averse to using injectable formulations [13, 14]. Transdermal sumatriptan, which has been linked with burns and scars at the application site [15] and has very limited efficacy (18% pain-free at 2 h [16]), has been voluntarily taken off the market. With the commercial formulation of sumatriptan intranasal spray (Imitrex® Nasal Spray, Imigran® Nasal Spray, GlaxoSmithKline), because the drug is not well absorbed through the nasal mucosa [17] ($T_{max}$ 0.88–1.75 h) [18]), its onset of action (30 – 45 min) is only slightly faster than oral sumatriptan [7]. Poor absorption is also a problem with intranasal zolmitriptan ($T_{max}$ ~3 h) [19], and sumatriptan nasal powder has reported a $T_{max}$ of 20 min to as long as 2 h [20, 21]. These important clinical limitations, particularly in light of the attributes of acute treatment that are most important to migraineurs (rapid onset of action, complete relief, no recurrence, lack of side effects [22–24]) highlight a gap in migraine pharmacotherapy and emphasize the unmet need for a safe and highly effective non-oral migraine medication with a rapid onset of action.

DFN-02 — sumatriptan 10 mg plus 0.20% 1-O-n-Dodecyl-β-D-Maltopyranoside (DDM), a permeation-enhancing excipient — is a new intranasal migraine treatment under clinical development that is designed to overcome many of the limitations to currently available acute medications. Sumatriptan is a well-known headache medicine that has been extensively studied and described [4, 5, 25]. DDM, on the other hand, belongs to a class of surfactants known as alkylglycosides, which are non-ionic and metabolized to simple carbohydrates and alcohols or acids that have shown promise as permeation enhancers for intranasal medication [26–28]. DDM appears to loosen cell-cell junctions and enhance paracellular movement through the nasal epithelium by altering mucosal viscosity and membrane fluidity, increasing blood flow, and inhibiting ciliary beat frequency and drug metabolizing enzymes [28–32].

In a pharmacokinetic (PK) study in healthy subjects, DFN-02 had a markedly more rapid sumatriptan absorption profile than commercial intranasal sumatriptan, systemic exposure was similar to 4 mg SC sumatriptan, and plasma sumatriptan concentration peaked 5 min earlier than 4 mg SC and 6 mg SC [33] — results that suggest it may have efficacy comparable to a 4-mg SC dose of sumatriptan, which has not yet been demonstrated in migraine patients. With efficacy expected based on PK equivalence data, the sole objective of this study was to evaluate the safety and tolerability of DFN-02's unique formulation in the acute treatment of migraine over a 6-month period, based on treatment-emergent adverse events (TEAEs), clinical laboratory results, and electrocardiograms.

## Methods

This was a multi-center, open-label, repeat-dose safety study in adults with episodic migraine with and without aura. The protocol, the patient information and consent form, and other relevant study documentation were approved by the Institutional Review Board (IRB) for each study center before initiation of the study. Protocol amendments were approved by the IRB before implementation or submitted to the IRB for information, as required. The study followed the Guidelines of the World Medical Association Declaration of Helsinki in its revised edition (Brazil, 2013), The International Council for Harmonisation guidelines for current Good Clinical Practice, the United States Food and Drug Administration Code of Federal Regulations, and the demands of national drug and data protection laws and other applicable regulatory requirements. Investigators and study staff recruited patients at the individual study sites; written consent to participate was provided after having been informed about the nature and purpose of the study, participation/termination conditions, and risks and benefits of treatment. The study was registered with Clinical-Trials.gov (NCT02279082).

## Subjects

To be enrolled in the study, subjects had to be adults aged 18 – 65 years diagnosed with acute migraine according to the criteria set forth in the International Classification of Headache Disorders, 2nd edition (ICHD-2)

[34]. They also had to have a history of 2 – 6 attacks with or without visual aura per month, with 14 or fewer headache days monthly and at least 48 h of headache-free time between attacks; when aura was present, it could not have lasted longer than 60 min. Females of childbearing potential had to have a negative urine pregnancy test, not be lactating, and agree to practice a reliable form of contraception or abstinence during the study. Males (with female partners) agreed to practice a reliable form of contraception or abstinence during the study. Subjects also had to be willing and able to return to the study site within 72 h of the first use of study medication; record each attack and each instance of the use of DFN-02 and rescue medication in a patient paper diary for the duration of the study; provide written informed consent; and use the DFN-02 intranasal spray device correctly after instruction.

Subjects were excluded if they had medication overuse headache (as defined by ICHD-2); used any botulinum toxin treatment within 180 days of screening; changed dosages of migraine preventive medications during the 30 days before and through screening; took mini-prophylaxis for menstrual migraine; had hemiplegic migraine or migraine with brain stem aura or other forms of neurologically complicated migraine; had a history of stroke, transient ischemic attack, migralepsy, seizure disorder, ischemic coronary artery disease, Wolff-Parkinson-White syndrome or arrhythmias associated with other cardiac accessory conduction pathway disorders, uncontrolled hypertension, peripheral vascular disease, ischemic bowel disease, neurological or psychiatric impairment, or cognitive dysfunction. They were also ineligible if they could not differentiate between a migraine attack and a tension-type or cluster headache; were intolerant to any formulation of sumatriptan or had experienced a significant adverse event related to any triptan; had a history of nonresponse to 2 or more triptans.

Subjects were also disqualified for any of the following: taking medications or having an illness likely to affect the physiology of the nasal mucosa; abnormal nasal physiology or pathology; intolerance to nasal sprays; severe renal impairment; serum total bilirubin > 2.0 mg/dL; serum aspartate aminotransferase, alanine aminotransferase, or alkaline phosphatase > 2.5 times the upper limit of normal; 1-year history of alcohol or substance abuse; positive urine drug screen for illicit drugs or unexplained prescription drugs; received treatment with an investigational drug or device within 4 weeks of the screening visit or participated in a central nervous system clinical trial in the 3 months before screening; tested positive for human immunodeficiency virus, hepatitis B surface antigen, or hepatitis C virus; any medical condition that would have confounded the objectives of the study.

## Treatment

DFN-02 was provided in a single-use intranasal spray device designed to deliver 100 µL/spray containing 10 mg of sumatriptan plus 0.20% DDM.

## Study conduct

The study involved 9 visits: screening (Day -21 to Day -1), enrollment (Day 0), initial follow up (within 72 h of treatment), and 6 monthly visits (every 30 ± 3 days). At the screening visit, subjects signed informed consent and underwent the following assessments: inclusion/exclusion criteria, demographics, medical history, physical examination, vital signs, serology, urine pregnancy test, clinical labs, urinalysis, urine drug test, 12-lead electrocardiogram (ECG), adverse event and concomitant medications review, and device training and medication instruction. Hematology, clinical chemistry, urinalysis, urine drug screen, and human immunodeficiency virus, Hepatitis B surface antigen, and Hepatitis C virus antibody analyses were performed at a central laboratory (ACM Global Central Laboratory, US, 160 Elmgrove Park, Rochester, NY 14624). At each visit, 3 ECG readings were collected, no less than 5 min apart, and reviewed initially by the investigator for any immediate concerns, and then by a central reader (ERT, 1818 Market St., Suite 1000, Philadelphia, PA 19103).

Subjects were observed for 21 days after the screening visit to evaluate whether they satisfied inclusion criteria and had no medication overuse headache. The screening period was shortened up to Day -1 if subjects met inclusion criteria before this time. Subjects continued to take their normal migraine medication during the screening period.

At enrollment, screening assessments (with the exception of demographics) were re-performed; DFN-02 devices (individually blister packed and labeled), an Instructions for Use document, and a paper diary were dispensed; and rescue medication was determined. The quantity of DFN-02 devices initially dispensed (6 or 12) was determined by the frequency of attacks (≤ 3/month = 6 devices; ≥ 4/ month = 12 devices); at subsequent resupply visits, unused devices were counted and additional devices were dispensed as needed. Throughout the study, additional instructions on the dispensation of the study medication were available through an interactive web-response system.

For the next 6 months, DFN-02 was self-administered once into 1 nostril (either right or left per subject's choice) at the onset of acute migraine pain; for attacks with aura, subjects were instructed to use DFN-02 at the onset of pain, not at the onset of aura. If pain relief at 1 h post-dose was insufficient, subjects were permitted to take either another dose of DFN-02 or rescue medication. If a second dose of DFN-02 was taken and relief was still inadequate after 2 h, rescue medication was permitted; the rescue medication was chosen with the investigator at screening and adjusted as necessary. No more than 2 doses of DFN-02 were permitted in a 24-h period.

During the treatment period, subjects recorded the migraine pain start and stop for each attack (date and time), use of DFN-02 (date and time), and use of rescue medication (date, time, name, and dose) in the paper diary dispensed to them at each study visit. The paper diary was reviewed by investigators, and its data were entered into the electronic case report form by study site personnel.

## Assessments

There were no efficacy variables in this study. Safety variables included the incidence of AEs, clinical laboratory data (hematology, chemistry, and urinalysis), vital sign measurements (sitting blood pressure, pulse, respiration rate, and body temperature), physical examination findings, 12-lead ECG readings, urine pregnancy test results, study medication use, and concomitant medication use. The primary endpoint was the incidence of TEAEs during the 6-month treatment period based on the incidence of TEAEs, clinical laboratory results, and ECG findings. The number of study medication doses taken within a migraine attack was determined based on dosing and migraine start/end dates and times recorded by the subjects; values were corroborated by the site staff. These data were also reconciled with data in the Drug Accountability Log, which recorded all used and unused study medication.

Adverse events were coded by using the Medical Dictionary for Regulatory Activities (MedDRA, version 17.0) and classified by severity (mild, moderate, severe) and causality (not related, possibly related, probably related, definitely related). Treatment-emergent AEs were defined as AEs with a start date on or after the initial dose and up to 5 days after the last dose of DFN-02 or events that became worse in severity on or after the date of the first DFN-02 dose. Severe AEs were defined as AEs that prevented normal everyday activities and usually needed treatment or other intervention. Investigators also characterized the seriousness of AEs, and serious AEs (SAE) were defined as any untoward medical occurrences or effects that, at any dose, resulted in death or were life-threatening; required or prolonged in-patient hospitalization, resulted in persistent or significant disability/incapacity, or were congenital anomaly/birth defects. Severe AEs were not necessarily SAEs.

## Statistics

All analyses and summaries were produced using SAS version 9.3 or above (SAS Institute, Cary, NC). The study populations for analysis included all subjects who were screened (for disposition) and all subjects who received at least 1 dose of study medication (for all safety endpoints). Continuous variables were summarized using the number of observations (n), mean, standard deviation (SD), median, minimum, and maximum. Categorical variables were summarized using frequency and percentages of subjects. If there were multiple valid results at a given visit, the first value at each visit window was used, unless a test was repeated and the result suggested that the initial value was an error, in which case the last observation within the visit window was used.

Unless otherwise specified, baseline assessment was the latest available valid measurement taken prior to the initial dose administration of study medication, generally Day 0. Missing safety data were not imputed in this study.

No formal sample size calculation was performed. It was estimated that at least 150 subjects would need to be enrolled to ensure that at least 100 subjects completed the 6-month study period.

## Results

Twenty-five US investigator sites participated in the study. The first subject was enrolled into the study on 06 October 2014, and the last subject completed the study on 19 August 2015.

### Subjects

A total of 229 subjects was screened, 173 subjects met inclusion criteria, 167 subjects received at least 1 dose of study drug and were evaluable for safety (96.5%), 134 subjects (77.5%) completed the 6-month treatment period, and 39 subjects (22.5%) discontinued early from the study (Fig. 1). The majority of subjects were female and white (n = 136, 81.4% for both variables). The median age was 45.0 (19–64) years, and the mean body mass index was 28.7 (7.0) kg (Table 1). During the 6-month treatment period, 167 subjects had 2211 attacks, averaging 13.2 attacks per subject and 2.4 attacks per month. Those who completed the study (n = 134) experienced 2036 attacks, averaging 15.2 attacks per subject and 2.5 attacks monthly.

### Medication usage

The median duration of DFN-02 exposure was 181 days. Over the course of the study, subjects treated 2190 attacks with 3292 doses of DFN-02, averaging 1.5 doses of DFN-02 per attack. An average of approximately one third (32%) of attacks per subject was treated with more than 1 dose of DFN-02. Each month, subjects took a mean of 3.6 DFN-02 doses, for a 6-month total of 19.7 doses; among those completing the study, the mean

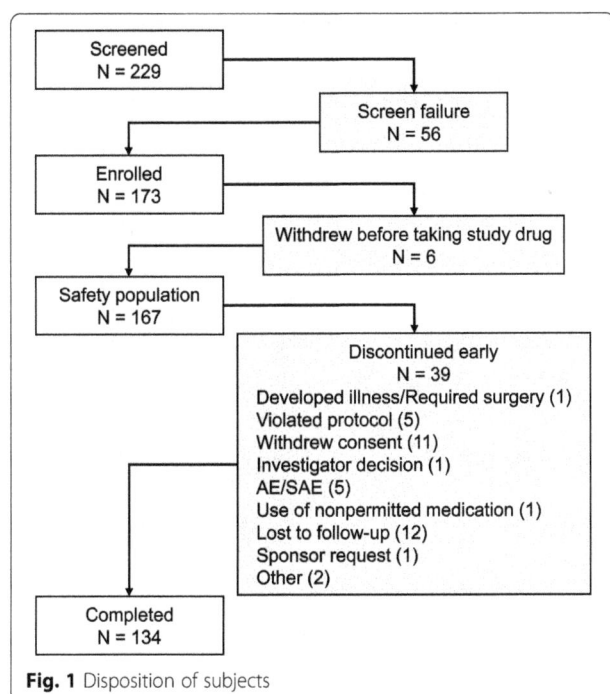

**Fig. 1** Disposition of subjects

Screened
N = 229

Screen failure
N = 56

Enrolled
N = 173

Withdrew before taking study drug
N = 6

Safety population
N = 167

Discontinued early
N = 39
Developed illness/Required surgery (1)
Violated protocol (5)
Withdrew consent (11)
Investigator decision (1)
AE/SAE (5)
Use of nonpermitted medication (1)
Lost to follow-up (12)
Sponsor request (1)
Other (2)

Completed
N = 134

**Table 2** Extent of DFN-02 exposure overall and in subjects who completed the study

| | Safety population (N = 167) | Completers (n = 134) |
|---|---|---|
| Days[a] | | |
| Mean (SD) | 163.3 (48.9) | |
| Median | 181 | |
| Range | 3–241 | |
| Months[b,] | | |
| Mean (SD) | 5.4 (1.6) | |
| Median | 6.0 | |
| Range | 0.1–8.0 | |
| Doses taken | 3292 | 3031 |
| Doses per patient | | |
| Mean (SD) | 19.7 (13.0) | 22.6 (12.1) |
| Median | 18.0 | 20.5 |
| Range | (1–61) | (2–61) |
| Doses per patient (monthly)[c] | | |
| Mean (SD) | 3.6 (2.1) | 3.7 (2.0) |
| Median | 3.3 | 3.4 |
| Range | 0.3–10.2 | 0.3–10.2 |

SD standard deviation
[a]Date of study completion or early termination – date of enrollment +1
[b]Number of days in the study/30
[c]Number of total doses taken/number of months in the study

number of DFN-02 doses per month was 3.7, and the per-subject total was 22.6 (Table 2).

Most subjects (58%, 97/167) used rescue medication at least once in 6 months. The mean total doses per subject was 2.4 for 6 months, and the mean monthly average dose per subject was 0.5. The most commonly used rescue medications were ibuprofen (21%, 35/167); fixed combinations of aspirin-acetaminophen-caffeine (16.8%, 28/167) and aspirin-butalbital (5.4%, 9/167); and acetaminophen (5.4%, 9/167).

**Table 1** Demographics

| Characteristic | Total (N = 167) n (%) |
|---|---|
| Sex | |
| Male | 31 (18.6) |
| Female | 136 (81.4) |
| Age (years)[a] | 45.0 (19–64) |
| BMI (kg)[b] | 28.7 (7.0) |
| Race | |
| American Indian or Alaska Native | 0 |
| Asian | 2 (1.2) |
| Black or African American | 25 (15.0) |
| Native Hawaiian or Other Pacific Islander | 1 (0.6) |
| White | 136 (81.4) |
| Other | 3 (1.8) |

BMI body mass index
[a]Median (range)
[b]Mean (SD)

## Safety

In total, 71.9% (120/167) of subjects reported 1264 TEAEs in up to 6 months of treatment. About half of subjects who reported TEAEs (61/120) had mild TEAEs; only 9 had TEAEs at a level of discomfort that were determined by the investigator as severe. The severe TEAEs included dyspepsia, hiatus hernia, application site pain, gastroenteritis, diverticulitis, sinusitis, post-traumatic pain (worsening of pain from right shoulder injury noted in medical history), myalgia (transient entire body myalgia associated with each occurrence of study medication dosing), bladder injury (noted during an open hysterectomy procedure), and menometrorrhagia; each severe TEAE affected 1 subject, except for bladder injury and menometrorrhagia, both of which occurred in the same subject.

A total of 52.7% of subjects (88/167) experienced study medication-related events, with TEAEs in 35.9% of subjects (60/167) considered definitely related, in 11.4% of subjects (19/167) considered probably related, and in 5.4% of subjects (9/167) considered possibly related. One migraine TEAE and 3 headache TEAEs were considered related to study drug. Table 3 lists AEs related to treatment with DFN-02 that affected at least 2% of subjects.

**Table 3** Treatment-emergent adverse events: total and those occurring in ≥2% of subjects by incidence, severity, and relationship to study medication[a] (N = 167)

| | Subjects | Mild | Moderate | Severe | Not related | Possibly related | Probably related | Definitely related |
|---|---|---|---|---|---|---|---|---|
| Overall | 120 (71.9) | 61 (36.5) | 50 (29.9) | 9 (5.4) | 32 (19.2) | 9 (5.4) | 19 (11.4) | 60 (35.9) |
| Application site pain | 51 (30.5) | 38 (22.8) | 12 (7.2) | 1 (0.6) | 0 | 2 (1.2) | 9 (5.4) | 40 (24.0) |
| Dysgeusia | 35 (21.0) | 30 (18.0) | 5 (3.0) | 0 | 0 | 4 (2.4) | 7 (4.2) | 24 (14.4) |
| Application site reaction | 9 (5.4) | 7 (4.2) | 2 (1.2) | 0 | 0 | 1 (0.6) | 2 (1.2) | 6 (3.6) |
| Application site irritation | 7 (4.2) | 7 (4.2) | 0 | 0 | 0 | 1 (0.6) | 0 | 6 (3.6) |
| Throat irritation | 8 (4.8) | 6 (3.6) | 2 (1.2) | 0 | 0 | 1 (0.6) | 2 (1.2) | 5 (3.0) |
| Chest discomfort | 4 (2.4) | 4 (2.4) | 0 | 0 | 1 (0.6) | 0 | 0 | 3 (1.8) |
| Nausea | 7 (4.2) | 2 (1.2) | 5 (3.0) | 0 | 1 (0.6) | 1 (0.6) | 2 (1.2) | 3 (1.8) |
| Dizziness | 6 (3.6) | 4 (2.4) | 2 (1.2) | 0 | 0 | 3 (1.8) | 1 (0.6) | 2 (1.2) |
| Paresthesia | 4 (2.4) | 3 (1.8) | 1 (0.6) | 0 | 1 (0.6) | 1 (0.6) | 1 (0.6) | 1 (0.6) |
| Vomiting | 4 (2.4) | 2 (1.2) | 2 (1.2) | 0 | 2 (1.2) | 0 | 2 (1.2) | 0 |
| Diarrhea | 4 (2.4) | 3 (1.8) | 1 (0.6) | 0 | 3 (1.8) | 0 | 1 (0.6) | 0 |
| Gastroenteritis viral | 6 (3.6) | 3 (1.8) | 3 (1.8) | 0 | 6 (3.6) | 0 | 0 | 0 |
| Influenza | 4 (2.4) | 1 (0.6) | 3 (1.8) | 0 | 4 (2.4) | 0 | 0 | 0 |
| Nasopharyngitis | 12 (7.2) | 10 (6.0) | 2 (1.2) | 0 | 12 (7.2) | 0 | 0 | 0 |
| Sinusitis | 11 (6.6) | 4 (2.4) | 6 (3.6) | 1 (0.6) | 10 (6.0) | 1 (0.6) | 0 | 0 |
| Upper respiratory tract infection | 18 (10.8) | 15 (9.0) | 3 (1.8) | 0 | 18 (10.8) | 0 | 0 | 0 |
| Urinary tract infection | 5 (3.0) | 3 (1.8) | 2 (1.2) | 0 | 5 (3.0) | 0 | 0 | 0 |

[a]Values are n (%)

The most common TEAEs were application site pain, dysgeusia, application site reaction, upper respiratory tract infection, nasopharyngitis, and sinusitis (Table 3). Application site pain (including verbatim of nasal or nostril burning or stinging) was most common, affecting 30.5% of subjects (51/167) at least once over the 6-month study period; of those who reported application site pain, about three quarters (38/51) experienced mild pain, nearly one quarter (12/51) experienced moderate pain, and 1 subject experienced severe pain. The next most common TEAE, dysgeusia, was reported by 21% of subjects (35/167); the vast majority (30/35) of these subjects had mild dysgeusia, and 5 had moderate dysgeusia. Severe dysgeusia was not reported.

In the study, there were a total of 94 triptan-related TEAEs in 32 subjects (19.2%) (Table 3); three quarters of these subjects (24/32) had mild triptan-related TEAEs, and one quarter (8/32) had moderate events. Twelve subjects experienced triptan-related TEAEs that were considered by the investigator to be definitely related to study medication. An additional 12 subjects experienced triptan-related TEAEs that were considered probably related to study medication, 7 subjects experienced TEAEs that were considered possibly related to study medication, and 1 subject experienced a TEAE that was considered not related to study medication. The most common triptan-related TEAEs were dizziness and nausea (3.6%, 6 subjects each).

Four subjects experienced 5 SAEs; diverticulitis, cholecystitis, and menometrorrhagia each affected 1 subject, and a fourth had both pyelonephritis and myocardial infarction. Three SAEs were treatment-emergent (diverticulitis, pyelonephritis, and menometrorrhagia each affected 1 subject), but all 5 SAEs were considered not related to study medication.

Five subjects experienced a total of 10 TEAEs leading to discontinuation from study medication. These TEAEs included dizziness (1.2%), which affected 2 subjects, and diarrhea, dyspepsia, nausea, vomiting, feeling jittery, pain, lethargy, and dyspnea, each of which occurred in 1 subject (0.6%). Another subject was discontinued due to cholecystitis, an SAE requiring hospitalization, but it was not treatment-emergent and was considered not related to the study medication. There were no clinically meaningful trends in mean changes from baseline or individual changes for any clinical laboratory variable, vital sign, or ECG.

## Discussion

In this 6-month, multicenter, open-label safety study — during which study medication was used to treat more than 2000 migraine attacks — DFN-02 was safe and tolerable for the acute treatment of patients with episodic migraine with and without aura. Adverse events with DFN-02 were similar in pattern, frequency, and severity to those seen in previous research with triptans and nasally administered medications [17, 35], and no novel safety signals were seen. As expected, dysgeusia and application site pain were the most commonly reported tolerability issues; most TEAEs were mild, however, which may have been a factor in the high rate of study completion (77.5%).

Although there were no efficacy assessments completed in this study, findings on other measures indicate that subjects using DFN-02 appear to have experienced migraine relief. For example, the vast majority of subjects completed the study, treating multiple attacks over the 6-month study period, and rescue medication was only used in about 18% of attacks (2.4 doses for an average of 13 attacks). Moreover, although repeat dosing of DFN-02 was permitted at least 1 h after the initial dose, approximately two thirds of qualifying attacks were treated with a single dose of DFN-02. Since subjects were provided with multiple canisters of DFN-02 and could repeat the dose as needed to control their symptoms, the high proportion of attacks treated with a single dose suggests that DFN-02, which contains only 10 mg sumatriptan, provided most subjects with adequate migraine relief.

Previous research with the commercial formulation of intranasal sumatriptan 20 mg demonstrated good safety and tolerability; the incidence of individual AEs was similar to placebo [17, 35]. The persistent exception is bad, bitter, or unpleasant taste, which affected 19–36% of subjects in randomized, placebo-controlled studies [35] and 22%–27% of subjects in a pooled analysis [17]. With DFN-02, dysgeusia was similarly common (21% of subjects), but symptoms were mostly mild, and no subjects cited it as a reason for discontinuation. Application site pain with DFN-02 was more common than in previous research with intranasal formulations (30.5% vs 4% [17, 35]); these events may be related to the presence of the permeation enhancer DDM in DFN-02. In clinical practice, however, the kinetics of DFN-02 have been shown to be about the same as sumatriptan 4 mg SC [33], with migraine patients expected to experience similar times to onset of action and rates of pain freedom, which suggests that the risk of site reactions with DFN-02 could be about 30% lower than with comparable acute treatments, such as 4 mg SC (30.5% vs 43% [36]). Since most TEAEs were mild, the study completion rate was high, and few subjects withdrew, the relative frequency of application site pain does not seem a likely barrier to care with DFN-02.

This study provides clinically useful data but has some limitations. Subject eligibility was based on ICHD-2, while the current version is ICHD-3 (beta). At the time of the study set-up, ICHD-3 (beta) [1] was newly available and still collecting feedback from experts; therefore, the study proceeded using the previous version.

Nevertheless, ICHD-2 and ICHD-3 (beta) are identical with respect to diagnosis of acute episodic migraine. Lacking a placebo control, the true incidence of AEs related to DFN-02 could not be determined. Additionally, in the absence of a direct comparison of DFN-02 with the commercially available intranasal formulation of sumatriptan, it was not possible to assess the relative safety of DFN-02 and marketed products. Given the well-established safety profile of intranasal sumatriptan, however, it is unlikely that any of these factors influenced the generalizability of these results or the long-term safety outcomes seen with DFN-02.

Sumatriptan is widely used and has been available in oral tablet, nasal spray, and injectable formulations for decades [25]. However, nearly 30% of migraineurs report dissatisfaction with acute therapies [37], with the most common complaint being that pain relief takes too long [22]; close to 90% of patients express a willingness to try new acute treatments [23, 24]. Because the PK of DFN-02 are compatible with a possible rapid onset of action and a favorable safety profile without the disadvantages associated with oral or SC therapies, DFN-02 may be useful for patients who prefer not to treat their condition with injectable medications, as well as patients in whom nonresponse, dysphagia, nausea, or vomiting preclude the use of orally administered drugs. As seen with similar triptan delivery systems [38, 39], ease of use may make DFN-02 especially convenient for treatment at home, work, and while traveling [35].

## Conclusions

In this multicenter, open-label safety study, DFN-02, a novel intranasal spray formulation composed of sumatriptan 10 mg and a permeation-enhancing excipient DDM, was safe and tolerable for the acute treatment of episodic migraine over a 6-month study. Adverse events with DFN-02 were similar in pattern, frequency, and severity to those seen in previous research with intranasal sumatriptan.

### Abbreviations

AE: Adverse event; DDM: 1-O-n-Dodecyl-β-D-Maltopyranoside; ECG: Electrocardiogram; ICHD: International Classification of Headache Disorders; IRB: Institutional Review Board; MedDRA: Medical Dictionary for Regulatory Activities; SAE: Serious adverse event; SC: Subcutaneous; SD: Standard deviation; TEAE: Treatment-emergent adverse event

### Acknowledgements

The authors acknowledge Kendra Gulbronson (Dr. Reddy's Laboratories, Princeton, NJ) for assisting with the conduct of this study. Medical writing services were provided by Christopher Caiazza. DRL Publication #791.

### Funding

This study was sponsored by Dr. Reddy's Laboratories Ltd., which developed and manufactures DFN-02.

## Authors' contributions

SM, ELHS, RKC, and AMR conceived and designed the study. SM, EBS, and KA analyzed the data. SM and EBS wrote the paper, and all authors revised and approved the final manuscript.

## Competing interests

This study was supported and funded by Dr. Reddy's Laboratories Ltd, manufacturer of DFN-02. SM is employed by and owns stocks of Dr. Reddy's Laboratories Ltd.; EBS and KA are employees of Dr. Reddy's Laboratories Ltd.; and ELHS, RKC, and AMR were paid consultants of Dr. Reddy's Laboratories Ltd.

## Author details

[1]Dr. Reddy's Laboratories Ltd., 107 College Road East Princeton, Princeton, NJ 08540, USA. [2]Dental Medicine Headache & Face Pain Program Tufts Medical Center, Craniofacial Pain Center Tufts University School, 800 Washington Street Boston, Boston, MA 02111, USA. [3]Clinvest/A Division of Banyan Inc., 3805 S Kansas Expy Springfield, Springfield, MO 65807, USA. [4]David Geffen School of Medicine at UCLA, Los Angeles, CA, USA.

## References

1. International Headache Society (2013) The International Classification of Headache Disorders, 3rd edition (beta version). Cephalalgia 33:629–808
2. Silberstein SD (2000) Practice parameter: evidence-based guidelines for migraine headache (an evidence-based review): report of the Quality Standards Subcommittee of the American Academy of Neurology. Neurology 55:754–762
3. Mathew NT, Loder EW (2005) Evaluating the triptans. Am J Med 118(Suppl 1):28s–35s
4. Lionetto L, Negro A, Casolla B et al (2012) Sumatriptan succinate : pharmacokinetics of different formulations in clinical practice. Expert Opin Pharmacother 13:2369–2380
5. Napoletano F, Lionetto L, Martelletti P (2014) Sumatriptan in clinical practice: effectiveness in migraine and the problem of psychiatric comorbidity. Expert Opin Pharmacother 15:303–305
6. Derry CJ, Derry S, Moore RA. Sumatriptan (oral route of administration) for acute migraine attacks in adults. Cochrane Database Syst Rev. 2012:Cd008615
7. IMITREX (sumatriptan succinate) tablets [Prescribing information]. Available at: https://www.gsksource.com/pharma/content/dam/GlaxoSmithKline/US/en/Prescribing_Information/Imitrex_Tablets/pdf/IMITREX-TABLETS-PI-PIL.PDF. Accessed 29 Dec 2016.
8. Aurora S, Kori S, Barrodale P et al (2007) Gastric stasis occurs in spontaneous, visually induced, and interictal migraine. Headache 47:1443–1446
9. Aurora SK, Kori SH, Barrodale P et al (2006) Gastric stasis in migraine: more than just a paroxysmal abnormality during a migraine attack. Headache 46:57–63
10. Boyle R, Behan PO, Sutton JA (1990) A correlation between severity of migraine and delayed gastric emptying measured by an epigastric impedance method. Br J Clin Pharmacol 30:405–409
11. Mathew NT, Dexter J, Couch J et al (1992) Dose ranging efficacy and safety of subcutaneous sumatriptan in the acute treatment of migraine. US Sumatriptan Research Group. Arch Neurol 49:1271–1276
12. IMITREX (sumatriptan succinate) injection [Prescribing Information]. Available at: https://www.gsksource.com/pharma/content/dam/GlaxoSmithKline/US/en/Prescribing_Information/Imitrex_Tablets/pdf/IMITREX-TABLETS-PI-PIL.PDF. Accessed 29 Dec 2016.
13. Silberstein SD, Marcus DA (2013) Sumatriptan : treatment across the full spectrum of migraine. Expert Opin Pharmacother 14:1659–1667
14. Rapoport A (2011) New frontiers in headache therapy. Neurol Sci 32(Suppl 1):S105–109
15. FDA Drug Safety Communication: FDA evaluating the risk of burns and scars with Zecuity (sumatriptan) migraine patch. Available at: http://www.fda.gov/Drugs/DrugSafety/ucm504588.htm. Accessed 29 Dec 2016.
16. Goldstein J, Smith TR, Pugach N et al (2012) A sumatriptan iontophoretic transdermal system for the acute treatment of migraine. Headache 52:1402–1410
17. Derry CJ, Derry S, Moore RA. Sumatriptan (intranasal route of administration) for acute migraine attacks in adults. Cochrane Database Syst Rev. 2012:Cd009663
18. IMITREX (sumatriptan succinate) nasal spray [Prescribing Information]. Available at: https://www.gsksource.com/pharma/content/dam/GlaxoSmithKline/US/en/Prescribing_Information/Imitrex_Nasal_Spray/pdf/IMITREX-NASAL-SPRAY-PI-PIL.PDF. Accessed 29 Dec 2016.
19. ZOMIG (zomlitriptan) nasal spray [Prescribing Information]. Available at: http://www.astrazeneca-us.com/cgi-bin/az_pi.cgi?product=zomig_nasal&country=us&popup=no. Accessed 29 Dec 2016.
20. Luthringer R, Djupesland PG, Sheldrake CD et al (2009) Rapid absorption of sumatriptan powder and effects on glyceryl trinitrate model of headache following intranasal delivery using a novel bi-directional device. J Pharm Pharmacol 61:1219–1228
21. ONZETRA Xsail (sumatriptan nasal powder) [Prescribing Information]. Available at: http://onzetrahcp.com/sites/default/files/onzetra_xsail_prescribing_information.pdf. Accessed 29 Dec 2016.
22. Lipton RB, Hamelsky SW, Dayno JM (2002) What do patients with migraine want from acute migraine treatment? Headache 42(Suppl 1):3–9
23. Macgregor EA, Brandes J, Eikermann A (2003) Migraine prevalence and treatment patterns: the global Migraine and Zolmitriptan Evaluation survey. Headache 43:19–26
24. Malik SN, Hopkins M, Young WB et al (2006) Acute migraine treatment: patterns of use and satisfaction in a clinical population. Headache 46:773–780
25. Martelletti P (2015) The therapeutic armamentarium in migraine is quite elderly. Expert Opin Drug Metab Toxicol 11:175–177
26. Pillion DJ, Hosmer S, Meezan E (1998) Dodecylmaltoside-mediated nasal and ocular absorption of lyspro-insulin: independence of surfactant action from multimer dissociation. Pharm Res 15:1637–1639
27. Ahsan F, Arnold J, Meezan E et al (2001) Enhanced bioavailability of calcitonin formulated with alkylglycosides following nasal and ocular administration in rats. Pharm Res 18:1742–1746
28. Pillion DJ, Ahsan F, Arnold JJ et al (2002) Synthetic long-chain alkyl maltosides and alkyl sucrose esters as enhancers of nasal insulin absorption. J Pharm Sci 91:1456–1462
29. Mustafa F, Yang T, Khan MA et al (2004) Chain length-dependent effects of alkylmaltosides on nasal absorption of enoxaparin. J Pharm Sci 93:675–683
30. Maggio ET (2006) Intravail: highly effective intranasal delivery of peptide and protein drugs. Expert Opin Drug Deliv 3:529–539
31. Eley JG, Triumalashetty P (2001) In vitro assessment of alkylglycosides as permeability enhancers. AAPS PharmSciTech 2:E19
32. Tirumalasetty PP, Eley JG (2005) Evaluation of dodecylmaltoside as a permeability enhancer for insulin using human carcinoma cells. J Pharm Sci 94:246–255
33. Munjal S, Gautam A, Offman E et al (2016) A randomized trial comparing the pharmacokinetics, safety, and tolerability of DFN-02, an intranasal sumatriptan spray containing a permeation enhancer, with intranasal and subcutaneous sumatriptan in healthy adults. Headache 56:1455–1465
34. International Headache Society (2004) The International Classification of Headache Disorders: 2nd edition. Cephalalgia 24(Suppl 1):9–160
35. Ryan R, Elkind A, Baker CC et al (1997) Sumatriptan nasal spray for the acute treatment of migraine. Results of two clinical studies. Neurology 49:1225–1230
36. Wendt J, Cady R, Singer R et al (2006) A randomized, double-blind, placebo-controlled trial of the efficacy and tolerability of a 4-mg dose of subcutaneous sumatriptan for the treatment of acute migraine attacks in adults. Clin Ther 28:517–526
37. Walling AD, Woolley DC, Molgaard C et al (2005) Patient satisfaction with migraine management by family physicians. J Am Board Fam Pract 18:563–566
38. Gawel M, Aschoff J, May A et al (2005) Treatment satisfaction with zolmitriptan nasal spray for migraine in a real life setting: results from phase two of the REALIZE study. J Headache Pain 6:405–411
39. Weidmann E, Unger J, Blair S et al (2003) An open-label study to assess changes in efficacy and satisfaction with migraine care when patients have access to multiple sumatriptan succinate formulations. Clin Ther 25:235–246

# Validation of the Social support and Pain Questionnaire (SPQ) in patients with painful temporomandibular disorders

Songlin He[1,2,3] and Jinhua Wang[1,2,3]*

## Abstract

**Background:** The present study aimed to validate of Social support and Pain Questionnaire (SPQ) for use in Chinese patients with painful temporomandibular disorders (TMD).

**Methods:** The Chinese version of SPQ was produced by translation and cross-culturally adaptation of the original English version according to international guidelines. The Chinese version of SPQ was then distributed to a total of 118 patients with painful TMD. Reliability of the SPQ was evaluating using internal consistency and test-retest methods and validity of the SPQ was determined by construct validity and convergent validity. The exploratory factor analysis (EFA) was used to assess the construct validity of SPQ. And convergent validity was assessed by correlating the SPQ scores with the score of a global oral health question.

**Results:** The Chinese version of SPQ has a high internal consistency (Cronbach's alpha value, 0.926) and good test-retest reliability ((intraclass correlation coefficient (ICC), 0.784). Construct validity was evaluated by EFA, extracting one factor, accounting for 74.8% of the variance. All factor loadings of the six items had exceeded 0.80. As regards convergent validity, the SPQ showed good correlation with the global oral health question.

**Conclusion:** These findings support that the Chinese version of SPQ can be used as a reliable and valid tool for Chinese patients with painful TMD.

**Keywords:** Validation, SPQ, Temporomandibular disorders

## Background

Temporomandibular disorders (TMD) are "a group of biopsychosocial illnesses characterized by chronic painful conditions and dysfunction in the muscles of mastication and the temporomandibular joint" [1]. It affects 14.9 to 17.9% of Chinese population [2, 3]. Pain is one of the most common clinical symptoms of TMD [4]. TMD pain involves not only the masticatory muscles and TMD, but also affects the adjacent structures such as ears, teeth, head and neck muscles [5]. Studies have shown that oral health-related quality of life (OHRQoL) is negatively affected by TMD pain [6–8].

In recent years, there is a growing interest in exploring the relationship between social support and pain behavior [9–11]. Several studies reported that social support plays an important role in overcoming pain-related disability [9, 12]. Other studies, however, have shown that social support has negative effects on mobility and physical function [13, 14]. To further explore the impact of social support on chronic pain may give us new insights into the treatment of pain-related diseases [15]. Most measures on social support are mainly concerned with social support in daily-life situations, rather than its relationship to pain [16, 17]. The West Haven-Yale Multidimensional Pain Inventory (MPI) is the widely used instrument to evaluate the chronic pain experience from the cognitive-behavioral perspective [18, 19]. It does concern support related to pain by one person. However, it fails to capture the social support from others, like friends and family [20].

* Correspondence: dentistwjh@163.com
[1]College of Stomatology, Chongqing Medical University, No. 426 Songshibei Road, Chongqing 401147, China
[2]Chongqing Key Laboratory of Oral Diseases and Biomedical Sciences, Chongqing, China
Full list of author information is available at the end of the article

Recently, the Social support and Pain Questionnaire (SPQ) was developed by the Academic Centre for Dentistry Amsterdam (ACTA) to measure satisfaction with social support related to pain [15]. It is a 6-item, one-factor structure, self-administered English instrument [15]. The SPQ is a reliable and valid tool to evaluate the patient's satisfaction with pain-related social support [15].

To make this instrument suitable for other languages and cultures, an internationally standardized evaluation procedure must be implemented. Therefore, the aim of our study is to validate a Chinese translation of the SPQ for patients with painful TMD.

## Methods
### Patients

A total of 118 consecutive patients were recruited from our university clinic between January 2015 and October 2015. The inclusion criteria were: at least 18 years of age, a diagnosis of painful TMD according to the Research Diagnostic Criteria for Temporomandibular Disorders [21], complaint of pain for at least 3 months, and sufficient ability to fill in the questionnaire. The exclusion criteria included: had a history of psychiatric illness, had acute pain for less than 3 months, a systemic disease, dental pain, and were reluctant to sign informed consents. For the sample size, it was determined according to the quality criteria for health status questionnaires [22]. The criteria suggested that a study should recruit at least 100 patients for reliability and validity analysis [22]. Before completing the SPQ, patients were instructed how to fill in the questionnaire. When necessary, they can consult interviewer at any time.

All the patients signed the written informed consent, and the present study was approved by the Ethics Committee of Chongqing Medical University.

### The SPQ

The original SPQ is composed of 6 items: *the support that I get from the people around me, the advice that I get from the people around me, how much opportunity I have to discuss the pain with the people around me, how much care I receive, how much understanding the people around me show and the practical help people around me give.* The response is scored using a Likert scale from 0 to 4 (0 = very dissatisfied, 1 = dissatisfied, 2 = neutral, 3 = satisfied, 4 = very satisfied). In general, higher scores indicate more satisfaction with social support related to pain. Additionally, to assess the convergent validity, an extra global question ("*In general, how would you rate your social support related to pain* ") was added at the end of instrument. The question is scored with the following options: (1 = very good, 2 = good, 3 = fair, 4 = poor, 5 = very poor).

### Translation and cross-cultural adaptation

The process of translation and cross-cultural adaptation of the original SPQ was carried out according to Guillemin's guidelines [23].

1. Translation into Chinese: the original SPQ was firstly translated into Chinese by two bilingual translators independently. One translator was a linguist and the other one was a clinical psychology expert.
2. Back translation into English: the two other bilingual translators who had no knowledge of the original SPQ translated the Chinese version into English. They were native English speakers and fluent in Chinese.
3. Expert committee compared the two versions: the two versions were compared and assessed by an expert committee (two public health experts and two dental experts) to assure that there were no differences in the meaning of the items. The initial Chinese version of SPQ was then obtained.
4. Pilot test: a pilot test of the initial Chinese version of SPQ with 20 painful TMD patients was carried out to ensure that the formulation of items was clear. The expert committee reevaluated all of findings and then approved the final Chinese version of SPQ.

### Statistical analysis
#### Reliability

A Cronbach's alpha between 0.70 and 0.95 and an Intraclass Correlation Coefficients (ICC) value over 0.70 were used to determine the internal consistency and test-retest reliability, respectively [22]. The ICC vales were analyzed by asking 30 patients to complete the Chinese SPQ again after a period of 2-week.

#### Validity

Validation of the Chinese SPQ included the assessment of the construct validity and convergent validity.

Construct validity was examined using exploratory factor analysis (EFA). The Kaiser–Meyer–Olkin test and Bartlett's sphericity test were firstly carried out to determine if the data was suitable for performing the EFA [24]. The EFA followed by varimax rotation method was carried out to evaluate the dimensionality of the Chinese SPQ. Significance was defined as a loading higher than 0.40.

Convergent validity was assessed by correlating the SPQ scores with the score of the global oral health question. The correlation values were categorized as follows: poor correlation (0–0.20), fair correlation (0.21–0.40), moderate correlation (0.41–0.60), good correlation (0.61–0.80), and excellent correlation (0.81–1.0) [25].

All the statistical analysis were performed using version 20.0 of the SPSS software (IBM Corp. 2011; NY; USA). In the present study, the $p$ value of <0.05 was considered statistically significant.

## Results

### Patient characteristics

A total of 118 patients with painful TMD were recruited from a university-affiliated dental clinic. All the patients declared that the questions were easy to understand and completed the questionnaire fully. Patient characteristics are shown in Table 1. Of the 118 patients selected, 56.8% were female, with the mean age of 46.4 ± 14.7 years old. The majority of patients were employed (72.9%), and half of them had been educated in middle school (54.2%). The pain were classified into joint pain (32.2%), muscle pain (36.4%) and mixed pain (31.4%). The mean scores, corrected item-total correlations and Cronbach's alpha if item deleted results for the SPQ are presented in Table 3.

### Reliability

As displayed in Table 2, Cronbach's alpha for the SPQ was 0.926. The test-retest reliability of the instrument was also acceptable, with the ICC value of 0.87 (Table 2).

### Validity

The result of the KMO test was 0.788 and Bartlett's test of sphericity was 716.2 (df = 15, $P < 0.001$). These results suggested that EFA of the sample was appropriate. Table 3 shows the results of the EFA for the SPQ. The factor loadings of all items had exceeded the recommended 0.40. A one-factor model, accounted for 74.8% of the explanatory variance, was retained.

In term of convergent validity, it was assessed by correlating the SPQ scores with the score of the global oral health question. The result showed that the correlation was good (Table 2).

**Table 1** Characteristics of patients (n = 118)

| | | Value |
|---|---|---|
| Age (years) | Mean (SD) | 46.4 ± 14.7 |
| Gender (n) | Male | 51 (43.2%) |
| | Female | 67 (56.8%) |
| Employment (n) | Employed | 86 (72.9%) |
| | Unemployed | 32 (27.1%) |
| Education history (n) | Primary School | 25 (21.2%) |
| | Middle school | 64 (54.2%) |
| | Bachelor degree or above | 29 (24.6%) |
| Classification of pain (n) | joint pain | 38 (32.2%) |
| | muscle pain | 43 (36.4%) |
| | mixed pain | 37 (31.4%) |

**Table 2** Internal consistency, test–retest reliability and convergent validity of the SPQ

| Scale | Internal consistency (n = 118) | Test–retest (ICC, 95% CI) (n = 30) | $r_s$* (95% CI) (n = 118) |
|---|---|---|---|
| Total score | 0.926 | 0.784 (0.648–0.893) | 0.624 (0.554–0.719)** |

ICC Intraclass correlation coefficient
*Spearman's rank correlation coefficient
**$P < 0.001$

## Discussion

In the present study, the translation and validation of the Chinese version of SPQ is carried out. Statistical analysis showed that the 6-item Chinese version of SPQ with one-factor structure was reliable and valid. It can be used in Chinese population to evaluate the patient's satisfaction with pain-related social support.

In the current study, chronic TMD pain lasting for at least 3 months was used as a temporal criterion to recruit patients suffering from painful TMD. This was consistent with other previous studies [15, 26]. In order to get a semantically and conceptually similar version to the original SPQ, the process of translation and cross-cultural adaptation of the original SPQ was carried out. The Chinese version of SPQ was overall well received by the patients, and no problem or language difficulty existed.

In terms of reliability, both the internal consistency and test-retest reliability were proved to be good. The Cronbach's alpha for the SPQ was 0.926, indicating a high level of internal consistency. This value indicates high correlations among items of SPQ. And when each item was deleted, the values of Cronbach's alpha remained stable. The value of ICC (0.784, 90% CI: 0.648–0.893) was

**Table 3** Range, mean scores, corrected item-total correlations and factor analysis results for the SPQ

| Item | Mean (SD) | Corrected item-total correlation | Cronbach's alpha if item deleted | Factor loading |
|---|---|---|---|---|
| 1. the support that I get from the people around me | 2.25 (1.16) | 0.870 | 0.902 | 0.922 |
| 2. the advice that I get from the people around me | 2.15 (0.90) | 0.839 | 0.906 | 0.880 |
| 3. how much opportunity I have to discuss the pain with the people around me | 2.31 (1.17) | 0.729 | 0.925 | 0.880 |
| 4. how much care I receive | 1.99 (0.83) | 0.749 | 0.918 | 0.875 |
| 5. how much understanding the people around me show | 2.21 (0.84) | 0.809 | 0.911 | 0.820 |
| 6. the practical help people around me give | 2.09 (0.85) | 0.803 | 0.912 | 0.805 |

higher than the values in the original study, indicating good test-retest reliability [15]. For the selection of the time interval, previous study suggested that a period of 2 days to 2 weeks was thought to be suitable [27]. A period of 2 weeks was chosen in the present study. And in the original study, a maximal time interval of 8 weeks was adopted. The lower ICC value may be explained by the longer time interval in the original study [15].

Regarding factorial structure of the SPQ, the finding of EFA identified a one-factor structure of the SPQ. This result was consistent with previous study proposed by Van Der Lugt et al. [15]. Similar as the original study, the factor loadings of all items were above 0.80 [15]. As regards convergent validity, the Chinese version of SPQ had good correlation with the global oral health question. The finding was close to the values in the original study [15]. Overall, the Chinese version of SPQ had adequate validity for using in patients with painful TMD.

However, the present study has two limitations which requiring further assessment. Firstly, all patients were enrolled from a single university-affiliated hospital, and thus may not be able to represent all Chinese population affected by painful TMD. Secondly, the current study does not contain long-term follow-up analyses, and therefore the sensitivity and responsiveness of the Chinese version of SPQ could not be evaluated.

## Conclusion

The present study supports that the Chinese version of Social support and Pain Questionnaire (SPQ) can be used as a reliable and valid tool for Chinese patients with painful TMD.

### Abbreviations

EFA: Exploratory factor analysis; ICC: Intraclass correlation coefficient; KMO: Kaiser–Meyer–Olkin test; RDC/TMD: Research diagnostic criteria for temporomandibular disorders; SPQ: The Social support and Pain Questionnaire; TMD: Temporomandibular disorders

### Acknowledgments

The authors wish to thank all the patients for participating in the current study.

### Funding

This research is funded by the Chongqing Municipal Commission of Health and Family Planning Grants(No. 20142052), the Program for Innovation Team Building at Institutions of Higher Education in Chongqing in 2016 and the Chongqing Municipal Key Laboratory of Oral Biomedical Engineering of Higher Education.

### Authors' contributions

SL and JH designed the study and prepared the draft manuscript. SL collected and analyzed the data. All authors read and approved the final manuscript.

### Competing interests

The authors declare that they have no competing interests.

### Author details

[1]College of Stomatology, Chongqing Medical University, No. 426 Songshibei Road, Chongqing 401147, China. [2]Chongqing Key Laboratory of Oral Diseases and Biomedical Sciences, Chongqing, China. [3]Chongqing Municipal Key Laboratory of Oral Biomedical Engineering of Higher Education, Chongqing, China.

### References

1. Ozdemir-Karatas M, Peker K, Balik A, Uysal O, Tuncer EB (2013) Identifying potential predictors of pain-related disability in Turkish patients with chronic temporomandibular disorder pain. J Headache Pain 14:17.
2. Wu N, Hirsch C (2010) Temporomandibular disorders in German and Chinese adolescents. J Orofac Orthop 71(3):187–198.
3. Deng YM, Fu MK, Hagg U (1995) Prevalence of temporomandibular joint dysfunction (TMJD) in Chinese children and adolescents. A cross-sectional epidemiological study. Eur J Orthod 17(4):305–309.
4. Gil-Martinez A, Grande-Alonso M, Lopez-de-Uralde-Villanueva I, Lopez-Lopez A, Fernandez-Carnero J, La Touche R (2016) Chronic Temporomandibular disorders: disability, pain intensity and fear of movement. J Headache Pain 17(1):103.
5. Suvinen TI, Reade PC, Kemppainen P, Kononen M, Dworkin SF (2005) Review of aetiological concepts of temporomandibular pain disorders: towards a biopsychosocial model for integration of physical disorder factors with psychological and psychosocial illness impact factors. Eur J Pain 9(6):613–633.
6. Almoznino G, Zini A, Zakuto A, Sharav Y, Haviv Y, Hadad A, Chweidan H, Yarom N, Benoliel R (2015) Oral health-related quality of life in patients with Temporomandibular disorders. J Oral Facial Pain Headache 29(3):231–241.
7. Tjakkes GH, Reinders JJ, Tenvergert EM, Stegenga B (2010) TMD pain: the effect on health related quality of life and the influence of pain duration. Health Qual Life Outcomes 8:46.
8. He S, Wang J, Ji P (2016) Validation of the Tampa scale for Kinesiophobia for Temporomandibular disorders (TSK-TMD) in patients with painful TMD. J Headache Pain 17(1):109.
9. Evers AW, Kraaimaat FW, Geenen R, Jacobs JW, Bijlsma JW (2003) Pain coping and social support as predictors of long-term functional disability and pain in early rheumatoid arthritis. Behav Res Ther 41(11):1295–1310.
10. Ledoux E, Dubois JD, Descarreaux M (2012) Physical and psychosocial predictors of functional trunk capacity in older adults with and without low back pain. J Manip Physiol Ther 35(5):338–345.
11. Romano JM, Jensen MP, Schmaling KB, Hops H, Buchwald DS (2009) Illness behaviors in patients with unexplained chronic fatigue are associated with significant other responses. J Behav Med 32(6):558–569.
12. Kornblith AB, Herndon JE 2nd, Zuckerman E, Viscoli CM, Horwitz RI, Cooper MR, Harris L, Tkaczuk KH, Perry MC, Budman D, Norton LC, Holland J, Cancer, & Leukemia Group, B (2001) Social support as a buffer to the psychological impact of stressful life events in women with breast cancer. Cancer 91(2):443–454.
13. Kristensen MT (2013) Hip fracture-related pain strongly influences functional performance of patients with an intertrochanteric fracture upon discharge from the hospital. PM R 5(2):135–141.
14. Romano JM, Turner JA, Jensen MP, Friedman LS, Bulcroft RA, Hops H, Wright SF (1995) Chronic pain patient-spouse behavioral interactions predict patient disability. Pain 63(3):353–360.
15. Van Der Lugt CM, Rollman A, Naeije M, Lobbezoo F, Visscher CM (2012) Social support in chronic pain: development and preliminary psychometric assessment of a new instrument. J Oral Rehabil 39(4):270–276.
16. van den Akker-Scheek I, Stevens M, Spriensma A, van Horn JR (2004) Groningen Orthopaedic social support scale: validity and reliability. J Adv Nurs 47(1):57–63.
17. Suurmeijer TP, Doeglas DM, Briancon S, Krijnen WP, Krol B, Sanderman R, Moum T, Bjelle A, Van Den Heuvel WJ (1995) The measurement of social support in the 'European research on incapacitating diseases and social Support': the development of the social support questionnaire for transactions (SSQT). Soc Sci Med 40(9):1221–1229.
18. Kerns RD, Turk DC, Rudy TE (1985) The West Haven-Yale Multidimensional pain inventory (WHYMPI). Pain 23(4):345–356.
19. Eklund A, Bergstrom G, Bodin L, Axen I (2016) Do psychological and behavioral factors classified by the West Haven-Yale Multidimensional pain inventory (Swedish version) predict the early clinical course of low back pain in patients receiving chiropractic care? BMC Musculoskelet Disord 17:75.

20. Turner RJ, Marino F (1994) Social support and social structure: a descriptive epidemiology. J Health Soc Behav 35(3):193–212.

21. Schiffman E, Ohrbach R, Truelove E, Look J, Anderson G, Goulet JP, List T, Svensson P, Gonzalez Y, Lobbezoo F, Michelotti A, Brooks SL, Ceusters W, Drangsholt M, Ettlin D, Gaul C, Goldberg LJ, Haythornthwaite JA, Hollender L, Jensen R, John MT, De Laat A, de Leeuw R, Maixner W, van der Meulen M, Murray GM, Nixdorf DR, Palla S, Petersson A, Pionchon P, Smith B, Visscher CM, Zakrzewska J, Dworkin SF, International Rdc/Tmd Consortium Network, I. a. f. D. R., & Orofacial Pain Special Interest Group, I. A. f. t. S. o. P (2014) Diagnostic criteria for Temporomandibular disorders (DC/TMD) for clinical and research applications: recommendations of the international RDC/TMD consortium network* and Orofacial pain special interest Groupdagger. J Oral Facial Pain Headache 28(1):6–27.

22. Terwee CB, Bot SD, de Boer MR, van der Windt DA, Knol DL, Dekker J, Bouter LM, de Vet HC (2007) Quality criteria were proposed for measurement properties of health status questionnaires. J Clin Epidemiol 60(1):34–42.

23. Guillemin F, Bombardier C, Beaton D (1993) Cross-cultural adaptation of health-related quality of life measures: literature review and proposed guidelines. J Clin Epidemiol 46(12):1417–1432.

24. Bartlett MS (1950) Tests of significance in factor analysis. Br J Stat Psychol 3(2):77–85.

25. Peter MF, David M (2000) Quality of life assessment, analysis and interpretation. John Wiley and Sons, Inc, Chichester.

26. Matos M, Bernardes SF (2013) The Portuguese formal social support for autonomy and dependence in PAIN inventory (FSSADI_PAIN): a preliminary validation study. Br J Health Psychol 18(3):593–609.

27. Marx RG, Menezes A, Horovitz L, Jones EC, Warren RF (2003) A comparison of two time intervals for test-retest reliability of health status instruments. J Clin Epidemiol 56(8):730–735.

# Onabotulinumtoxin A for the management of chronic migraine in current clinical practice: results of a survey of sixty-three Italian headache centers

Cristina Tassorelli[1,2*], Marco Aguggia[3], Marina De Tommaso[4], Pierangelo Geppetti[5], Licia Grazzi[6], Luigi Alberto Pini[7], Paola Sarchielli[8], Gioacchino Tedeschi[9], Paolo Martelletti[10†] and Pietro Cortelli[11,12†]

## Abstract

**Background:** Chronic migraine is a complex clinical condition often undertreated. Onabotulinumtoxin A (OBT-A) was approved in Italy in 2013 for symptom relief in patients with chronic migraine who have failed, or do not tolerate, oral prophylactic treatments. However, the impact of OBT-A in clinical practice remains to be defined.

**Methods:** To investigate the current management of chronic migraine with OBT-A in clinical practice, a web-based survey was conducted among clinicians working in third-level headache centers across Italy. A 26-item questionnaire was designed and developed by a group of 10 Italian headache specialists to address the following issues: treatment paradigm and OBT-A injection intervals, frequency of treatment and retreatment, definition of responders/non-responders, satisfaction with treatment potential impact of early treatment with OBT-A. Ninety-six headache centers were selected and contacted via e-mail. The online survey was anonymous and carried out using a secure website.

**Results:** Overall, 64 of the 96 centers (66.7%) completed the questionnaire. Most centers (98.4%) had been using OBT-A for >1 year. OBT-A was administered according to the PREEMPT paradigm in most centers (88.9%). While during the first year of prophylaxis with OBT-A most clinicians (93.6%) repeated OBT-A treatment every 3 months, as recommended, in the following years interval duration was variable. Response to OBT-A was defined as a ≥ 50% reduction in the headache days by 58.7% of the clinicians, and as a ≥ 30% reduction by 25.4% of them. Almost 60% of the clinicians considered OBT-A as a long-lasting therapy, while for one-third of them treatment could be discontinued in patients showing a benefit for ≥6 months. According to 80% of the clinicians, early administration of OBT-A after the onset of chronic migraine was associated with better outcomes, and 47.6% felt that OBT-A should be recommended as a first-line option.

**Conclusions:** This survey indicates that in third-level headache centers in Italy OBT-A is used in good compliance with current recommendations. There is agreement about the definition of response as a reduction in headache days by 30% to 50%. Additional effort is required to define response to OBT-A and to establish optimal treatment duration.

**Keywords:** Botox, Chronic migraine, Headache, Migraine prophylaxis, Onabotulinumtoxin A

* Correspondence: cristina.tassorelli@unipv.it
†Equal contributors
[1]Headache Science Center, National Neurological Institute C. Mondino, Pavia, Italy
[2]Department of Brain and Behavioral Sciences, University of Pavia, Via Mondino 2, 27100 Pavia, Italy
Full list of author information is available at the end of the article

## Background

Migraine is a neurologic disorder characterized by attacks of severe pulsating unilateral headache [1]. Episodic migraine can progress to chronic migraine (CM), which is defined as headache on ≥15 days/month for ≥3 months of which ≥8 days meet criteria for migraine or respond to migraine-specific treatments [1]. CM is estimated to affect 0.9% to 2.2% of the general population and its burden on affected individuals is considerable [2–5]. The management of patients with CM poses a major challenge to headache specialists because of the complex comorbidities frequently associated with this condition, including drug overuse, anxiety, and depressive disorders [6, 7]. Furthermore, patients with CM are often poor responders to prophylactic treatments [2, 8–10].

Few evidence-based treatment options are available for CM [11–13]. In recent years, the efficacy of Onabotulinumtoxin A (OBT-A) for the prophylaxis of CM has been demonstrated in two well-designed phase III clinical trials, the Phase III Research Evaluating Migraine Prophylaxis Therapy-1 (PREEMPT) 1 and 2 trials [14, 15]. A pooled analysis of these trials showed that OBT-A was significantly more effective than placebo in reducing the mean frequency of days with headache and headache episodes [16]. The PREEMPT clinical program also established the standardized paradigm for OBT-A administration for CM prophylaxis that is currently recommended for the first 56 weeks of treatment [14, 15]. This paradigm involves the intramuscular injection of a dose of 155 U of OBT-A, administered to 31 injection sites across 7 head and neck muscles (5 U in 0.1 mL for each injection). The addition of up to 40 U OBT-A, administered to 8 additional injection sites across 3 head and neck muscles, is allowed using a follow-the-pain approach. Based on the evidence from the PREEMPT program, OBT-A was granted authorization for the prophylaxis of CM by the US Food and Drug Administration (FDA) and the European Medicines Agency (EMA) in 2010. The use of OBT-A for the prophylaxis of CM has also been endorsed by several international societies, usually as second-line treatment [17–21].

The performance of a drug, as well as the possible issues associated with its use, may vary considerably from randomized clinical trials (RCTs) to the real-world setting [22–24]. In the strictly controlled environment of RCTs, the characteristics and comorbidities of the study population, the setting, and the conditions under which a given drug is administered may differ from those typically encountered in clinical practice. Due to the relatively recent approval of OBT-A for CM, real-world data, essential for establishing the effectiveness of a novel treatment, are just beginning to emerge [25–28]. The evidence so far available supports the results from the PREEMPT clinical program [25, 29]. In Italy, OBT-A was approved in 2013 for symptom relief in patients with CM who have failed, or do not tolerate, oral prophylactic treatments [30]. Since then, several Italian headache centers have adopted OBT-A for the routine management of CM and some of them have confirmed the efficacy of this new approach as assessed by conventional outcome measures, including headache frequency, pain intensity, use of medications for symptom relief, headache-related disability, and health-related quality of life (HR-QoL) [26, 31–35]. However, data are lacking concerning the practical challenges that clinicians may have to face when using OBT-A in real life, or concerning the effectiveness of this treatment based on their judgment as well as on patient reports.

In this context, we set out to conduct a web-based survey to describe the current management of CM with OBT-A in the everyday practice of headache centers in Italy. Surveys have long been recognized as a useful tool in clinical research [36, 37]. Electronic surveys have several advantages over conventional ones (e.g., postal and telephone surveys), including the practical convenience associated with the direct storage of responses in a database, the possibility of easily contacting large samples of participants, and the rapidity of data collection [36, 37]. The specific objectives of our survey were to investigate the opinion of clinicians about the efficacy of the treatment of migraine with OBT-A, to identify unmet needs from the clinician and/or patient perspective, and to collect other practice-related suggestions to be used for further optimizing the prophylaxis of CM with OBT-A. This article presents the results of our survey.

## Methods

This was an independent survey investigating the current management of migraine treatment with OBT-A. The survey was designed and developed over the course of 2016, during two meetings organized and attended by a group of 10 Italian experts in the treatment of CM, under the auspices of the board of the *Associazione Italiana per la Ricerca sulle Cefalee* (ANIRCEF) and the *Società Italiana per lo Studio delle Cefalee* (SISC). The first meeting was virtual and took place via a web-conference, the second was a face-to-face meeting. The main objectives of the meetings were to develop a questionnaire addressing practical and controversial issues of CM treatment with OBT-A to be used for a survey, to decide, based on consensus, the methodology of the survey, and to identify the characteristics of headache centers to be invited to participate in the survey.

The questionnaire was developed based on the experience of the 10 headache experts in the management of CM in clinical practice, and on the review and discussion of the available scientific evidence concerning OBT-A for CM. During the first meeting, the following issues were discussed and identified as relevant for the current management of CM: treatment paradigm and OBT-A injection intervals, frequency of treatment and retreatment, definition of responders/non-responders, satisfaction with treatment, potential impact of early treatment with OBT-A, and availability of resources. Such issues were addressed in the questionnaire, which consisted of 26 questions (available in Additional file 1). A set of questions concerned the characteristics of the responding centers (number of patients treated, qualifications, number of years of experience). For most items, we adopted close-ended, single-choice questions. Two questions (8 and 9) allowed multiple answers and the participants were asked to rank their answers according to importance. Two other questions (23 and 24) were about the degree of satisfaction with OBT-A treatment assessed on a scale from 0 (no satisfaction) to 10 (highest satisfaction). Contents and questions of the survey were developed following published recommendations for the design and set-up of web-based surveys [38–40].

The experts agreed on the use of a web-based methodology that invited participants via an e-mail message containing a personalized link for accessing the online questionnaire. The centers to be invited to participate in the survey were identified from the registries of the two Italian scientific headache societies (ANIRCEF and SISC) [41, 42]. The following requirements had to be satisfied by the centers in order to be eligible for the survey: i) qualification as third-level headache centers (i.e., hospital-based centers in which advanced multidisciplinary care is delivered by headache specialists) [43]; ii) certification of training in the use of OBT-A in CM according to the PREEMPT paradigm obtained after attendance of the specialized courses of Continuing Medical Education delivered in Italy; iii) at least one year of experience in the use of OBT-A for the treatment of CM; and iv) routine use of a headache diary to monitor patients' symptoms [20, 44]. Care was taken to ensure that the participating centers were located over the entire national territory so as to be representative of clinical practice across the various regions of Italy. Overall, 96 centers using OBT-A for CM and fulfilling the inclusion requirements were identified.

In April 2016, a cover letter was sent by e-mail to the chairs of the selected centers explaining the rationale and objective of the survey, and providing a personalized link to access the questionnaire and instructions on how to complete it. The questionnaire was accessible online for a period of 3 weeks. After this period, a reminder was sent by e-mail to those clinicians who had not yet responded to the survey, allowing them an additional week to complete the questionnaire. The online survey was carried out using a secure survey website (www.surveymonkey.com). In order to avoid duplication of data, we adopted the Verisign

certificate version 3 and 128-bit encryption, which strictly associated a single link to a single questionnaire. The questionnaires were rigorously anonymous and did not foresee the collection of sensitive data, including identifiers of the respondents, demographic data, identifiable patient information, and geographic location. In addition, to further ensure privacy protection, questionnaires were dissociated from the original link before being processed for data analysis.

With regard to ethical issues, given the independent nature of the survey, the measures taken to ensure anonymity, and the absence of sensitive patients data in the questionnaire, and in accordance with Italian regulations, no formal approval of the survey was required from the Institutional Review Boards of the participating centers.

The results of the survey were analyzed by descriptive statistics, summarized in tables and figures as percentages. During a face-to-face meeting held in Rome in July 2016, the expert panel discussed the results of the survey.

## Results

### Response rate and characteristics of the participating centers

Of the 96 selected centers, 46 (47.9%) responded to the survey after 3 weeks. Sending a reminder improved the response rate to 66.7%, with a total of 64 out of 96 centers completing the questionnaire. All the questionnaires received were completely filled, but one center reported less than 1 year of experience with OBT-A. Answers from this center were therefore excluded from further analysis.

Most centers (61.9%) were treating moderate numbers of patients (5-20 per month) (Table 1). All centres included in the analysis had been using OBT-A for the prophylaxis of CM for more than 1 year, and 38.1% for more than 3 years. More than 80% of the centers had a dedicated facility for the administration of OBT-A to patients with CM and the majority of them (71.4%) used an electronic data recording system in their everyday practice.

### Treatment characteristics

Most centers (88.9%) administered OBT-A exclusively according to the PREEMPT paradigm (Fig. 1a). The PREEMPT paradigm was followed frequently by 7.9% of the centers, while only 3.2% used it rarely. The follow-the-pain approach was used very frequently, with only a minority of centers never resorting to it (Fig. 1b). The interval of 3 months between treatment cycles was adopted by the large majority of the centers (93.6%) during the first year (Fig. 2a). The proportion of centers that adopted the 3-month interval decreased to 54.0% during

**Table 1** Characteristics of the centers that participated in the survey

| Answer options | n (%) |
|---|---|
| Number of patients treated on a monthly basis with Onabotulinumtoxin A (OBT-A) | |
| < 5 patients | 15 (23.8) |
| 5–10 patients | 21 (33.3) |
| 10–20 patients | 18 (28.6) |
| 20–40 patients | 5 (7.9) |
| > 40 patients | 4 (6.4) |
| Years of experience with OBT-A for chronic migraine | |
| > 1 year and ≤3 years | 39 (61.9) |
| > 3 years | 24 (38.1) |
| Longest follow-up of patients treated with OBT-A for chronic migraine | |
| 1 year | 13 (20.6) |
| 2 years | 24 (38.1) |
| 3 years | 18 (28.6) |
| ≥ 4 years | 8 (12.7) |
| Availability of electronic data recording system | |
| Yes | 45 (71.4) |
| No | 18 (28.6) |
| Availability of a facility dedicated to the treatment of chronic migraine with OBT-A | |
| Yes | 51 (81.9) |
| No | 12 (19.1) |

the second year of treatment (Fig. 2b). During the third year, the centers mostly relied on the information contained in the patient clinical diary to make decisions concerning the timing of retreatment (58.7%) and, with the exception of 11.1% of them, they no longer adhered strictly to the 3-month interval between cycles (Fig. 2c).

### Indicators of treatment efficacy

According to the participants in the survey, the most relevant indicator of efficacy of the prophylaxis with OBT-A was the reduction in the number of days with headache, followed by the reduction in the number of days with migraine and by patient satisfaction/improvement in QoL (Fig. 3a). The clinicians completing the questionnaire had the perception, based on the feedback and comments received from their patients, that patients evaluated treatment efficacy slightly differently, with satisfaction/improvement in QoL being the most important outcome, followed by the reduction in headache days and the decrease in headache pain intensity (Fig. 3b).

### Definition of response to OBT-A

Data concerning the definition of response to OBT-A and related issues are summarized in Table 2. For nearly 60% of the participants in the survey, response to OBT-A corresponded to a ≥ 50% reduction in the number of days with headache. Notably, 1 out of 4 clinicians also considered patients who experienced a reduction in the number of headache days ≥30% as responders. Furthermore, a small proportion of clinicians also felt that a reduction <30% in headache days could be clinically relevant if associated with at least another subjective or objective indicator of improvement. According to 55.6% of the clinicians, patients should be classified as non-responders after the failure of at least 3 cycles of treatment, while about 40% of the clinicians felt that the failure of 4 or more treatment sessions is needed before classifying a patient as a non-responder. More than half of the participants (58.7%) considered the treatment with OBT-A as a therapy that should be maintained in the long-term in responders, while about one-third thought

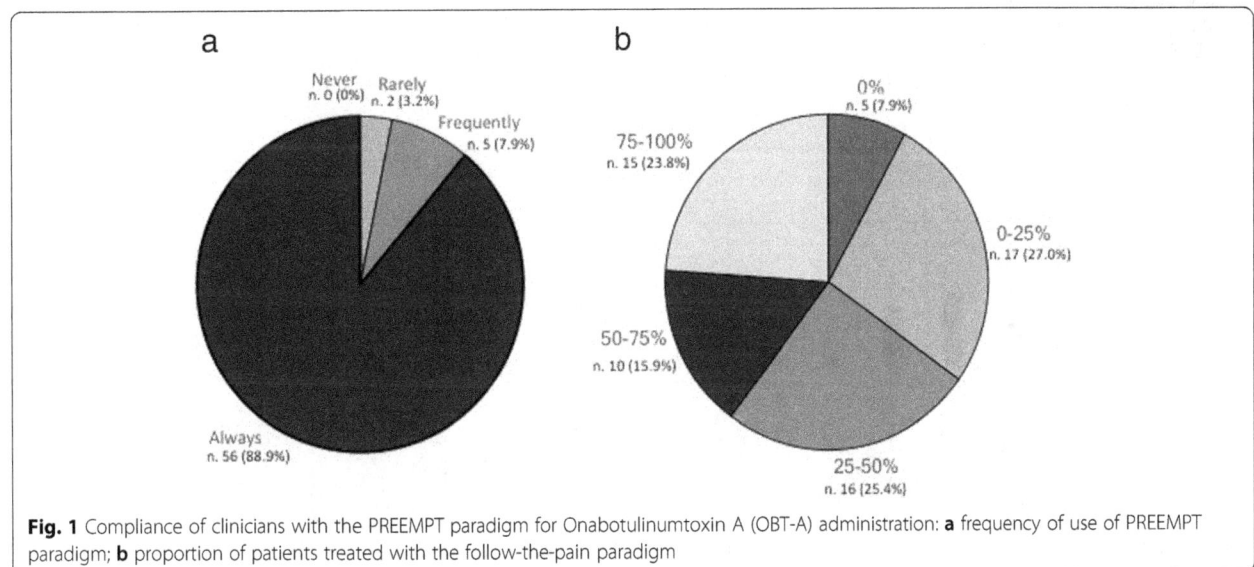

**Fig. 1** Compliance of clinicians with the PREEMPT paradigm for Onabotulinumtoxin A (OBT-A) administration: **a** frequency of use of PREEMPT paradigm; **b** proportion of patients treated with the follow-the-pain paradigm

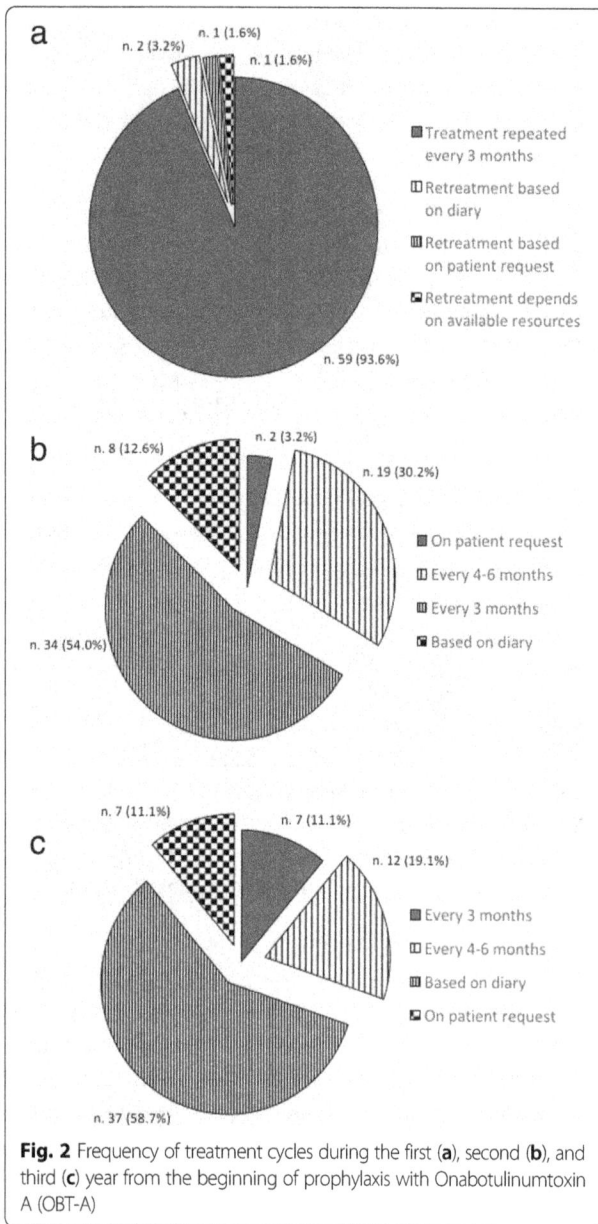

**Fig. 2** Frequency of treatment cycles during the first (**a**), second (**b**), and third (**c**) year from the beginning of prophylaxis with Onabotulinumtoxin A (OBT-A)

that the treatment could be discontinued in those patients showing a benefit persisting for at least 6 months (Table 2).

## OBT-A and other prophylactic treatments

OBT-A treatment was offered by 60.3% of the clinicians after the failure of more than 3 oral prophylactic agents (Table 3). However, in most centers (71.4%), OBT-A was frequently associated with one or more additional prophylactic treatments (Table 3). Most clinicians (69.8%) considered OBT-A to be more favorable than the available oral prophylactic therapies because of a better safety profile. In addition, 80% frequently had the perception that the efficacy of OBT-A was greater when the treatment was administered earlier after the onset of CM (Table 3). Thus, almost half of the participants (47.6%) felt that OBT-A should be recommended as a first-line option for the treatment of CM.

## Satisfaction with OBT-A treatment

Satisfaction with treatment was high among clinicians, as suggested by the great proportion of participants (77.8%) with a satisfaction score ≥ 7 on a scale from 0 (totally unsatisfied) to 10 (maximum satisfaction) (Fig. 4a). Satisfaction with OBT-A treatment appeared to be high also among patients, according to the clinicians' perception (Fig. 4b). Indeed, 76.2% of the clinicians estimated that their patients would rate treatment satisfaction with a score ≥ 7.

## Impact of resources on treatment

Overall, the centers participating in the survey reported sufficient resources to meet current and future demand (Table 4). In those centers with insufficient resources, the impact on patients was variable and ranging from longer waiting times for the first visit or follow-up visits to difficulties in respecting the exact schedule of drug administration leading, in a few cases, to the referral of patients to other centers for treatment.

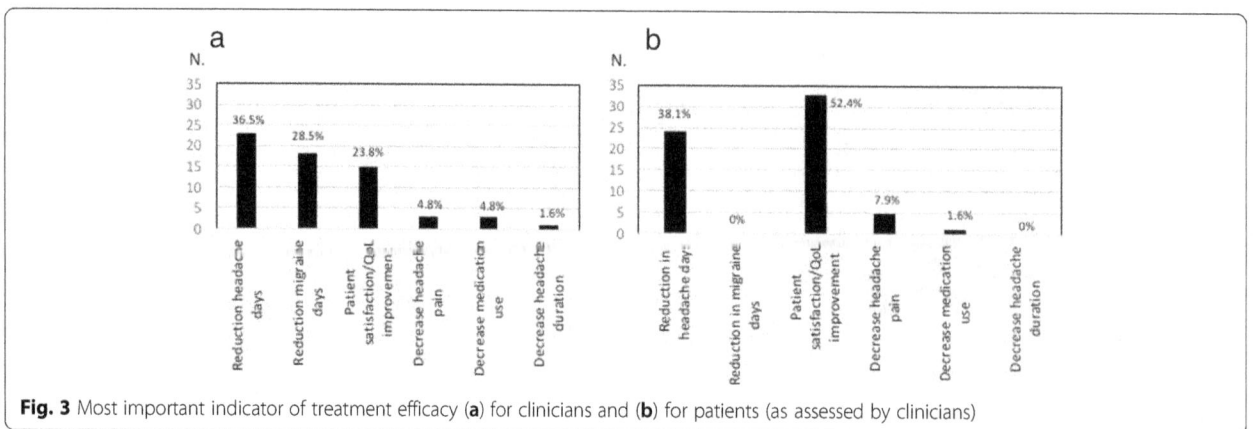

**Fig. 3** Most important indicator of treatment efficacy (**a**) for clinicians and (**b**) for patients (as assessed by clinicians)

**Table 2** Definition of response to treatment with Onabotulinumtoxin A (OBT-A) and treatment duration in chronic migraine

| Answer options | n (%) |
|---|---|
| Reduction in the number of headache days required to define response to OBT-A | |
| ≥ 30% | 16 (25.4) |
| ≥ 50% | 37 (58.7) |
| < 30% provided that at least one of the following improves: | 10 (15.9) |
| • patient satisfaction with treatment and QoL | |
| • intensity of headache pain | |
| • use of medications for symptom relief | |
| • duration of headache attacks | |
| Number of treatment cycles administered before considering a patient as a non-responder and discontinuing OBT-A | |
| 2 | 1 (1.6) |
| 3 | 35 (55.6) |
| 4 | 14 (22.2) |
| > 4 | 13 (20.6) |
| Criteria adopted for discontinuing OBT-A in responders | |
| None, as treatment should be maintained in the long-term | 37 (58.7) |
| Benefits for ≥6 months | 21 (33.3) |
| After 5 treatment cycles | 3 (4.8) |
| Achievement of <15 days/month with headache | 2 (3.2) |

*QoL* quality of life

**Table 3** Onabotulinumtoxin A (OBT-A) in the context of other prophylactic therapies for chronic migraine and timing of OBT-A initiation

| Answer options | n (%) |
|---|---|
| Frequency of combination of OBT-A with other prophylactic therapies | |
| Never | 3 (4.8) |
| Rarely | 14 (22.2) |
| Frequently | 45 (71.4) |
| Always | 1 (1.6) |
| Number of prophylactic therapies used before initiating OBT-A | |
| 0 | 1 (1.6) |
| 1 | 2 (3.2) |
| 2-3 | 22 (34.9) |
| > 3 | 38 (60.3) |
| Rating of tolerability profile of OBT-A vs. oral prophylactic therapies | |
| More favorable | 57 (90.5) |
| Comparable | 5 (7.9) |
| Less favorable | 1 (1.6) |
| Rating of efficacy/safety ratio of OBT-A vs. oral prophylactic therapies | |
| More favorable | 44 (69.8) |
| Comparable | 18 (28.6) |
| Less favorable | 1 (1.6) |
| Impression of greater efficacy of OBT-A when initiated early in the course of chronic migraine | |
| Never | 0 |
| Rarely | 9 (14.3) |
| Frequently | 51 (80.9) |
| Always | 3 (4.8) |
| Recommendation of OBT-A as first-line treatment based on the pharmacological profile | |
| Yes | 30 (47.6) |
| No | 33 (52.4) |

## Discussion

CM is a highly disabling condition that affects as much as 2% of the general population [3, 5], responds poorly to prophylactic therapies [8–10], and is associated with significant costs for affected individuals and society [2, 4, 45]. A better knowledge of the use of OBT-A for migraine prophylaxis in real-life practice is of paramount importance to further optimize the effectiveness of this treatment. This survey investigated the experience acquired by third-level headache centers in Italy in the use of OBT-A since its approval.

To our knowledge, this is the first survey in the field of CM to be conducted among expert clinicians. The survey reveals the very good compliance of Italian headache centers with current recommendations on the use of OBT-A for the prophylaxis of CM, as shown by the fact that 89% of the centers participating in the survey always used the recommended PREEMPT paradigm for OBT-A administration, and 94% repeated the treatment at 3-month intervals during the first year of prophylaxis. Our findings also show that clinicians were generally satisfied with OBT-A treatment and that, in their opinion, patients as well were satisfied with it.

The survey suggests a difference between clinicians and patients in the relevance given to the various measures of efficacy. For clinicians, the most important indicator of efficacy was represented by the reduction in the number of days with headache, in agreement with the efficacy measures used in the clinical trials and in real-life studies evaluating OBT-A in CM [14, 15, 28, 31, 34, 35]. In the case of patients, the impression of clinicians was that they valued OBT-A efficacy mostly in terms of changes in QoL, a secondary outcome measure in the PREEMPT program [14, 15] which has not been extensively investigated in real-life studies. Of note, a *post-hoc* analysis of the PREEMPT studies showed a significantly positive impact of OBT-A treatment on patient health-related QoL [46].

The present survey also suggests that a number of issues related to the use of OBT-A remain unsolved in clinical practice. An important unsettled issue is how long treatment should be continued after the first year

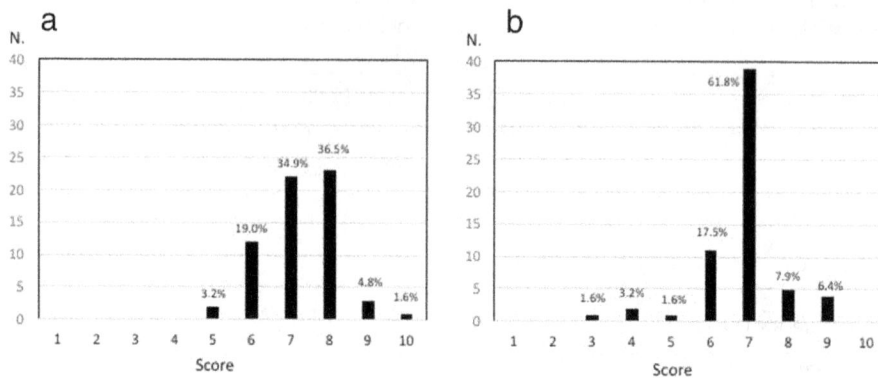

**Fig. 4** Satisfaction with Onabotulinumtoxin A (OBT-A) treatment: **a** treatment satisfaction of clinicians; **b** treatment satisfaction of patients (as perceived by clinicians). Treatment satisfaction was rated on a scale from 0 (no satisfaction) to 10 (highest satisfaction)

of prophylaxis with OBT-A. The survey shows that, after the first year, treatment schedules became variable with time intervals between treatment cycles ranging from 3 to 6 months. This behavior indicates a tendency of clinicians to explore whether OBT-A treatment may be gradually discontinued, while being ready to start it again if relapses occur. This tendency was more evident during the third year from the commencement of OBT-A, when only 10% of the clinicians maintained the 3-month interval between treatment cycles, nearly 20% of them extended the interval duration to 4-6 months, while the majority relied on the pattern of headache reported in the patients' headache diaries to make decisions about treatment timing. Schedule variability after the first year of prophylaxis with OBT-A likely reflects the clinicians' intention to comply with current

**Table 4** Resources for patient management

| Answer options | Percent |
| --- | --- |
| Evaluation of adequacy of available resources (equipment and personnel) at center | |
| Able to meet current and expected future demand | 33 (52.4) |
| Able to meet current demand, but not expected future demand | 23 (36.5) |
| Unable to meet current and future demand | 5 (7.9) |
| Other | 2 (3.2) |
| Impact of inadequate resources on patient management | |
| Scheduled visits are postponed or cancelled | 2 (3.2) |
| Treatment not administered according to recommended schedule | 8 (12.7) |
| Patients not monitored with recommended timing | 13 (20.6) |
| Long waiting times for first visit | 24 (38.1) |
| Long waiting times for follow-up visits | 10 (15.9) |
| Referral of new patients to other centers to avoid increase in waiting times | 2 (3.2) |
| Other | 4 (6.4) |

recommendations, according to which OBT-A treatment should be interrupted when CM reverts to an episodic pattern (i.e., < 15 days with headache/month) [11, 19] and, at the same time, the fear that treatment discontinuation might revert episodic migraine to chronicity.

Identification of the best timing for treatment discontinuation is crucial for the therapeutic program with OBT-A. The PREEMPT study showed a progressive increase in the efficacy of OBT-A over time [15], but the relatively short treatment duration (14 months) of the trial did not provide data about long-term outcomes. In a recent real-life study, Guerzoni and coworkers have shown that the benefits in terms of headache days and QoL progressively increased during at least 7 cycles (18 months) of treatment with OBT-A [31]. Progressively increasing benefits for up to 24 months in terms of reduced number of headache days and decreased use of acute medications have been reported also by Negro and coworkers [32]. The limited evidence currently available suggests that treatment discontinuation performed once the frequency of headache days is <15 days/month, as currently recommended [19], results in worsening of headache, decrease in QoL [31] and the need to reinitiate treatment [47]. The decision to discontinue treatment has a heavy burden of consequences, given that CM can be highly refractory to treatment, disabling, and associated with comorbidities including depression, anxiety, and medication overuse [6, 7].

The need for a precise definition of response to treatment is another critical issue emerging from the survey. According to current guidelines for clinical trials in migraine [48], response to treatment for migraine is defined by a reduction ≥50% in the number of headache days. However a reduction ≥30% can also be clinically meaningful for CM [49]. Other authors have suggested different scores. Khalil and coworkers, for example, define as a responder any patient with either a 50% reduction in headache or migraine days or an increment in crystal clear days twice that of the baseline in a 30-day period (Hull criteria) [25]. According to our survey, 25% of the clinicians considered as a clinically meaningful response a ≥ 30% reduction in the number of the headache days. Furthermore, a smaller, but not irrelevant, percentage of clinicians (15.9%) felt that also a smaller reduction in the number of headache days (< 30%) might be worth considering when evaluating clinical response, provided that such reduction is associated with at least another indicator of improvement, including patient satisfaction with treatment, improvement of QoL, reduction in pain intensity, decrease in the number of medications used to relieve symptoms, or reduced duration of headache attacks. These findings, along with data from the literature [50], suggest that multiple efficacy measures should be considered to fully reflect clinical relevance, not only in regulatory clinical trials but also, and more importantly, in the real-life setting.

With regard to the definition of non-responders, the survey shows good agreement with the definition emerging from the literature (i.e., failure of at least 3 cycles of treatment) [50]. This finding also suggests that clinicians are aware of the putative mechanism of action of OBT-A, which is likely to require a prolonged time interval to revert the changes associated with the progression of migraine to chronicity [51].

Not surprisingly, the survey indicates that the treatment with OBT-A is usually initiated after the failure of several types of prophylactic agents (> 3 agents, according to 60% of clinicians), as current guidelines recommend OBT-A only for patients who have failed to respond to, or have not tolerated at least 3 prior pharmacologic prophylactic therapies [19]. However, according to our findings, most clinicians claimed, based on their experience, that the efficacy of OBT-A seems greater when the treatment is administered earlier in the course of CM. This impression is in agreement with previously published data. The pooled analysis of the PREEMPT 1 and 2 trials, for example, showed an increased benefit in patients who initiated OBT-A earlier compared to those who were treated 6 months later [16]. Furthermore, Castrillo and colleagues, in a real-life study, reported a negative correlation between the reduction in pain intensity and the number of drug treatments received before initiating OBT-A [52]. Along with the data from the literature, our findings indicate that further effort is required to define whether the early administration of OBT-A is associated with increased efficacy in CM. Currently we can only speculate about the reasons why early treatment may be more beneficial. It is generally accepted that recurring migraine attacks induce peripheral and central sensitization [53]. In CM, sensitization phenomena are associated with progressive and more pervasive functional and neuroanatomical changes [54]. Early treatment with OBT-A, via the direct inhibition of peripheral neurotransmitter and neuropeptide release, and the possible interaction with the surface expression of relevant membrane receptors, may counteract these changes when they are only partially expressed thus preventing their consolidation [54]. At the same time, we cannot exclude that early-stage CM may be more likely to undergo spontaneous fluctuations and/or to improve spontaneously than long-term CM. The potential benefits of early administration are relevant, not only to alleviate migraine pain, but also to prevent the loss of productivity and the increased use of healthcare resources typically associated with CM [55, 56]. Appropriate studies are required to establish whether OBT-A should be a first-line option in the management of patients with CM as 47.6% of the clinicians in the present survey recommend.

The cost-effectiveness of OBT-A in CM has yet to be defined in ad hoc prospective, long-term studies. Evidence suggests that the use of OBT-A may be associated with a decrease in resource use. An observational study in 35 patients initiating prophylaxis with OBT-A found that the new treatment was associated with a reduction in visits to the emergency department by 87% [57]. A retrospective study based on a health care claims database has shown that OBT-A treatment is associated with a significantly lower likelihood of headache-related visits to the emergency department and of hospitalizations [58]. Furthermore, analysis of data from the PREEMPT program, using a Markov model applied to the UK health care system, led to the conclusion that OBT-A treatment in CM represents a cost-effective use of resources [59].

Notably, the present survey reported a better tolerability profile and a more favorable efficacy/safety ratio of OBT-A compared with other prophylactic agents for migraine. The favorable tolerability/safety profile of OBT-A has been supported by comparative trials with oral drugs for the prophylactic treatment of CM [60, 61], and by its extended use in clinical practice in other indications [62].

The present study has a number of limitations. The response rate to our survey (65%), although in line with the mean response rates of physicians to mailed questionnaires reported in the literature, was slightly below the threshold of 70% generally considered desirable for ensuring survey validity [37]. Despite these inherent limitations, we believe that the selection of survey participants, based on the proven expertise in the management of headache disorders, ensured that the source of information was reliable and qualified. Of note, most survey participants had several years of experience in the use of OBT-A for CM; in some cases, the duration of OBT-A use extended beyond the approval date (2013) of OBT-A in Italy, probably because of the off-label use of the drug or the participation in RCTs [63]. Our findings, which describe the status of OBT-A use in Italy, may not be applicable to the clinical practice in other countries. However, most items in the questionnaire addressed unresolved issues of general interest in the field of CM, and were articulated in a way that avoided the constraints of national regulations. We believe that the information produced by our survey may be useful for the design of appropriate studies in the near future.

## Conclusions

At three years from the approval of OBT-A for the prophylaxis of CM in Italy, this novel therapeutic option appears to be used in accordance with current recommendations. The majority of clinicians in the survey considered the efficacy/safety profile of OBT-A more favorable than that of oral prophylactic agents. Satisfaction with this approach was high among clinicians and, according to almost 50% of them, OBT-A should be offered as first-line treatment. Additional effort from the headache community is required to define response to treatment and to establish the optimal duration of prophylaxis with OBT-A. Such effort is crucial to further improve the therapeutic approach to CM.

## Abbreviations

ANIRCEF: Associazione Italiana per la Ricerca sulle Cefalee; EMA: European Medicines Agency; FDA: US Food and Drug Administration; HR-QoL: Health-related quality of life; OBT-A: Onabotulinumtoxin A; PREEMPT: Phase III Research Evaluating Migraine Prophylaxis Therapy-1; QoL: Quality of life; RCTs: Randomized clinical trials; SISC: Società Italiana per lo Studio delle Cefalee

## Acknowledgments

The authors are deeply grateful to the clinicians who filled in the online questionnaire with the data representing their practice. The survey participants were blinded to funding sources for this survey. Editorial assistance during manuscript preparation was provided by HPS, Health Publishing & Services, Srl, Italy, and medical writer assistance was supported by Allergan SpA-Italy.

## Authors' contributions

All authors were involved in the conception and design of the survey and in the collection, analysis, and interpretation of the data. The manuscript was drafted by CT. All authors reviewed and approved the final manuscript.

## Competing interests

CT has participated in advisory boards for Allergan and, ElectroCore. She has received research grants for preclinical studies from MSD and FB Health. She is PI or collaborator in RCTs for ElectroCore, Eli-Lilly, Teva, Alder. She is PI or partner in Projects funded by the EU Commission, the Italian Ministry of Health and the Italian Ministry of University. LG has participated in advisory boards for Allergan & Electrocore; PI in RCTS for Electrocore and Alder; collaborator in RCTs for Eli-Lilly and Teva. PG has participated in advisory boards for Allergan, Evidera and Electro-Core; has received research grants for preclinical studies from MSD; is PI of RCTs for ElectroCore, Eli-Lilly, Teva, Novartis. PM has participated in advisory boards or has received research or educational grants from ACRAF, Allergan, Amgen, Electro-core, ElytraPharma, Novartis, Sanofi, SpringerNature, Teva.

## Author details

[1]Headache Science Center, National Neurological Institute C. Mondino, Pavia, Italy. [2]Department of Brain and Behavioral Sciences, University of Pavia, Via Mondino 2, 27100 Pavia, Italy. [3]Headache Center, Neurology Department, Asti Hospital, Asti, Italy. [4]Applied Neurophysiology and Pain Unit, SMBNOS Department, Polyclinic General Hospital, Bari Aldo Moro University, Bari, Italy. [5]Headache Center, Department of Health Sciences, University of Florence, Florence, Italy. [6]Headache and Neuroalgology Unit, Neurological Institute "C. Besta" IRCCS Foundation, Milan, Italy. [7]Center for Neuroscience and Neurotechnology, Polyclinic Hospital, University of Modena and Reggio Emilia, Modena, Italy. [8]Neurology Clinic, University Hospital of Perugia, Perugia, Italy. [9]Department of Medical, Surgical, Neurological, Metabolic and Aging Sciences, University of Campania "Luigi Vanvitelli", Naples, Italy. [10]Department of Clinical and Molecular Medicine, Sapienza University of Rome and Regional Referral Headache Center, Sant'Andrea Hospital, Rome, Italy. [11]Department of Biomedical and Neuromotor Sciences, University of Bologna, Bologna, Italy. [12]IRCCS Institute of Neurological Sciences of Bologna, Bellaria Hospital, Bologna, Italy.

## References

1. Headache Classification Committee of the International Headache Society (IHS) (2013) International classification of headache disorders, 3rd edition (beta version). Cephalalgia 33:629–808

2. Bigal ME, Serrano D, Reed M, Lipton RB (2008) Chronic migraine in the population: burden, diagnosis, and satisfaction with treatment. Neurology 71:559–566

3. Natoli JL, Manack A, Dean B, Butler Q, Turkel CC, Stovner L, Lipton RB (2010) Global prevalence of chronic migraine: a systematic review. Cephalalgia 30: 599–609

4. Manack AN, Buse DC, Lipton RB (2011) Chronic migraine: epidemiology and disease burden. Curr Pain Headache Rep 15:70–78

5. Buse DC, Manack AN, Fanning KM, Serrano D, Reed ML, Turkel CC, Lipton RB (2012) Chronic migraine prevalence, disability, and sociodemographic factors: results from the American migraine prevalence and prevention study. Headache 52:1456–1470

6. Ruscheweyh R, Muller M, Blum B, Straube A (2014) Correlation of headache frequency and psychosocial impairment in migraine: a cross-sectional study. Headache 54:861–871

7. Bendtsen L, Munksgaard S, Tassorelli C, Nappi G, Karsarava Z, Lainez M, Leston J, Fadic R, Spadafora S, Stoppini A, Jensen R, COMOESTAS Consortium (2014) Disability, anxiety and depression associated with medication-overuse headache can be considerably reduced by detoxification and prophylactic treatment. Results from a multicentre, multinational study (COMOESTAS project). Cephalalgia 34:423–433

8. Irimia P, Carmona-Abellán M, Martínez-Vila E (2012) Chronic migraine: a therapeutic challenge for clinicians. Expert Opin Emerg Drugs 17:445–447

9. Hepp Z, Dodick DW, Varon SF, Gillard P, Hansen RN, Devine EB (2015) Adherence to oral migraine-preventive medications among patients with chronic migraine. Cephalalgia 35:478–488

10. Hepp Z, Bloudek LM, Varon SF (2014) Systematic review of migraine prophylaxis adherence and persistence. J Manag Care Pharm 20:22–33

11. Gooriah R, Ahmed F (2015) Onabotulinumtoxin a for chronic migraine: a critical appraisal. Ther Clin Risk Manage 11:1003–1013

12. Silberstein SD, Lipton RB, Dodick DW, Freitag FG, Ramadan N, Mathew N, Brandes JL, Bigal M, Saper J, Ascher S, Jordan DM, Greenberg SJ, Hulihan J, Topiramate Chronic Migraine Study Group (2007) Efficacy and safety of topiramate for the treatment of chronic migraine: a randomized, double-blind, placebo-controlled trial. Headache 47:170–180

13. Diener HC, Bussone G, Van Oene JC, Lahaye M, Schwalen S, Goadsby PJ, TOPMAT-MIG-201(TOP-CHROME) Study Group (2007) Topiramate reduces headache days in chronic migraine: a randomized, double-blind, placebo-controlled study. Cephalalgia 27:814–823

14. Aurora SK, Dodick DW, Turkel CC, DeGryse RE, Silberstein SD, Lipton RB, Diener HC, Brin MF, PREEMPT 1 Chronic Migraine Study Group (2010) OnabotulinumtoxinA for treatment of chronic migraine: results from the double-blind, randomized, placebo-controlled phase of the PREEMPT 1 trial. Cephalalgia 30:793–803

15. Diener HC, Dodick DW, Aurora SK, Turkel CC, DeGryse RE, Lipton RB, Silberstein SD, Brin MF, PREEMPT 2 Chronic Migraine Study Group (2010)

OnabotulinumtoxinA for treatment of chronic migraine: results from the double-blind, randomized, placebo-controlled phase of the PREEMPT 2 trial. Cephalalgia 30:804–814

16. Aurora SK, Winner P, Freeman MC, Spierings EL, Heiring JO, DeGryse RE, VanDenburgh AM, Nolan ME, Turkel CC (2011) OnabotulinumtoxinA for treatment of chronic migraine: pooled analyses of the 56-week PREEMPT clinical program. Headache 51:1358–1373

17. Simpson DM, Hallett M, Ashman EJ, Comella CI, Green MW, Gronseth GS, Armostrong MJ, Gloss D, Potrebic S, Jankovic J, Karp BR, Naumann M, So YT, Yablon SA (2016) Practice guideline update summary: Botulinum neurotoxin for the treatment of blepharospasm, cervical dystonia, adult spasticity, and headache. Neurology 86:1818–1826

18. Guias diagnoticas y terapeuticas de la Sociedad Espanola de Neurologia (2015) Guia oficial de practica clinica en cefeleas. Ezpeleta D and Pozo Rosich P editors. Available via http://www.sen.es/noticias/78-noticias-sen/1204-guia-oficial-de-practica-clinica-en-cefaleas-2015. Accessed 19 Dec 2016

19. National Institute for Health and Care Excellence (2012) Botulinum toxin type a for the prevention of headache in adults with chronic migraine. Available at https://www.nice.org.uk/guidance/ta260/resources/botulinum-toxin-typea-for-the-prevention-of-headaches-in-adults-with-chronic-migraine-82600545273541. Accessed 19 Dec 2016

20. Sarchielli P, Granella F, Prudenzano MP, Pini LA, Guidetti V, Bono G, Pinessi L, Alessandri M, Antonaci F, Fanciullacci M, Ferrari A, Guazzelli M, Nappi G, Sances G, Sandrini G, Savi L, Tassorelli C, Zanchin G (2012) Italian guidelines for primary headaches: 2012 revised version. J Headache Pain 13(Suppl):S31–S70

21. Agenas: linee guida nazionali di riferimento per la prevenzione e terapia delle cefalee nell'adulto (2012). Available at http://matera.fimmg.org/Linee%20guida/Cefalea%20nell'adulto%20.pdf. Accessed 19 Dec 2016

22. Flather M, Delahunty N, Collinson J (2006) Generalizing results of randomized trials to clinical practice: reliability and cautions. Clin Trials 3:508–512

23. Zarbin MA (2016) Challenges in applying the results of clinical trials to clinical practice. JAMA Ophthalmol 134:928–933

24. Martelletti P, Curto M (2016) Headache: cluster headache treatment – RCTs versus real-world evidence. Nat Rev Neurol 12:557–558

25. Khalil M, Zafar HW, Quarshie V, Ahmed F (2014) Prospective analysis of the use of Onabotulinumtoxin a (BOTOX) in the treatment of chronic migraine; real-life data in 254 patients from Hull, UK. J Headache Pain 15:54

26. Grazzi L, Usai S (2015) Onabotulinumtoxin a (Botox) for chronic migraine treatment: an Italian experience. Neurol Sci 36(Suppl1):S33–S35

27. Cernuda-Morollon E, Ramon C, Larrosa D, Alvarez R, Riesco N, Pascual J (2015) Long-term experience with onabotulinumtoxinA in the treatment of chronic migraine: what happens after one year? Cephalalgia 35:864–868

28. Kollewe K, Escher CM, Wulff DU, Fathi D, Paracka L, Mohammadi B, Karst M, Dressler D (2016) Long-term treatment of chronic migraine with Onabotulinumtoxin a: efficacy, quality of life and tolerability in a real-life setting. J Neural Transm 123:533–540

29. Khalil M, Zafar H, Ahmed F (2015) Hull prospective analysis of Onabotulinumtoxin a (Botox®) in the treatment of chronic migraine; real-life data in 465 patients; an update. Presented at the 17th Congress of the International Headache Society (IHC), Valencia, Spain, 14-17 May, 2015

30. Botox. Riassunto delle caratteristiche del prodotto. Available at https://farmaci.agenziafarmaco.gov.it/aifa/servlet/PdfDownloadServlet?pdfFileName=footer_000753_034883_RCP.pdf&retry=0&sys=m0b1l3. Accessed 19 Dec 2016

31. Guerzoni S, Pellesi L, Beraldi C, Pini LA (2016) Increased efficacy of regularly repeated cycles with Onabotulinumtoxin a in MOH patients beyond the first year of treatment. J Headache Pain 17:48

32. Negro A, Curto M, Lionetto L, Martelletti P (2016) A two years open-label prospective study of Onabotulinumtoxin a 195 U in medication overuse headache: a real-world experience. J Headache 17:1

33. Russo M, Manzoni GC, Taga A, Genovese A, Veronesi L, Pasquarella C, Sansebastiano GE, Torelli P (2016) The use of Onabotulinumtoxin a (Botox®) in the treatment of chronic migraine at the Parma headache Centre: a prospective observational study. Neurol Sci 37:1127–1131

34. Aicua-Rapun I, Martínez-Velasco E, Rojo A, Hernando A, Ruiz M, Carreres A, Porqueres E, Herrero S, Iglesias F, Guerrero AL (2016) Real-life data in 115 chronic migraine patients treated with Onabotulinumtoxin a during more than one year. J Headache Pain 17:112

35. Vikelis M, Argyriou AA, Dermitzakis EV, Spingos KC, Mitsikostas DD (2016) Onabotulinumtoxin-a treatment in Greek patients with chronic migraine. J Headache Pain 17:84

36. Eysenbach G, Wyatt J (2002) Using the internet for surveys and health research. J Med Internet Res 4:e13

37. Burns KEA, Duffett M, Kho ME, Meade MO, Adhikari NK, Sinuff T, Cook DJ, ACCADEMY Group (2008) A guide for the diagnosis and conduct of self-administered surveys of clinicians. CMAJ 179:245–252

38. Klabunde CN, Willis GB, McLeod CC, Dillman DA, Johnson TP, Greene SM, Brown ML. Improving the quality of surveys of physicians and medical groups: a research agenda. Eval Health Prof. 2012;35(4):477–506

39. Thorpe C, Ryan B, McLean S, Burt A, Stewart M, Brown J, Reid GJ, Harris S (2009) How to obtain excellent response rates when surveying physicians. Fam Pract 26:65–68

40. Boynton PM, Greenhalgh T (2004) Selecting, designing, and developing your questionnaire. BMJ 328:1312–1315

41. Società Italiana per lo Studio delle Cefalee. Strutture delle Cefalee. Available at: http://www.sisc.it/ita/centri-cefalee-in-italia_2.html. Accessed 19 Dec 2016

42. Associazione Neurologica Italiana per la Ricerca sulle Cefalee. Centri per la cura delle cefalee. Available at: http://www.anircef.it/opencms/sezioni/pazienti/centri/. Accessed 19 Dec 2016

43. Steiner TJ, Antonaci F, Jensen R, Lainez MJ, Lanteri-Minet M, Valade D, European Headache Federation, Global Campaign against Headache (2011) Recommendations for headache service organisation and delivery in Europe. J Headache Pain 12:419–426

44. Jensen R, Tassorelli C, Rossi P, Allena M, Osipova V, Steiner T, Sandrini G, Olesen J, Nappi G, Basic Diagnostic Headache Diary Study Group (2011) A basic diagnostic headache diary (BDHD) is well accepted and useful in the diagnosis of headache. A multicentre European and Latin American study. Cephalalgia 31:1549–1560

45. Stovner LJ, Andree C (2008) Impact of headache in Europe: a review for the Eurolight project. J Headache Pain 9:139–146

46. Lipton RB, Rosen NL, Ailani J, DeGryse RE, GillardPJ VSF (2016) Onabotulinumtoxin a improves quality of life and reduces impact of chronic migraine over one year of treatment: pooled results from the PREEMPT randomized clinical trial program. Cephalalgia 36:899–908

47. Zafar H, Khalil M, Ahmed F (2014) How long to continue botox in chronic migraine patients? A two-year follow up of 85 patients treated in Hull, UK. Presented at the 4th European headache Migraine Trust international congress, Copenhagen, Denmark, 18-21 September 2014

48. Tfelt-Hansen P, Block G, Dahlöf C, Diener HC, Ferrari MD, Goadsby PJ, Guidetti V, Jones B, Lipton RB, Massiou H, Meinert C, Sandrini G, Steiner T, Winter PB, International Headache Society Clinical Trials Subcommittee (2000) Guidelines for controlled trials of drugs in migraine: second edition. Cephalalgia 20:765–786

49. Silberstein S, Tfelt-Hansen P, Dodick DW, Limmroth V, Lipton RB, Pascual J, Wang SJ, Task Force of the International Headache Society Clinical Trials Subcommittee (2008) Guidelines for controlled trials of prophylactic treatment of chronic migraine in adults. Cephalalgia 28:484–495

50. Silberstein SD, Dodick DW, Aurora SK, Diener HC, DeGryse RE, Lipton RB, Turkel CC (2015) Percent of patients with chronic migraine who responded per Onabotulinumtoxin a treatment cycle: PREEMPT. J Neurol Neurosurg Psychiatry 86:996–1001

51. Burstein R, Zhang XC, Levy D, Aoki KR, Brin MF (2014) Selective inhibition of meningeal nociceptors by botulinum neurotoxin type a: therapeutic implications for migraine and other pains. Cephalalgia 34:853–869

52. Castrillo Sanz A, Morollon Sanchez-Mateos N, Simonet Hernandez C, Fernandez Rodriguez B, Cerdan Santacruz D, Mendoza Rodriguez A, Rodriguez Sanz MF, Tabernero Garcia C, Guerrero Becerra P, Ferrero Ros M, Duate Garcia-Luis J (2016) Experiencia con toxina botulinica en la migrana cronica. Neurologia. doi: 10.1016/j.nrl.2016.09.004. [Epub ahead of print]

53. Dodick S, Silberstein S (2006) Central sensitization theory of migraine: clinical implications. Headache 46(Suppl 4):S182–S191

54. Aurora SK, Brin MF (2017) Chronic migraine: an update on physiology, imaging, and the mechanism of action of two pharmacologic therapies. Headache 57:109–125

55. Steiner TJ, Stovner LJ, Katsarava Z, Lainez JM, Lampl C, Lantéri Minet M, Rastenyte D, Ruiz de la Torre E, Tassorelli C, Barré J, Andrée C (2014) The impact of headache in Europe: principal results of the Eurolight project. J Headache Pain 15:31. doi:10.1186/1129-2377-15-31

56. Allena M, Steiner TJ, Sances G, Carugno B, Balsamo F, Nappi G, Andrée C, Tassorelli C (2015) Impact of headache disorders in Italy and the public-health and policy implications: a population-based study with the Eurolight project. J Headache Pain 16:100

57. Oterino A, Ramón C, Pascual J (2011) Experience with onabotulinumtoxinA (BOTOX) in chronic refractory migraine: focus on severe attacks. J Headache Pain 12:235–238

58. Hepp Z, Rosen NL, Gillard PG, Varon SF, Mathew N, Dodick DW (2016) Comparative effectiveness of onabotulinumtoxinA versus oral migraine prophylactic medications on headache-related resource utilization in the management of chronic migraine: retrospective analysis of a US-based insurance claims database. Cephalalgia 36:862–874

59. Batty AJ, Hansen RN, Bloudek LM, Varon SF, Hayward EJ, Pennington BW, Lipton RB, Sullivan SD (2013) The cost-effectiveness of onabotulinumtoxinA for the prophylaxis of headache in adults with chronic migraine in the UK. J Med Econ 16:877–887

60. Blumenfeld AM, Schim JD, Chippendale TJ (2008) Botulinum toxin type a and divalproex sodium for prophylactic treatment of episodic or chronic migraine. Headache 48:210–220

61. Mathew NT, Jaffri SF (2009) A double-blind comparison of onabotulinumtoxina (BOTOX) and topiramate (TOPAMAX) for the prophylactic treatment of chronic migraine: a pilot study. Headache 49: 1466–1478

62. Colosimo C, Tiple D, Berardelli A (2012) Efficacy and safety of long-term botulinum toxin treatment in craniocervical dystonia: a systematic review. Neurotox Res 22:265–273

63. Sandrini G, Perrotta A, Tassorelli C, Torelli P, Brighina F, Sances G, Nappi G (2011 Aug) Botulinum toxin type-a in the prophylactic treatment of medication-overuse headache: a multicenter, double-blind, randomized, placebo-controlled, parallel group study. J Headache Pain 12(4):427–433

# Is topiramate effective for migraine prevention in patients less than 18 years of age?

Kai Le, Dafan Yu, Jiamin Wang, Abdoulaye Idriss Ali and Yijing Guo[*] ⓘ

## Abstract

**Background:** Mainly based on evidence of success in adults, various medications are commonly used to prevent pediatric migraines. Topiramate has been approved for migraine prevention in children as young as 12 years of age. In this meta-analysis, we aimed to assess the currently published data pertaining to the efficacy of topiramate for migraine prevention in patients less than 18 years of age.

**Methods:** We searched PubMed/Medline, Embase and the Cochrane Library (from inception to April 2017) for randomized controlled trials (RCTs) published in English. Two independent investigators performed data extraction and quality evaluation using the Cochrane Collaboration's tool. The data extracted were analyzed by Review Manager 5.3 software.

**Results:** A total of four RCTs matching the inclusion criteria were included, with an aggregate of 465 patients. Of these patients, 329 were included in the topiramate group, and 136 were included in the placebo group. This meta-analysis revealed that compared with placebo, topiramate failed to decrease the number of patients experiencing a $\geq$ 50% relative reduction in headache frequency ($n = 465$, RR = 1.26, 95% CI = [0.94,1.67], Z = 1.55, $P = 0.12$) or the number of headache days ($n = 465$, MD = −0.77, 95% CI = [−2.31,0.76], Z = 0.99, $P = 0.32$) but did reduce PedMIDAS scores ($n = 205$, MD = −9.02, 95% CI = [−17.34, −0.70], Z = 2.13, $P = 0.03$). Higher rates of side effects and adverse events in the topiramate group than in the placebo group were observed in the included trials.

**Conclusions:** Topiramate may not achieve a more effective clinical trial endpoint than placebo in the prevention of migraines in patients less than 18 years of age, and topiramate may lead to more side effects or adverse events in the included patients.

**Keywords:** Topiramate, Pediatric, Adolescent, Children, Migraine, Prevention

## Background

Migraine is the most common cause of headache in pediatric neurology outpatient clinics, and it has been recognized as one of the most prevalent neurological disorder in children and adolescents worldwide, affecting 5–10% of the pediatric population in multiple areas of life. Because patients miss school and social activities, migraines can impair the development of friendships that are vital to social development and self-esteem and may destroy family harmony [1, 2]. The mean age of onset of migraine is 7.2 years in boys and 10.9 years in girls [3], and the prevalence of migraine increases with age, as demonstrated by clinical studies. The diagnostic criteria for migraine headaches have developed over time; modern migraine classification includes frequency as a criterion, with episodic headaches occurring up to 14 days per month, and chronic migraine is defined as the persistence of headache without aura for at least 15 days per month and for at least 3 consecutive months without medication overuse (ICHD-II) [4]. Because of the diversity of symptoms, the diagnosis of migraines in children

* Correspondence: 975607384@qq.com
Department of Neurology, Affiliated ZhongDa Hospital, School of Medicine, Southeast University, Nanjing, Jiangsu 210009, People's Republic of China

and adolescents needs to be refined even further. Due to the harm caused by migraines, reducing the number of migraine attacks to the greatest extent possible should be a priority.

At present, a variety of prophylactic therapy options are available to reduce the frequency or severity of headaches [5]. Topiramate is an antiepileptic drug with positive efficacy and safety for older children and adults with epilepsy [6], and it has been approved for migraine prevention in adults in Europe since 2003 and in the United States since 2004 [7]. The exact mechanism of topiramate in the treatment of migraine is unknown, although it may be associated with the influence of topiramate on pain transmission in the trigeminocervical complex and the third-order neurons in the ventroposteromedial thalamus [8]. Several case series and open-label trials [9–13] have shown that topiramate served as a preventive treatment for pediatric migraines, while the research of Scott W [14] indicated that there were no significant differences between topiramate and placebo in the prevention of pediatric migraine. Hence, in the present study, we performed a meta-analysis of randomized controlled trials (RCTs) to evaluate the efficacy of topiramate for the prevention of migraine in patients less than 18 years of age.

## Methods
### Protocol registration
The protocol registration number was CRD42017062287 (http://www.crd.york.ac.uk/Prospero).

### Data sources and search strategies
We searched using the following databases: PubMed/Medline, Embase and the Cochrane Library (inception to April 2017) to retrieve the RCTs of topiramate in migraine prevention for patients less than 18 years of age. The following search terms were used in combination: ("topiramate" OR "topamax") AND ("migraine disorders" OR "migraine" OR "migraineur" OR "migraineurs" OR "migrain" OR "sick headache") AND ("pediatric" OR "adolescent" OR "adolescence" OR "child" OR "children" OR "childhood" OR "teen" OR "youth"). The references of eligible studies, relevant systematic reviews, and meta-analysis were also manually retrieved. The publication language was restricted to English.

### Study selection
The automatically retrieved studies were evaluated by two independent investigators and included in the meta-analysis based on the criteria presented below. The reviewers resolved any differences by consensus. The investigators selected the retrieved studies that matched the inclusion and exclusion criteria.

### Inclusion criteria
Studies were included in the meta-analysis if they fulfilled the following criteria: (1) the study was a trial comparing topiramate with placebo in migraine patients, (2) the study had similar diagnostic criteria for migraine or definition of migraine, (3) the age of the participants was less than 18 years, (4) the study was a clinical RCT, (5) the intent-to-treat population numbers in the topiramate and placebo groups were provided, and (6) the number of participants showing ≥50% reduction in headache frequency, baseline and follow-up data of headache days or PedMIDAS scores were available.

### Exclusion criteria
Studies were excluded according to the following exclusion criteria: (1) the study was not a RCT but a review, case report, letter, editorial or other type of publication not describing original research, (2) the full text was not available, (3) the study did not afford extractable outcomes, (4) the control group of the trial did not contain placebo (for example, the trial only used propranolol or sodium valproate as a control), and (5) the trial involved adults and children, but the characteristics or outcomes of the pediatric subgroup were unavailable or unextractable.

### Risk of bias in individual studies
The methodological quality of RCTs was evaluated according to the risk of bias tool described in the Cochrane Handbook for Systematic Reviews of Interventions [15]. Seven quality elements that contain random sequence generation, allocation concealment, blinding of participants and personnel, blinding of outcome assessment, incomplete outcome data, selective reporting and baseline balance bias were assessed. Study selection, data extraction and risk bias assessment were conducted by two researchers (Kai Le and Dafan Yu) independently; in case of discrepancies consensus was reached by discussion with a third party (Yijing Guo).

### Data extraction
Our primary outcome was a relative reduction in the number of headache days of 50% or more in the comparison of the 28-day baseline period with the last 28 days. Secondary outcomes included headache days and PedMIDAS scores. The PedMIDAS score, which is used to ascertain a change in headache-related disability [16] between the beginning and the end of the trial and the decrease in the number of headache days from the 28-day baseline period to the final 28-day period of treatment were recorded. The main information, including the numbers of participants in the topiramate and placebo groups, the diagnostic tool, the dose and duration of topiramate, the numbers of patients experiencing a ≥ 50% relative reduction in headache

frequency, the mean headache days per 28-day period and the mean PedMIDAS score in both groups, was extracted. Additional information was also abstracted, such as publication year, first author, age and sex. Side effects and adverse events after drug administration were also recorded if they occurred. The two investigators (Kai Le and Dafan Yu) extracted all the data independently. If there was any disagreement between the two reviewers, they resolved it by discussion and consensus, with a third party participating if necessary.

## Statistical analysis

The meta-analysis was conducted using Review Manager 5.3 software (Cochrane Collaboration, Copenhagen, Denmark). Continuous data are presented as the mean difference (MD) with a 95% confidence interval (CI) and inverse variance (IV). Dichotomous outcomes were analyzed by pooled risk ratio (RR) with a 95% CI to present effect estimate and Mantel-Haenszel test. The heterogeneity among eligible trials was quantified using a chi-squared-based $Q$-statistic test ($P < 0.1$, suggesting the existence of heterogeneity). An $I^2$ statistic was alsoused to quantify the inconsistency across studies, with $I^2 > 50\%$ considered statistically significant. When there was no statistically significant heterogeneity, we used a fixed-effects model for pooling the results; otherwise, a random-effects model was used. A 2-sided $P$ value <0.05 was taken to indicate statistical significance for 1 comparison group over the other. The results of the meta-analysis were visualized using forest plots. Visual inspection of funnel plots was used to assess possible publication bias if more than 10 trials were identified that reported on the same outcome [17].

## Results

### Search results

A total of 541 articles were identified from among 56 listed in PubMed/Medline, 429 in Embase and 56 in the Cochrane Library. After excluding 82 duplicates, 459 potentially eligible articles were selected. Of these articles, 401 were excluded through titles and abstracts, leaving 58 articles for further evaluation. The reasons for exclusion during full-text review were "studies involved adults only" ($n = 15$), "studies included adults and children" ($n = 14$), "conference abstract" ($n = 2$), "editorial" ($n = 3$), "not controlled" ($n = 6$), "no placebo" ($n = 9$), "insufficient data" ($n = 4$) and "protocol" ($n = 1$). Finally, 4 prospective RCTs [14, 18–20] were included in our meta-analysis. The research process is shown in Fig. 1.

### Characteristics of the included RCTs

The 4 included studies were published between 2005 and 2017. Study sample sizes ranged from 42 to 163, with a total of 465 randomized patients, including 329

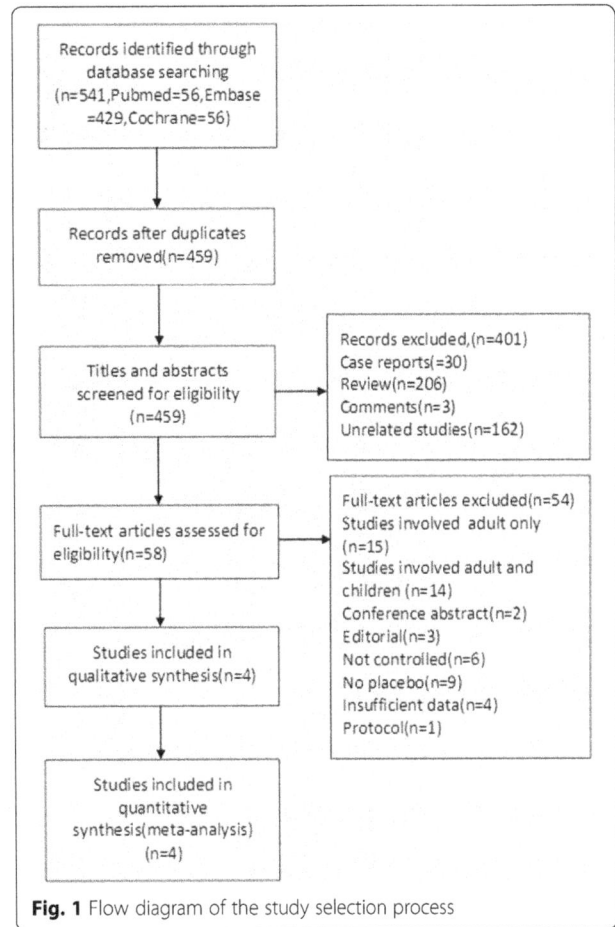

**Fig. 1** Flow diagram of the study selection process

patients in the topiramate group and 136 in the placebo group, and the age of the participants varied from 8 to 17 years old. To diagnose a migraine, one trial [20] employed the International Headache Society (IHS) diagnostic criteria for pediatric migraine and 3 trials [14, 18, 19] used the International Classification of Headache Disorders, 2nd Edition (ICHD-II) [21]. One trial [18] used 2 doses of topiramate versus placebo. Another trial [14] used amitriptyline and topiramate as the two treatment arms, and we extracted the results of topiramate versus placebo. The duration of the included trials consisted of titration and maintenance periods: 2 trials [18, 19] lasted 16 weeks, one trial [20] lasted 20 weeks, and one trial [14] lasted 24 weeks. The detailed characteristics of the studies included in the meta-analysis are listed in Table 1.

### Risk of bias of the included trials

All RCTs described the procedure of randomization and blinded participants and researchers, and all trials reported allocation concealment and blinding of outcome assessment. All outcome data were complete. Detailed information is shown in Fig. 2.

**Table 1** Characteristics of Studies Included in the Meta-Analysis

| First authors, year | Diagnostic tool | Topiramate | | | Dose & Duration | | Side effects/Adverse events | Placebo | | |
|---|---|---|---|---|---|---|---|---|---|---|
| | | N | Age (years), mean ± SD | Gender (male:female,%) | Titration | Maintenance | | N | Age (years), mean ± SD | Gender (male:female,%) |
| Paul Winner, 2005 | International Headache Society (IHS) diagnostic criteria for pediatric migraine | 108 | 11.3 ± 2.5 | 50.9:49.1 | 8-week: Week 1 = 15 mg/d, Week 2 = 30 mg/d, Week 3 = 50 mg/d (dose increased to 2–3 mg/kg/d) | 12-week: 2–3 mg/kg/d | upper respiratory tract infection, anorexia, weight decrease, gastroenteritis, paresthesia, somnolence | 49 | 10.7 ± 2.6 | 53.1:46.9 |
| C. V. S. Lakshmi, 2007 | International Classification of Headache Disorders, 2nd Edition (ICHD-II) | 21 | 10.95 ± 1.53 | 85.7:14.3 | 1-month: 25-mg incremented to 100 mg/d | 3-month: 100 mg/d | weight loss, lack of concentration in school, parasthesia, sedation, loss of appetite, pain in abdomen | 21 | 10.14 ± 1.35 | 52.4:47.6 |
| Donald Lewis, 2009 | International Classification of Headache Disorders, 2nd Edition (ICHD-II) | 70† | 14.2 ± 1.54 | 40:60 | 4-week: 25-mg incremented to 50 or 100 mg/d† | 12-week: 50 or 100 mg/d | upper respiratory tract infection, paresthesia, abdominal pain, anorexia, injury, rhinitis, coughing, viral infection, pharyngitis, fatigue, nausea, dizziness, taste perversion, insomnia, back pain, conjunctivitis, sinusitis, asthma, pneumonia, fever, allergy, vomiting, nervousness, somnolence, abnormal vision, eye pain | 33 | 14.4 ± 1.7 | 36:64 |
| Scott W. Powers, 2017[a] | International Classification of Headache Disorders, 2nd Edition (ICHD-II) | 145 | 14.2 ± 2.5 | 30:70 | 8-week: 2 mg/Kg.d, dose escalation occurred every 2 weeks | 16-week: average 1.93 ± 0.40 mg mg/Kg.d | aphasia, cognitive disorder, dizziness, memory impairment, paresthesia, general: fatigue, dry mouth, intussusception, streptococcal pharyngitis, upper respiratory tract infection, altered mood, suicide attempt, investigations: decreased weight, contusion, traumatic liver injury, respiratory: bronchospasm | 33 | 14.2 ± 2.2 | 32:68 |

*SD standard deviations, ¥ Total number in group*
[a]The analysis population included patients who ended trial early
†35 subjects treated with topiramate at 50 mg/day, 35 subjects treated with topiramate at 100 mg/day

Is topiramate effective for migraine prevention in patients less than 18 years...

107

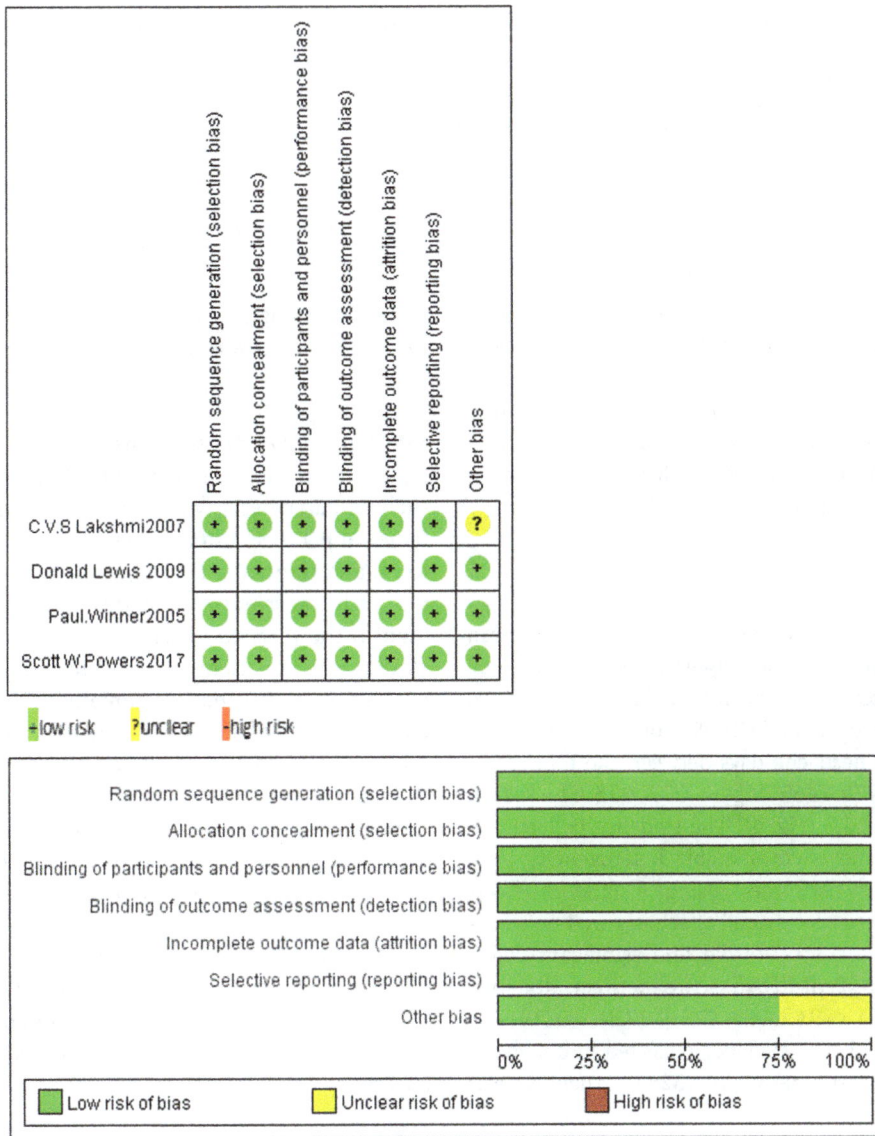

**Fig. 2** Risk of bias summary. Presentation of the risk of bias summary of the review authors

## Meta-analysis
### Primary outcome

As shown in Table 2, all 4 included trials investigated the effects of topiramate on migraine prevention via the

numbers of patients experiencing a ≥ 50% relative reduction in headache frequency. The results of our meta-analysis show that, there were no significant differences between the topiramate and placebo groups in terms

**Table 2** Trial outcomes of Studies Included in the Meta-Analysis

| First authors, year | Headache days per 28-day period (d), mean ± SD | | PedMIDAS score, mean ± SD | | ≥ 50% Relative reduction in headache frequency,n(%) | |
|---|---|---|---|---|---|---|
| | Topiramate | Placebo | Topiramate | Placebo | Topiramate | Placebo |
| Paul Winner,2005 | 3.1 ± 3 | 2.4 ± 2.8 | NA | NA | 59(54.63) | 23(46.94) |
| C. V. S. Lakshmi,2007 | 4.27 ± 1.95 | 7.48 ± 5.94 | 10.2 ± 6.39 | 23.7 ± 11.9 | 20(95.24) | 11(55) |
| Donald Lewis,2009 | 2.4 ± 3.11 | 3.5 ± 3.47 | NA | NA | 45(64.29) | 15(45.45) |
| Scott W.Powers,2017 | 4.6 ± 5.3 | 5.2 ± 6.5 | 14.4 ± 17.3 | 19.4 ± 20.8 | 72(55.38) | 20(60.61) |

*SD* standard deviations, *NA* not available

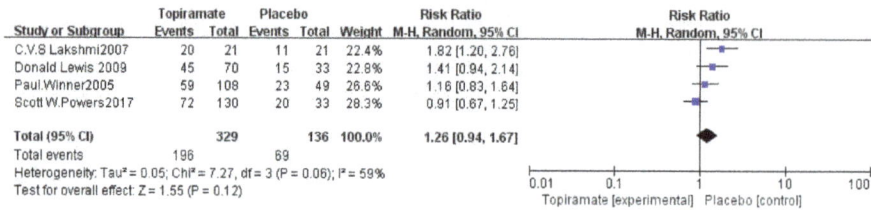

**Fig. 3** Forest plot of comparison:≥50% Relative reduction in headache frequency of topiramate versus placebo

of the numbers of patients experiencing a ≥ 50% relative reduction in headache frequency ($n$ = 465, RR = 1.26, 95% CI = [0.94, 1.67], $Z$ = 1.55, $P$ = 0.12) (Fig. 3). The evidence collected in our meta-analysis shows heterogeneity ($I^2$ = 59%). Analysis was performed by a random-effects model. The $z$-test result for overall effects showed no statistical significance ($P$ = 0.12).

### Secondary outcomes

All 4 trials included in our meta-analysis reported mean headache days from the 28-day baseline period to the final 28-day period of treatment, and 2 trials [14, 19] presented mean PedMIDAS scores (Table 2). We found no significant difference in mean headache days between the topiramate and placebo groups ($n$ = 465, MD = −0.77, 95% CI = [−2.31, 0.76], $Z$ = 0.99, $P$ = 0.32) (Fig. 4). The evidence collected in our meta-analysis shows considerable heterogeneity ($I^2$ = 70%). Analysis was performed using a random-effects model. The $z$-test result for overall effects showed no statistical significance ($P$ = 0.32). We did find significant differences in the mean PedMIDAS score between the two groups ($n$ = 205, MD = −9.02, 95% CI = [−17.34, −0.70], $Z$ = 2.13, $P$ = 0.03) (Fig. 5). The evidence collected in our meta-analysis shows heterogeneity ($I^2$ = 52%). Analysis was

performed suing a random-effects model. The $z$-test result for overall effects was statistically significant ($P$ = 0.03).

### Side effects and adverse events

All included trials reported side effects or adverse events such as paresthesia, weight decrease, anorexia, fever, fatigue, upper respiratory tract infection, somnolence, allergy, and traumatic liver injury. The overall incidence of most adverse events was higher in the topiramate group than in the placebo group, with ten of these events (including suicide attempts and other disabling events) occurring only in the topiramate group. Detailed side effects and adverse events and their frequency in both groups in the included studies are listed in Table 3. We also performed a meta-analysis of each side effect or adverse event that was reported in at least two RCTs. As shown in Fig. 6, there was a significant increase in paresthesia (Fig. 6a, n = 483, RR = 5.04, 95% CI = [2.13, 11.94]; $Z$ = 3.68, $P$ = 0.0002) and weight decrease (Fig. 6b, n = 380, RR = 4.38, 95% CI = [1.92, 10.01], $Z$ = 3.51, $P$ = 0.0005) in the topiramate group. The evidence collected in our meta-analysis shows no obvious heterogeneity ($I^2$ = 0%).Analysis was performed using a fixed-effects model.

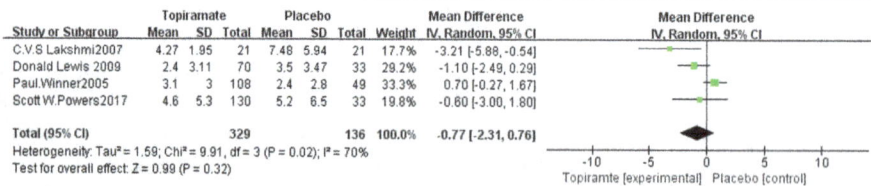

**Fig. 4** Forest plot of comparison: headache days per 28-day period of topiramate versus placebo

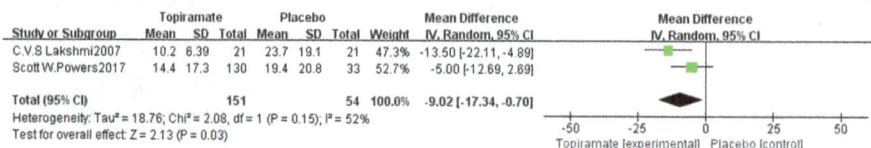

**Fig. 5** Forest plot of comparison: PedMIDAS score of topiramate versus placebo

**Table 3** Side effects/Adverse events occurring in any group and ranked by overall incidence

| Side effects/Adverse events | Topiramate N = 344 | Placebo N = 139 |
|---|---|---|
| Paresthesia | 71(20.64)[a] | 4(2.88) |
| Upper respiratory tract infection | 54(15.7) | 16(9.35) |
| Fatigue | 48(13.95) | 11(7.91) |
| Weight decrease | 39(11.34) | 5(3.59) |
| Abdominal pain | 22(6.40) | 12(8.63) |
| Anorexia | 26(7.56) | 7(5.03) |
| Dry mouth | 26(7.56) | 4(2.88) |
| Pharyngitis | 16(4.65) | 13(9.35) |
| Memory impairment | 24(6.98) | 3(2.16) |
| Injury | 16(4.65) | 11(7.91) |
| Cognitive disorder | 23(6.69) | 4(2.88) |
| Aphasia | 23(6.69) | 3(2.16) |
| Sinusitis | 14(4.07) | 7(5.03) |
| Nausea | 11(3.20) | 5(3.59) |
| Altered mood | 14(4.07) | 2(1.44) |
| Dizziness | 14(4.07) | 1(0.72) |
| Somnolence | 11(3.20) | 3(2.16) |
| Gastroenteritis | 10(2.91) | 3(2.16) |
| Fever | 10(2.91) | 2(1.44) |
| Influenza-like symptoms | 8(2.33) | 2(1.44) |
| Sedation | 4(1.16) | 2(1.44) |
| Rhintis | 5(1.45) | 1(0.72) |
| Insomnia | 4(1.16) | 1(0.72) |
| Viral infection | 4(1.16) | 1(0.72) |
| Back pain | 2(0.58) | 3(2.16) |
| Conjunctivitis | 4(1.16) | 1(0.72) |
| Lack of concentration in school# | 4(1.16) | 0(0) |
| Coughing# | 4(1.16) | 0(0) |
| Taste perversion# | 4(1.16) | 0(0) |
| Abnorma vision | 3(0.87) | 1(0.72) |
| Eye pain | 2(0.58) | 2(1.44) |
| Vomiting | 2(0.58) | 1(0.72) |
| Nervousness# | 3(0.87) | 0(0) |
| Asthma# | 2(0.58) | 0(0) |
| Pneumonia# | 2(0.58) | 0(0) |
| Allergy# | 2(0.58) | 0(0) |
| Respiratory:bronchospasm | 1(0.29) | 1(0.72) |
| Suicide attempt# | 1(0.29) | 0(0) |
| Intussusception# | 1(0.29) | 0(0) |
| Traumatic liver injury# | 1(0.29) | 0(0) |

An individual subject might have experienced more than one side effect or adverse event

[a]Values expressed as N (%)

#Reported only in the topiramate treatment group

## Publication bias

Since our meta-analysis included only four studies, a linear regression test of funnel plot asymmetry (Egger's test) could not be performed.

## Discussion

This meta-analysis examined the efficacy of topiramate in comparison with placebo for the prevention of migraines in patients less than 18 years of age. The IHS guidelines for conducting clinical trials indicate that a clinically meaningful end point in a migraine prevention trial is usually defined by a reduction in the total number of headache attacks in a 28-day period or the proportion of patients with a greater than 50% relative reduction in headache frequency [22].

Topiramate is a first-line option for the treatment of migraines in adults, and in March 2014, the U.S. Food and Drug Administration (FDA) approved topiramate for migraine prevention in the population aged 12 to 17 [23]. Moreover, this is the first and only medication currently approved for use in migraine patients 12 years and over. Nevertheless, neither the primary outcome of proportion of patients with a greater than 50% reduction in headache frequency nor the secondary outcome of reduced mean headache days in a 28-day period showed topiramate as more efficacious than placebo in our meta-analysis of four RCTs. According to the definition [22], topiramate showed no statistically significant benefit over placebo in reducing the number of headache days over the treatment period. In fact, the 50% response rate of the topiramate group in 2 trials [14, 20] was not statistically significant compared with the placebo group, and in another trial [18] a similar result was presented for the 50 mg/day topiramate treatment group. The finding conflicts with the outcomes of previous case series and open-label trials. There are at least three possible explanations for this finding. (1) Children tend to have a high placebo response rate, with younger patients in clinical trials demonstrating a greater tendency to respond to placebo. This age-dependent placebo response has ranged from 30% to 70% in migraine studies in general [24–27]. The outcome of our study shows that the average number of patients experiencing a $\geq 50\%$ relative reduction in headache frequency in the placebo group is 50.74% (69/136), which is higher than the rates reported in previous studies of topiramate preventing adult migraine (0–34.2%) [28–31]. Rothner et al. [32] suggested explanations for the higher placebo response rate in clinical trials with children and adolescents, such as the fact that they could not take medication while at school; "good doctor" effects; and the fact that if their symptoms relieved spontaneously, children and adolescents were more likely than adults to believe that they were receiving a drug that had a definite effect on

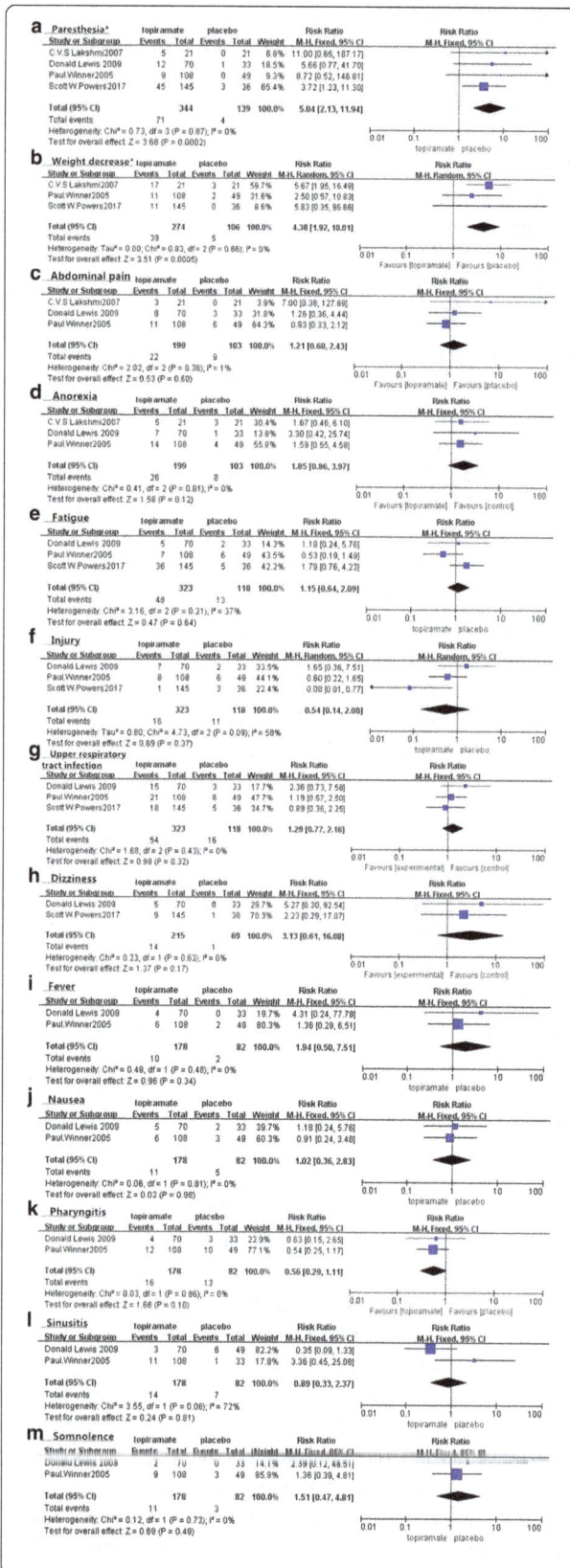

**Fig. 6** Forest plot of comparison: Side effects/adverse events (a-m, respectively, represent paresthesia, weight decrease, abdominal pain, anorexia, fatigue, injury, upper respiratory tract infection, dizziness, fever, nausea, pharyngitis, sinusitis and somnolence) of topiramate versus placebo(*There was a significant difference between topiramate and placebo groups)

headache. We speculate that this phenomenon is associated with at least the following factors: 1. Different psychological and neurobiological mechanisms exist in pediatric patients compared with adults. There are at least four psychological mechanisms associated with the placebo response: expectation, conditioning, therapeutic relationship and empowerment [33]; psychological mechanisms, especially the conditioning and expectation may guide people's behavior. The differential course of the maturation of different neurotransmitter systems may explain the differences. 2. The characteristics of migraine attacks are different [34]: migraine headaches in children and adolescents are often bilateral and may be of shorter duration than in adults. 3. Children/adolescents and adults have significantly different cognitive levels. The pain sensation is a highly subjective experience that is influenced by cognitive factors, and placebo analgesia is one of the most striking examples of cognitive regulation of pain [35, 36]. In addition, the lack of pediatric research and the shortage of experience in experimental design may lead to different outcomes. In short, the topic of the difference about placebo response between children/adolescents and adults deserves further discussion. (2) The minimum age at which topiramate was approved for treatment of migraine was 12 years old, but the minimum age of patients in the included trials was 8 years. It is often difficult to calculate the attacks of headache in younger children accurately, and the guardians generally interpret the attacks indirectly from the child's activity level [19]. (3) Our included patients included those with either episodic or chronic migraine [14], which may influence the results of our meta- analysis.

The second finding of our meta-analysis is that topiramate decreased PedMIDAS scores in migraine patients. PedMIDAS is often used to measure disability related to school absences and functioning, home functioning, and social absences and functioning [16]. This finding, which contradicts our first finding, may indicate that headache-related disability is alleviated by topiramate. However, mean PedMIDAS scores in both the topiramate group and the placebo group decreased between baseline and endpoint, and the fact that only two trials [14, 19] used this tool as a trial assessment may be the cause of the heterogeneity.

As with all antiepileptic drugs, topiramate has many potential side effects or adverse events, some of which may be serious and life-threatening [37]. The rate of adverse events in patients treated with topiramate was higher than that with placebo in our included trials. It has been reported that metabolic acidosis, renal calculi and nervous system effects, such as fatigue or somnolence, paresthesia, dizziness and cognitive disorder or aphasia, occurred in adults and pediatric patients taking topiramate in previous trials. Other adverse events, such as changes in visual acuity, including visual field deficits, acute myopia and secondary closed angle glaucoma, have also been reported. In addition, topiramate (100 mg/day) was related to modest increases in psychomotor reaction times [38]. Another more serious problem is the potential for suicidal behavior and ideation that has been observed in people taking antiepileptic drugs, including topiramate [39]. Thus, while the pathomechanism of migraine is not completely understood, the choice of medication for personalized therapy tailored to each patient needs to be made cautiously [40].

Some limitations in our meta-analysis must be acknowledged. First, because our analysis was limited to articles in the English language literature, we may have omitted some evidence. The secondary limitation is related to the data that we acquired from the four included trials. Three of the trials reported the baseline and follow-up data [14, 18, 19], and one reported baseline and change data [20]. We combined the follow-up and change data according to the research of da Costa, B. R [41]. In addition, one trial compared more than 1 dose [18]; it is likely that dose-finding pharmacologic studies are underrepresented and that additional unpublished industry trials exist. These situations might have resulted in ecological bias. Third, our data had obvious heterogeneity, and none of the variables we abstracted explained this variation. Because we only included four trials and because only three measurements were used in our study, therefore, our findings should be interpreted with caution. The variability in the selection criteria for RCTs and sample size, along with the incomplete reporting of intervention intensity, may also be limitations.

## Conclusions

This is the first meta-analysis of topiramate for migraine prevention in patients less than 18 years of age. We found that topiramate did not achieve a more effective clinical trial endpoint than placebo in the prevention of migraine in patients less than 18 years of age, and topiramate was associated with more adverse events in the included patients. It is possible that a high placebo response rate can be beneficial for children and adolescents with migraine and that drugs used to prevent pediatric migraine might be reconsidered. Because there was a significant placebo response, more placebo-controlled trials in the younger migraine population less than 12 years of age are needed.

## Acknowledgments
This study was supported by National Natural Science Foundation of China (NO. 81471187).
We also acknowledge all clinical investigators of the included studies and patients associated with these studies.

## Authors' contributions
Kai Le, Yijing Guo participated in the whole design of this study. Kai Le, Yijing Guo and Dafan Yu performed the database search, data extraction and analysis. Kai Le, Yijing Guo, Dafan Yu and Jiamin Wang wrote the draft and revised the whole manuscript. All authors read and approved the final version of the manuscript.

## Competing interests
The authors declare that they have no competing interests.

## References
1. Split W, Neuman W (1999) Epidemiology of migraine among students from randomly selected secondary schools in Lodz. Headache 39(7):494–501
2. Kacperski J (2015) Prophylaxis of migraine in children and adolescents. Paediatr Drugs 17(3):217–226. doi:10.1007/s40272-015-0125-5
3. Lewis D, Ashwal S, Hershey A, Hirtz D, Yonker M, Silberstein S (2004) Practice parameter: pharmacological treatment of migraine headache in children and adolescents: report of the American Academy of Neurology quality standards subcommittee and the practice Committee of the Child Neurology Society. Neurology 63(12):2215–2224
4. Lewis DW, Avener M, Gozzo Y (2005) Pediatric migraine, part 1: update on classification, diagnosis, and the evaluation. Headache Pain Diagn Challenges Curr Ther 16(2):81–88
5. Toldo I, De Carlo D, Bolzonella B, Sartori S, Battistella PA (2012) The pharmacological treatment of migraine in children and adolescents: an overview. Expert Rev Neurother 12(9):1133–1142. doi:10.1586/ern.12.104
6. French JA, Kanner AM, Bautista J, Abou-Khalil B, Browne T, Harden CL, Theodore WH, Bazil C, Stern J, Schachter SC et al (2004) Efficacy and tolerability of the new antiepileptic drugs II: treatment of refractory epilepsy: report of the therapeutics and technology assessment subcommittee and quality standards Subcommittee of the American Academy of neurology and the American Epilepsy Society. Neurology 62(8):1261–1273
7. Brandes JL, Saper JR, Diamond M, Couch JR, Lewis DW, Schmitt J, Neto W, Schwabe S, Jacobs D (2004) Topiramate for migraine prevention: a randomized controlled trial. JAMA 291(8):965–973. doi:10.1001/jama.291.8.965
8. Hoffmann J, Akerman S, Goadsby PJ (2014) Efficacy and mechanism of anticonvulsant drugs in migraine. Expert Rev Clin Pharmacol 7(2):191–201. doi:10.1586/17512433.2014.885835
9. Campistol J, Campos J, Casas C, Herranz JL (2005) Topiramate in the prophylactic treatment of migraine in children. J Child Neurol 20(3):251–253
10. Anand KS, Dhikav V, Aggarwal J (2012) Topiramate for migraine prophylaxis. Indian Pediatr 49(4):329–330. doi:10.1007/s13312-012-0040-6
11. Abbaskhanian ASHREAMS (2012) Effective dose of topiramate in pediatric migraine prophylaxis. In J Pediatr Neurosci 7:171–174
12. Fallah R, Divanizadeh MS, Karimi M, Mirouliaei M, Shamszadeh A (2013) Topiramate and propranolol for prophylaxis of migraine. Indian J Pediatr 80(11):920–924. doi:10.1007/s12098-013-0976-0
13. Hershey AD, Powers SW, Vockell ALB, LeCates S, Kabbouche M (2002) Effectiveness of topiramate in the prevention of childhood headaches. Headache 42(8):810–818. doi:10.1046/j.1526-4610.2002.02185.x
14. Powers SW, Coffey CS, Chamberlin LA, Ecklund DJ, Klingner EA, Yankey JW, Korbee LL, Porter LL, Hershey AD (2017) Trial of Amitriptyline, Topiramate, and placebo for pediatric migraine. N Engl J Med 376(2):115–124. doi:10.1056/NEJMoa1610384
15. Higgins JP, Green S (2011) Cochrane Handbook for Systematic Reviews of Interventions Version 5.1.0 (The Cochrane Collaboration).
16. Hershey AD, Powers SW, Vockell AL, LeCates S, Kabbouche MA, Maynard MK (2001) PedMIDAS: development of a questionnaire to assess disability of migraines in children. Neurology 57(11):2034–2039
17. Deeks JJ, Macaskill P, Irwig L (2005) The performance of tests of publication bias and other sample size effects in systematic reviews of diagnostic test accuracy was assessed. J Clin Epidemiol 58(9):882–893. doi:10.1016/j.jclinepi.2005.01.016

18. Lewis D, Winner P, Saper J, Ness S, Polverejan E, Wang S, Kurland CL, Nye J, Yuen E, Eerdekens M et al (2009) Randomized, double-blind, placebo-controlled study to evaluate the efficacy and safety of topiramate for migraine prevention in pediatric subjects 12 to 17 years of age. Pediatrics 123(3):924–934. doi:10.1542/peds.2008-0642

19. Lakshmi CVS, Singhi P, Malhi P, Ray M (2007) Topiramate in the prophylaxis of pediatric migraine: a double-blind placebo-controlled trial. J Child Neurol 22(7):829–835. doi:10.1177/0883073807304201

20. Winner P, Pearlman EM, Linder SL, Jordan DM, Fisher AC, Hulihan J (2005) Topiramate for migraine prevention in children: a randomized, double-blind, placebo-controlled trial. Headache 45(10):1304–1312. doi:10.1111/j.1526-4610.2005.00262.x

21. 2014) The International Classification of Headache Disorders: 2nd edition. Cephalalgia : an international journal of headache, 24 Suppl 1:9–160

22. Tfelt-Hansen P, Pascual J, Ramadan N, Dahlof C, D'Amico D, Diener HC, Hansen JM, Lanteri-Minet M, Loder E, McCrory D et al (2012) Guidelines for controlled trials of drugs in migraine: third edition. A guide for investigators. Cephalalgia Int J Headache 32(1):6–38. doi:10.1177/0333102411417901

23. 2014) FDA approves Topamax for migraine prevention in adolescents. J Pain Palliat Care Pharmacother, 28(2):191

24. Hershey AD (2010) Current approaches to the diagnosis and management of paediatric migraine. Lancet Neurol 9(2):190–204. doi:10.1016/s1474-4422(09)70303-5

25. Aaltonen K, Hamalainen M, Hoppu K (2000) Children's response to placebo in migraine attacks. Cephalalgia Int J Headache 20:385

26. Bendtsen L, Mattsson P, Zwart JA, Lipton RB (2003) Placebo response in clinical randomized trials of analgesics in migraine. Cephalalgia An Int J Headache 23(7):487–490. doi:10.1046/j.1468-2982.2003.00528.x

27. Faria V, Linnman C, Lebel A, Borsook D (2014) Harnessing the placebo effect in pediatric migraine clinic. J Pediatr 165(4):659–665. doi:10.1016/j.jpeds.2014.06.040

28. Silberstein SD, Hulihan J, Karim MR, Wu SC, Jordan D, Karvois D, Kamin M (2006) Efficacy and tolerability of topiramate 200 mg/d in the prevention of migraine with/without aura in adults: a randomized, placebo-controlled, double-blind, 12-week pilot study. Clin Ther 28(7):1002–1011. doi:10.1016/j.clinthera.2006.07.003

29. Diener HC, Bussone G, Van Oene JC, Lahaye M, Schwalen S, Goadsby PJ (2007) Topiramate reduces headache days in chronic migraine: a randomized, double-blind, placebo-controlled study. Cephalalgia : an international journal of headache 27(7):814–823. doi:10.1111/j.1468-2982.2007.01326.x

30. Freitag FG, Forde G, Neto W, Wang DZ, Schmitt J, Wu SC, Hulihan J (2007) Analysis of pooled data from two pivotal controlled trials on the efficacy of topiramate in the prevention of migraine. J Am Osteopath Assoc 107(7):251–258

31. Gupta P, Singh S, Goyal V, Shukla G, Behari M (2007) Low-dose topiramate versus lamotrigine in migraine prophylaxis (the Lotolamp study). Headache 47(3):402–412. doi:10.1111/j.1526-4610.2006.00599.x

32. Rothner AD, Wasiewski W, Winner P, Lewis D, Stankowski J (2006) Zolmitriptan oral tablet in migraine treatment: high placebo responses in adolescents. Headache 46(1):101–109. doi:10.1111/j.1526-4610.2006.00313.x

33. Antonaci F, Chimento P, Diener HC, Sances G, Bono G (2007) Lessons from placebo effects in migraine treatment. J Headache Pain 8(1):63–66. doi:10.1007/s10194-007-0360-4

34. Diener HC, Schorn CF, Bingel U, Dodick DW (2008) The importance of placebo in headache research. Cephalalgia Int J Headache 28(10):1003–1011. doi:10.1111/j.1468-2982.2008.01660.x

35. Kupers R, Faymonville ME, Laureys S (2005) The cognitive modulation of pain: hypnosis- and placebo-induced analgesia. Prog Brain Res 150:251–269. doi:10.1016/s0079-6123(05)50019-0

36. Ploghaus A, Becerra L, Borras C, Borsook D (2003) Neural circuitry underlying pain modulation: expectation, hypnosis, placebo. Trends Cogn Sci 7(5):197–200

37. Oakley CB, Kossoff EH (2014) Migraine and epilepsy in the pediatric population. Curr Pain Headache Rep 18(3):402. doi:10.1007/s11916-013-0402-3

38. Pandina GJ, Ness S, Polverejan E, Yuen E, Eerdekens M, Bilder RM, Ford L (2010) Cognitive effects of topiramate in migraine patients aged 12 through 17 years. Pediatr Neurol 42(3):187–195. doi:10.1016/j.pediatrneurol.2009.10.001

39. Fantasia HC (2014) Migraine headache prophylaxis in adolescents. Nurs Women's Health 18(5):420–424. doi:10.1111/1751-486X.12150

40. Tajti J, Szok D, Csáti A, Vécsei L (2016) Prophylactic drug treatment of migraine in children and adolescents: an update. Curr Pain Headache Rep 20(1):1–9. doi:10.1007/s11916-015-0536-6

41. da Costa BR, Nuesch E, Rutjes AW, Johnston BC, Reichenbach S, Trelle S, Guyatt GH, Juni P (2013) Combining follow-up and change data is valid in meta-analyses of continuous outcomes: a meta-epidemiological study. J Clin Epidemiol 66(8):847–855. doi:10.1016/j.jclinepi.2013.03.009

# The impact of onabotulinumtoxinA on severe headache days: PREEMPT 56-week pooled analysis

Manjit Matharu[1*], Rashmi Halker[2], Patricia Pozo-Rosich[3,4], Ronald DeGryse[5], Aubrey Manack Adams[5] and Sheena K. Aurora[6]

## Abstract

**Background:** OnabotulinumtoxinA has been shown to reduce headache-days among patients with chronic migraine (CM). The objective of this analysis was to determine whether onabotulinumtoxinA has an impact on headache-day severity in patients with CM among those patients who were deemed non-responders based on reduction in the frequency of headache days alone.

**Methods:** Data from the Phase 3 REsearch Evaluating Migraine Prophylaxis Therapy (PREEMPT) clinical trial program (a 24-week, 2-treatment cycle, double-blind, randomized, placebo-controlled, parallel-group phase, followed by a 32-week, 3-treatment cycle, open-label phase) were pooled for analysis. Patients kept a daily diary to record headache severity on a 4-point scale (from none to severe), and a 6-domain Headache Impact Test (HIT-6) was used to determine the clinical impact of headaches. Analysis was undertaken to assess whether the subset of patients that were headache-day frequency non-responders at week 24 (patients with <50% reduction in headache-day frequency) experienced a reduction in headache severity whilst receiving onabotulinumtoxinA.

**Results:** For headache-day frequency non-responders, significant reductions in the number of severe headache days, average daily headache severity, pooled percentage of severe headache days and headache severity score were observed at week 24 for patients who had received onabotulinumtoxinA compared with those who had received placebo. The between-group differences were reduced and non-significant at week 56. Similarly, headache-day frequency non-responders receiving onabotulinumtoxinA were found to have an improvement in the clinical impact of headaches using results from the HIT-6.

**Conclusions:** These results suggest that even those patients with CM who are deemed non-responders based on analysis of headache frequency alone experience clinically meaningful relief from headache intensity following treatment with onabotulinumtoxinA.

**Keywords:** Chronic migraine, OnabotulinumtoxinA, Headache severity, Hit-6, PREEMPT

## Background

Chronic migraine (CM; ≥15 headache days per month for ≥3 consecutive months and with ≥8 days/month of migraine-type headaches) [1] is associated with significant personal, societal, and economic burdens [2–5]. Compared with people with episodic migraine (EM; <15 headache days per month), those with CM experience greater headache intensity, increased pain severity and disability, [2] higher rates of comorbid medical conditions, [2, 4] reduced health-related quality of life, [2] greater economic burden, [6] and reduced productivity. [3, 6].

The Phase 3 REsearch Evaluating Migraine Prophylaxis Therapy (PREEMPT) clinical trial program established the safety and efficacy of onabotulinumtoxinA for CM [7–10]. In PREEMPT 1 and 2, patients were randomized to double-blind treatment with onabotulinumtoxinA or

---
* Correspondence: m.matharu@uclmail.net
[1]University College London (UCL) Institute of Neurology and The National Hospital for Neurology and Neurosurgery, Queen Square, London WC1N3BG, UK
Full list of author information is available at the end of the article

placebo (24 weeks), followed by open-label treatment with onabotulinumtoxinA (32 weeks) [7–10]. Treatment with onabotulinumtoxinA resulted in significant improvements in a variety of efficacy endpoints, including the change in frequency of headache days throughout the double-blind treatment period [10]. Nevertheless, anecdotal reports from treating clinicians have indicated that results from these trials do not fully reflect the patient benefits that are observed in clinical practice. Specifically, it has been suggested that onabotulinumtoxinA treatment may have an impact on other clinical characteristics such as headache-day severity.

In this analysis, we assessed the effect of onabotulinumtoxinA on headache-day severity in patients with CM using pooled data from the PREEMPT clinical trials. Our analysis placed a particular focus on the effect on patients who did not experience a clinically meaningful reduction in the frequency of headache days.

## Methods
Study details have been reported previously, [7, 8] and will be only summarized here.

### Study design
Briefly, PREEMPT 1 was conducted at 56 North American sites from January 2006 to July 2008 and PREEMPT 2 was conducted at 50 North American and 16 European sites from February 2006 to August 2008. The studies consisted of a 28-day baseline screening phase, followed by two 12-week treatment cycles over a 24-week randomized, double-blind, placebo-controlled phase (2 treatment cycles), and then a 32-week open-label phase in which all patients received onabotulinumtoxinA (3 treatment cycles).

The PREEMPT clinical trial program was conducted in accordance with the Declaration of Helsinki and Good Clinical Practice guidelines and was approved by an Independent Ethics Committee. All patients provided written informed consent prior to participation in the clinical trial (ClinicalTrials.gov identifiers: NCT00156910 and NCT00168428).

This post-hoc analysis reports pooled results of both PREEMPT 1 and PREEMPT 2 including data from the double-blind and open-label phases of the trials (a total of 56 weeks).

### Study participants
Men and women were eligible for inclusion if they had a history of migraine and met the *International Classification of Headache Disorders* (*2nd edition*; [*ICHD-2*]) migraine diagnostic criteria, with ≥15 headache days per month (headache day was defined as a calendar day with ≥4 continuous hours of headache), of which ≥50% were considered migraine-type headache days. Patients were excluded from the study if they were experiencing

continuous headaches, had taken headache prophylaxis in the 4 weeks before enrollment into the study or they had previously been treated with a botulinum toxin.

### Study treatment
Patients were randomized (1:1 in blocks of 4, stratified by frequency of acute pain medication use during the 28-day baseline period) [7, 8] to receive either onabotulinumtoxinA (155 U) or placebo for the first 2 treatment cycles. Therapy was administered via intramuscular injection in fixed dosages at 31 fixed-sites across 7 specific head and neck muscle areas. Up to 40 additional units of onabotulinumtoxinA could be administered according to a "follow the pain" strategy, up to a total dosage of 195 U per treatment cycle administered in up to 39 anatomical sites.

### Assessment of outcome measures
A patient daily telephone diary was kept using an interactive voice response system for the duration of the studies including the 28-day baseline screening period. Headache-day severity was collected on a daily basis via the patient diary and assessed every 4 weeks.

In the PREEMPT trials, pooled safety analyses were undertaken for all patients who received at least one dose of onabotulinumtoxinA or placebo.

#### Headache-day severity
In accordance with guidance for controlled trials, [11] the degree of headache severity was rated on a 4-point scale to indicate severe (3), moderate (2) or mild (1), or headache-free (0). The severity of headache days was determined by the maximum severity across all the headache reports for the day. For headaches that lasted >1 calendar day, the reported level of headache severity was applied to each day that the headache lasted for any given headache report. Diary days that were either without any reported headache or with a reported headache of <4 h continuous duration were defined as headache-free days.

Headache-day severity outcomes assessed the change from the baseline period in the number of days with severe headache (as assessed from patient dairies per 28-day period), pooled number of severe headache days (defined as the sum of severe headache days reported across all patients during the previous 28-day period), and the severity responder analysis. A severity responder was defined as a patient who achieved a ≥ 1 grade improvement in average daily headache severity (ADHS) score across the assessment period (e.g., a reduction in headache severity from severe to moderate).

Headache-day severity outcomes were then assessed among those patients who were considered headache-day frequency "non-responders". Headache-day frequency non-responders were defined as patients with <50% reduction in headache-day frequency from the 28-day baseline screening period to week 24, as defined by the number of patient diary-reported days per 28-day period with ≥4 continuous hours of headache.

The 6-Item Headache Impact Test (HIT-6), [12, 13] a 6-domain internet-based survey, was used to assess the impact of headaches on the patient. Response options for each of the 6 questions were: never (scored as 6), rarely (8), sometimes (10), very often (11), and always (13), giving a total possible score of between 36 and 78. If ≥50% of the questions were answered, the total score was extrapolated from the mean score across answered questions. If <50% of the questions were answered, the score was set to missing.

Using the HIT-6 outcomes, patient response was analyzed. Patients who had an improvement in headache severity from baseline (≥1-grade improvement in severity from baseline) and an improvement in their HIT-6 score of ≥5 points were considered to be "responders", as a reduction in HIT-6 scores of ≥5 points from baseline has previously been defined as clinically meaningful [14, 15].

### Statistical analyses
#### Headache-day severity
We assessed the change from baseline in the number of severe headache days. Missing counts were estimated using modified last observation carried forward (mLOCF) techniques. P-values for between-treatment comparisons were calculated using covariate analysis of variance (ANCOVA), with baseline values as the covariate. The main effects in the ANCOVA included treatment and medication-overuse strata, where the type III sum of squares was used.

Statistics were calculated for the number of severe headache days pooled across patients for each time period. Any missing time period data for a patient were estimated using mLOCF. Between-treatment comparisons of the percentage of severe headache days were determined by Pearson's chi-square or Fisher's exact tests (for this parameter and for others discussed below, if ≥25% of the expected cell counts were <5) for each headache-day severity category.

ADHS scores were the average severity score, as assessed by the patient, across all reported diary days, weighted to account for headache days without severity report and rounded to the nearest whole number. Improvement of ≥1 grade in ADHS (e.g. from severe to moderate) included patients with score reduction of at least 1. Statistics were calculated for the change from the baseline severity score. Missing values were estimated using mLOCF. Between-treatment comparisons of the percentage of patients with ≥1-grade improvement in ADHS were determined by Pearson's chi-square or Fisher's exact tests.

#### HIT-6 responder analysis
Similarly, statistics were calculated for baseline and change from baseline for HIT-6 scores to categorize HIT-6 responders, defined as patients with ≥5-point improvement in HIT-6 scores from baseline. For various time periods in the subset of headache-day frequency non-responders, whose headaches had reduced in severity by at least 1 grade by week 24, between-treatment comparisons of HIT-6 responders were determined by Pearson's chi-square or Fisher's exact tests.

### Results
#### Patient disposition and demographics
A total of 1384 patients received either onabotulinumtoxinA (n = 688) or placebo (n = 696) in the 24-week double-blind phase before receiving onabotulinumtoxinA in the open label phase. Baseline demographic and clinical characteristics were similar between the two overall treatment groups (Table 1). The mean patient age at baseline was 41 years, and the mean duration since the onset of CM was 19 years. More than 85% of the patients in both groups were female and more than 60% of patients were using prophylactic medications for migraine prior to enrollment into the study. Patient discontinuation across the 56-week study was 25.4% and 29.3% for the onabotulinumtoxinA and placebo study arms, respectively, with no major differences in the reasons for withdrawal from the study (Fig. 1).

Of the 645 patients that were classified as non-responders at week 24 (i.e. had <50% reduction in headache-day frequency), 285 patients had received onabotulinumtoxinA and 360 patients had received placebo. There were no statistically significant differences in the baseline demographic and clinical characteristics between the 2 non-responder groups (Table 1). The non-responder groups were also largely similar to the overall population; although a slightly higher percentage of the non-responders used prophylactic medications at baseline.

#### Changes in headache severity in headache-day frequency non-responders
Among those with a less than 50% reduction from baseline in headache-day frequency at week 24 (headache-day frequency non-responders), reduction from baseline in the number of severe headache days per 28-day period was significantly greater when treated with onabotulinumtoxinA compared with placebo throughout the 24-week double-blind period (Fig. 2). These between-group differences decreased and were no longer significant in the open-label phase of the study.

In addition, in headache-day frequency non-responders, the percentage of severe headache days pooled across patients was significantly lower throughout the 24-week double-blind period for those treated

**Table 1** Baseline demographic and clinical characteristics for overall PREEMPT group and the non-responder subgroup[a]

| Characteristic | Overall PREEMPT Group | | | Non-Responder Subgroup | | |
|---|---|---|---|---|---|---|
| | O/O (n = 688) | P/O (n = 696) | P-value[b] | O/O (n = 285) | P/O (n = 360) | P-value[b] |
| Mean (SD) age, y | 41.1 (10.4) | 41.5 (10.7) | 0.58 | 42.3 (10.4) | 42.8 (10.5) | 0.56 |
| Age ≥ 40 y, n (%) | 395 (57.4) | 408 (58.6) | 0.65 | 179 (62.8) | 224 (62.2.) | 0.94 |
| Sex, n (%) | | | | | | |
| Female | 603 (87.6) | 593 (85.2) | 0.19 | 242 (84.9) | 309 (85.8) | 0.74 |
| Race/Ethnicity, n (%) | | | 0.60 | | | 0.40 |
| White | 617 (89.7) | 630 (90.5) | | 257 (90.2) | 333 (92.5) | |
| Black | 34 (4.9) | 40 (5.7) | | 15 (5.3) | 17 (4.7) | |
| Hispanic | 27 (3.9) | 19 (2.7) | | 9 (3.2) | 9 (2.5) | |
| Other | 10 (1.5) | 7 (1.0) | | 4 (1.4) | 1 (0.3) | |
| Mean (SD) age of onset of CM, y | 21.2 (11.0) | 21.9 (11.9) | 0.46 | 21.3 (11.4) | 22.5 (12.1) | 0.19 |
| Mean (SD) CM duration, y | 19.4 (12.4) | 19.0 (12.7) | 0.49 | 20.4 (12.2) | 19.7 (12.8) | 0.46 |
| Mean (SD) headache days (≥4 h) per 28-day period | 19.9 (3.7) | 19.8 (3.7) | 0.52 | 20.5 (3.9) | 20.4 (4.0) | 0.61 |
| Prestudy headache prophylactic use, n (%) | 425 (61.8) | 454 (65.2) | 0.18 | 197 (69.1) | 263 (73.1) | 0.29 |
| Acute headache medicine overuse, n (%) | 446 (64.8) | 460 (66.1) | 0.62 | 195 (68.4) | 251 (69.7) | 0.73 |
| Mean (SD) HIT-6 score[c] | 65.5 (4.1) | 65.4 (4.3) | 0.64 | 65.4 (3.8) | 65.3 (4.4) | 0.84 |
| Patients with severe headache impact | | | | | | |
| (HIT-6 total score ≥ 60), %[c] | 93.5 | 92.7 | 0.57 | 93.7 | 92.8 | 0.75 |
| Mean (SD) MSQ score[d] | | | | | | |
| Role restrictive | 38.5 (16.6) | 38.7 (17.3) | 0.97 | 37.9 (16.7) | 38.4 (17.5) | 0.67 |
| Role preventive | 56.0 (21.2) | 56.1 (21.7) | 0.83 | 57.0 (21.9) | 56.1 (21.7) | 0.62 |
| Emotional functioning | 42.1 (24.1) | 42.4 (25.0) | 0.81 | 42.7 (23.6) | 44.6 (24.7) | 0.31 |

CM chronic migraine, HIT-6 6-item Headache Impact Test, MSQ Migraine-Specific Quality of Life Questionnaire, O/O onabotulinumtoxinA in double-blind phase and open-label phase, P/O placebo in double-blind phase and onabotulinumtoxinA in open-label phase, PREEMPT Phase 3 REsearch Evaluating Migraine Prophylaxis Therapy

[a]Nonresponder group = <50% reduction in headache-day frequency at week 24

[b]P-values are the pairwise t-test or the Fisher's exact test between the O/O vs the P/O groups for each respective population group

[c]HIT-6 scores of 36–49 indicate little or no impact; 50–55, some impact; 56–59, substantial impact; 60–78, severe impact

[d]MSQ v2.1 scores range from 0 (poor) to 100 (good)

with onabotulinumtoxinA than those receiving placebo (Fig. 3). These between-group differences decreased during the open-label phase of the trial when both groups of patients received onabotulinumtoxinA and the differences were no longer significant by week 40.

Patients who had at least a 1-grade improvement from baseline in the severity of their headaches based on patient diaries were considered to be severity responders. Among headache-day frequency non-responders, significant reductions in the severity of the headaches occurred more frequently in patients receiving onabotulinumtoxinA than in patients receiving placebo at week 24 (41.1% vs 31.4%; P = 0.011; Table 2). Once all patients were receiving onabotulinumtoxinA in the open-label phase of the trial, between-group differences disappeared and were not significant at week 56 (64.6% vs 65.6%; P = 0.792).

## Analysis based on HIT-6 scores

Separate analysis was undertaken to assess whether HIT-6 scores demonstrated a positive response to treatment (≥5-point increase in HIT-6 scores from baseline, as has previously been deemed to be a positive response to treatment [14, 15]) in patients whose headaches reduced in severity (≥1 grade change in severity). The results were similar to those reported above. At week 24, HIT-6 responder rates were significantly higher for onabotulinumtoxinA than for placebo (62.2% vs 43.5%; P < 0.001), and at week 56, the response rates were similar between treatment groups (74.4% vs 72.0%; P = 0.601; Table 2).

## Safety

The results of the PREEMPT trials previously published confirmed that onabotulinumtoxinA is safe and well tolerated for the long-term prophylactic treatment of CM [9]. Treatment-related adverse events (TRAEs) were consistent with the known safety profile of onabotulinumtoxinA. In the double-blind phase of the study, neck pain (6.7%), muscular weakness (5.5%), eyelid ptosis (3.3%), injection-site pain (3.2%), headache (2.9%),

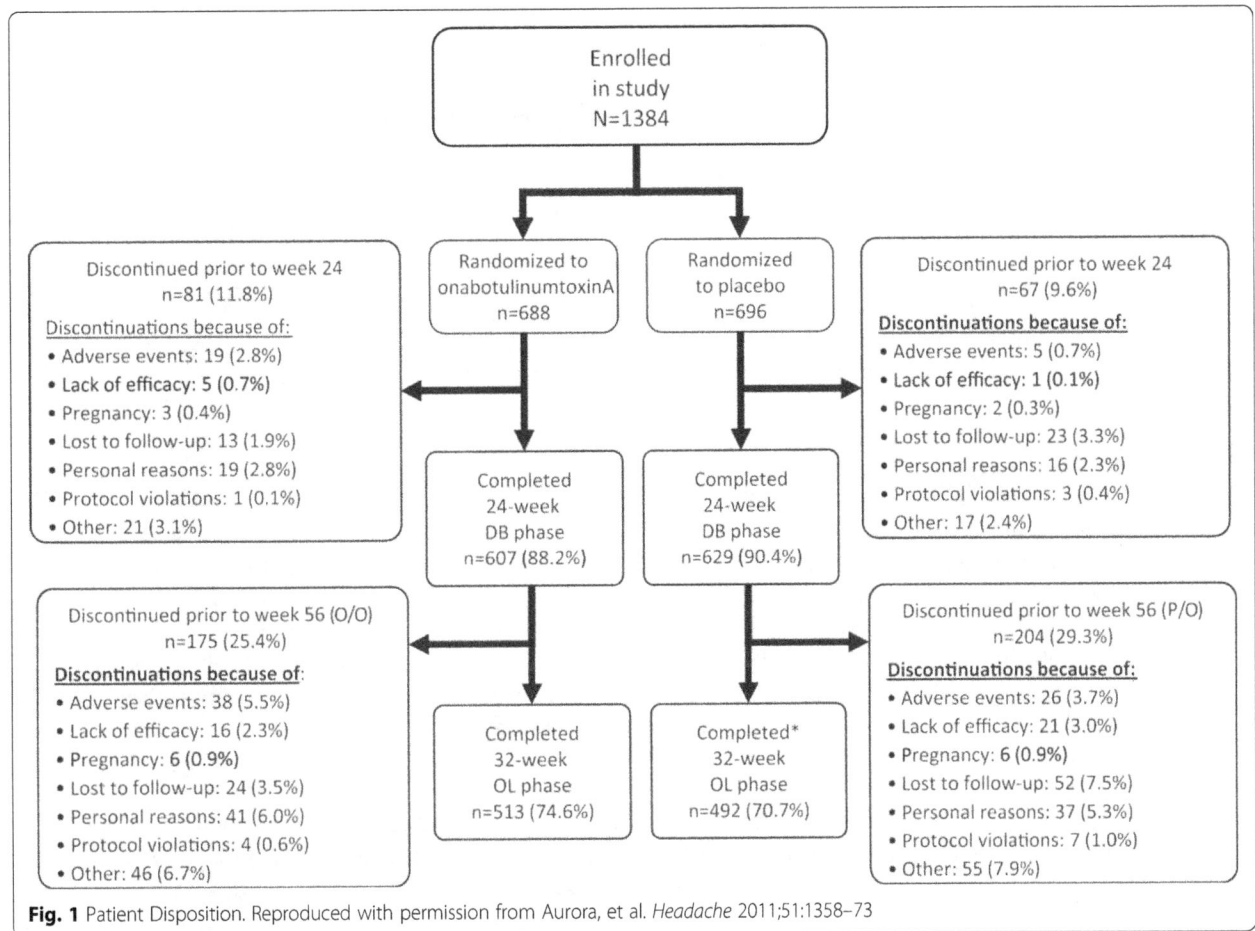

**Fig. 1** Patient Disposition. Reproduced with permission from Aurora, et al. *Headache* 2011;51:1358–73

myalgia (2.6%), musculoskeletal stiffness (2.3%), and musculoskeletal pain (2.2%) were reported by ≥2% of patients receiving onabotulinumtoxinA. TRAE decreased in the open-label phase of the study with neck pain (4.6%), muscular weakness (3.9%), eyelid ptosis (2.5%), muscle tightness (2.2%) and injection site pain (2.0%) the only TRAEs occurring in ≥2% of patients. Serious

TRAEs were rare occurring in 1 patient (0.1%) in both the double-blind and open-label phases of the PRE-EMPT trials.

**Discussion**

In an earlier analysis of the PREEMPT data, it was observed that 49% of patients treated with onabotulinumtoxinA

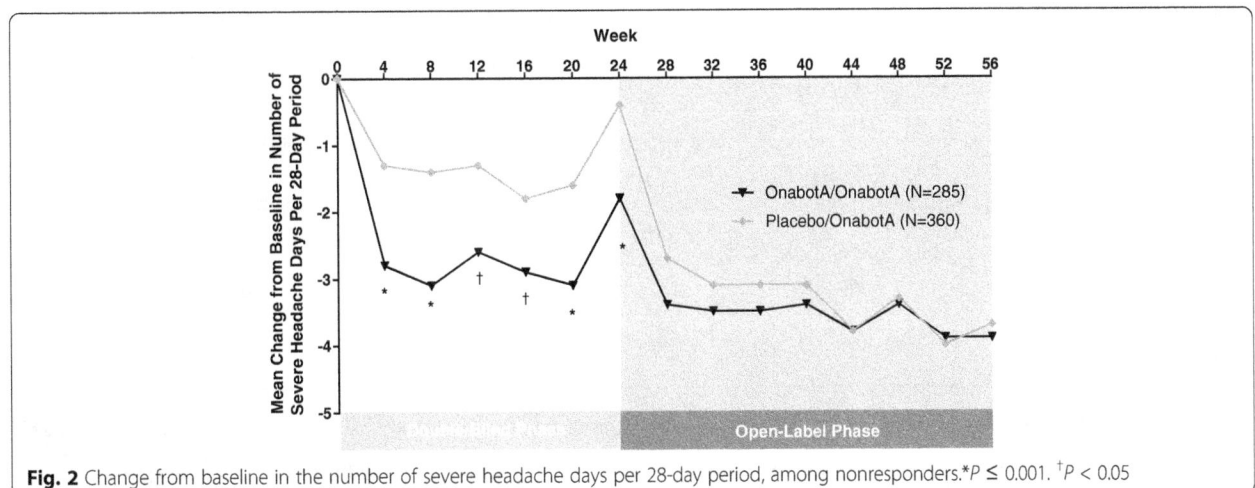

**Fig. 2** Change from baseline in the number of severe headache days per 28-day period, among nonresponders.*$P \leq 0.001$. †$P < 0.05$

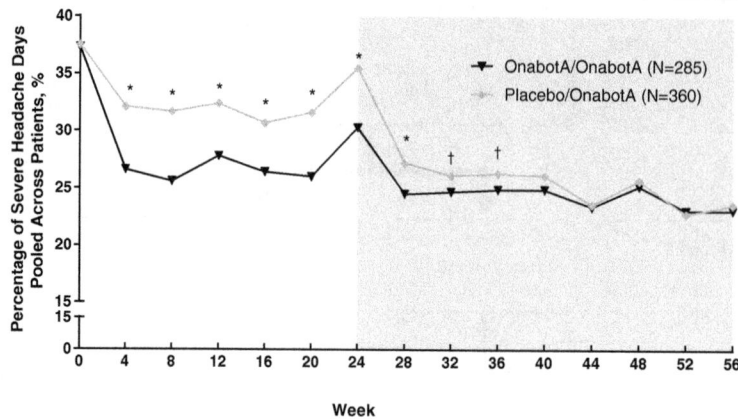

**Fig. 3.** Pooled number of severe headache days, among nonresponders. *$P \leq 0.001$. †$P < 0.05$

demonstrated a ≥ 50% reduction in headache-day frequency after 1 treatment cycle, and an additional 11% who did not respond after the first treatment cycle responded after treatment cycle 2 [16]. In the current analysis, we present data for the effect of onabotulinumtoxinA on headache-day severity among those with CM who did not have a reduction in headache-day frequency after two cycles of treatment (non-responders defined as <50% reduction in headache-day frequency at week 24). During the randomized, placebo-controlled, double-blind phase, patients treated with onabotulinumtoxinA demonstrated a greater reduction from baseline in the number of severe headache days per 28-day period than did those receiving placebo. In addition, compared with the placebo group, there were a lower percentage of patients receiving onabotulinumtoxinA with an ADHS score of severe, a lower percentage of severe headache days pooled across all patients within the onabotulinumtoxinA group, and a higher rate of at least 1-grade improvement in headache severity from baseline (severity responders). Among all severity responders, the proportion of HIT-6 responders (≥5-point improvement from baseline) was greater for the onabotulinumtoxinA group than the placebo group at the end of the double-blind phase.

The headache-day severity endpoints showed a noteworthy peak at week 24 in both onabotulinumtoxinA and placebo treatment groups. The key reason for this non-response peak is the selection criteria, since the population of interest was predefined as those without adequate treatment response in relation to headache-day frequency at week 24. It is interesting that in this group of non-responders, there was some response at other time points both before the arbitrary 24-week non-response point and after that time point.

Open-label results where both groups were receiving onabotulinumtoxinA generally demonstrated lesser between-group differences, with no significant differences between the groups observed by the end of the 56-week study. Conversely, headache-day frequency, as previously reported by Aurora et al., [9] was significantly reduced by onabotulinumtoxinA in the double-blind phase and continued to show between-group differences through to week 56, making a case for early treatment with onabotulinumtoxinA in patients with CM. This observation suggests that treatment with onabotulinumtoxinA produces significant reduction in headache-day severity that may compliment a reduction in headache-

**Table 2** Severity and HIT-6 Responder Analysis

*Proportion of severity responders, among headache-day frequency non-responders[a]*

|  | OnabotulinumtoxinA/ OnabotulinumtoxinA n = 285 | Placebo / OnabotulinumtoxinA n = 360 | P-value |
|---|---|---|---|
| Week 24 | 41.1% | 31.4% | 0.011 |
| Week 56 | 64.6% | 65.6% | 0.792 |

*Proportion of HIT-6 responders, among severity responders[b]*

|  | OnabotulinumtoxinA/ OnabotulinumtoxinA n = 246 | Placebo / OnabotulinumtoxinA n = 161 | P-value |
|---|---|---|---|
| Week 24 | 62.2% | 43.5% | <0.001 |
| Week 56 | 74.4% | 72.0% | 0.601 |

*HIT-6* 6-item Headache Impact Test
[a]Patients with severity response (≥1-grade improvement from baseline in severity), among patients with <50% reduction from baseline in headache-day frequency at week 24
[b]Patients with a HIT-6 response (≥5-point improvement from baseline), among patients with ≥1-grade reduction from baseline in headache-day severity at week 24

day frequency, since onabotulinumtoxinA treatment in the open-label phase was able to eliminate between-group differences in severity, but not frequency. These findings are worthy of further investigation to fully understand the potential therapeutic benefit of early treatment with onabotulinumtoxinA.

Importantly, the current analysis demonstrated reduced headache-day severity at the first post-baseline assessment (week 4) in patients who were headache-day frequency non-responders at week 24, suggesting an important clinical response to treatment not captured by the measure of headache-day frequency reduction. Furthermore, the alignment of the HIT-6 response with the severity response suggests that the reduction in headache-day severity of at least 1 grade was clinically meaningful. Further study is required to determine whether this clinical response translates into a reduction in healthcare resource utilization and broader economic benefits.

The large number of patients with CM included in these double-blind placebo-controlled studies makes these results particularly robust. The use of the voice interactive daily telephone diary encouraged high patient compliance with diary record keeping and captured data without the need for reliance on long-term recall. This would be expected to result in more accurate capture of patient data, as others have shown that current health status can have an impact upon a patient's recollection of the past [17].

The study is not without its limitations. The lack of an active comparator is a potential limitation. However, the lack of any approved prophylactic treatment for CM makes it difficult to identify an appropriate comparator. The time point to determine headache-day frequency nonresponse was set at week 24, which was an arbitrary time point. The selection of a different time point for the definition of non-response may have resulted in different outcomes. Further clinical trials may be required to understand if a different time point for the determination of headache-day frequency non-response has any clinically meaningful impact on the interpretation of the data presented here.

Similarly, no optimal responder rate for the reduction from baseline in headache-day frequency has been defined for the CM population. Although both 30% and 50% cutoffs for headache measures have been suggested to be clinically meaningful, [11] a 50% cutoff is more commonly used in migraine studies, and provided the rationale for the definition of non-responders for the current analysis. Analysis of the current data using a <30% reduction in headache-day frequency as the definition for non-response produced similar results to those reported here, with those classified as non-

responders achieving a significant reduction in headache severity (Additional file 1: Table S1, and Figures S1 and S2). This additional analysis using <30% as the cutoff further strengthens the findings of this analysis.

The International Headache Society has published guidelines for clinical trial assessment of prophylactic treatment for CM, including guidelines on the selection of outcome measures [11]. The primary end-point outcomes recommended by these international experts include headache days with moderate or severe intensity, migraine days, or frequency of migraine episodes. However, despite this international accord on the selection of outcome measures to encourage robust clinical trials, the outcomes may not fully align with the patient's expectation of therapy. This study demonstrates that frequency day response alone may not be sufficient to determine a clinically meaningful response to therapy, and highlights the need for further work on developing key patient-endorsed outcome measures for the assessment of prophylactic treatment of chronic migraine in particular and headache disorders in general.

## Conclusions

Patients from the PREEMPT clinical trial program who received onabotulinumtoxinA and met our definition for headache-day frequency non-response (<50% reduction in headache-day frequency at week 24) demonstrated significantly reduced headache-day severity (compared with those receiving placebo). Among those who showed reduced headache-day severity, onabotulinumtoxinA also produced greater reduction in headache impact scores. These results suggest that patients with CM experience clinically meaningful relief from headache intensity following treatment with onabotulinumtoxinA, even among those who may not experience a clinically meaningful reduction in the frequency of their headaches.

**Abbreviations**
ADHS: Average daily headache severity; ANCOVA: Analysis of covariance; CM: Chronic migraine; HIT-6: 6-Item Headache impact test; *ICHD-2: International classification of headache disorders (2nd Edition)*; mLOCF: Modified last observation carried forward; PREEMPT: Phase 3 REsearch Evaluating Migraine Prophylaxis Therapy; TRAE: Treatment-related adverse event

**Acknowledgments**
Editorial support for development of this manuscript was provided by Amanda Kelly, MPhil, MSHN, and Lee Hohaia, PharmD, of Complete Healthcare Communications. LLC (Chadds Ford, PA), a CHC Group company, and funded by Allergan plc (Dublin, Ireland). All authors met the ICMJE

authority criteria. Neither honoraria nor payments were made for authorship.

## Funding

Allergan plc (Dublin, Ireland) funded the study.

## Authors' contributions

Drs. Matharu, Halker, Pozo-Rosich, Manack Adams, and Aurora made substantial contributions to conception and design, or acquisition of data, or analysis and interpretation of data. All authors have been involved in drafting the manuscript or revising it critically for important intellectual content. All authors have given final approval of the version to be published. Each author has participated sufficiently in the work to take public responsibility for appropriate portions of the content.
Dr. Matharu has agreed to be accountable for all aspects of the work in ensuring that questions related to the accuracy or integrity of any part of the work are appropriately investigated and resolved.

## Competing interests

**Dr. Matharu** has received consulting fees/honoraria from Allergan plc, Saint Jude Medical, Medtronic and electroCore. **Dr. Halker** has received honoraria from Medlink Neurology, New England Journal of Medicine Journal Watch Neurology, and Current Neurology and Neuroscience Reports. **Dr. Pozo-Rosich** has received consulting fees/honoraria from Allergan plc. **Mr. DeGryse** and **Dr. Manack Adams** are employees of Allergan plc and may own stock in the company. **Dr. Aurora** is a full-time employee of Lilly and has received consulting fees/honoraria from Allergan plc, eNeura, Merck, and Teva and speaker's bureau participation for Allergan plc.

## Author details

[1]University College London (UCL) Institute of Neurology and The National Hospital for Neurology and Neurosurgery, Queen Square, London WC1N3BG, UK. [2]Mayo Clinic, Department of Neurology, 5777 East Mayo Blvd, Phoenix, AZ 85054, USA. [3]Headache and Pain Research Group, Institut de Recerca, Universitat Autònoma de Barcelona, Barcelona, Spain. [4]Neurology Department, Vall d'Hebron University Hospital, P.de la Vall d'Hebron, 119-129 08035 Barcelona, Spain. [5]Allergan plc, 2525 Dupont Dr, Irvine, CA, USA. [6]Formerly of the Department of Neurology, Stanford University, 300 Pasteur Dr. Room A301 MC 5325, Stanford, CA, USA.

## References

1. Headache Classification Committee of the International Headache Society (2013) The international classification of headache disorders, 3rd edition (beta version). Cephalalgia 33:629–808. doi:10.1177/0333102413485658
2. Blumenfeld AM, Varon SF, Wilcox TK, Buse DC, Kawata AK, Manack A, Goadsby PJ, Lipton RB (2011) Disability, HRQoL and resource use among chronic and episodic migraineurs: results from the international burden of migraine study (IBMS). Cephalalgia 31:301–315. doi:10.1177/0333102410381145
3. Bigal ME, Serrano D, Reed M, Lipton RB (2008) Chronic migraine in the population: burden, diagnosis, and satisfaction with treatment. Neurology 71:559–566. doi:10.1212/01.wnl.0000323925.29520.e7
4. Buse DC, Manack Adams A, Serrano D, Turkel C, Lipton RB (2010) Sociodemographic and comorbidity profiles of chronic migraine and episodic migraine sufferers. J Neurol Neurosurg Psychiatry 81:428–432. doi: 10.1136/jnnp.2009.192492
5. Manack Adams A, Serrano D, Buse DC, Reed ML, Marske V, Fanning KM, Lipton RB (2015) The impact of chronic migraine: the chronic migraine epidemiology and outcomes (CaMEO) study methods and baseline results. Cephalalgia 35:563–578. doi:10.1177/0333102414552532
6. Munakata J, Hazard E, Serrano D, Klingman D, Rupnow MF, Tierce J, Reed M, Lipton RB (2009) Economic burden of transformed migraine: results from the American migraine prevalence and prevention (AMPP) study. Headache 49:498–508. doi:10.1111/j.1526-4610.2009.01369.x
7. Aurora SK, Dodick DW, Turkel CC, DeGryse RE, Silberstein SD, Lipton RB,

Diener HC, Brin MF (2010) OnabotulinumtoxinA for treatment of chronic migraine: results from the double-blind, randomized, placebo-controlled phase of the PREEMPT 1 trial. Cephalalgia 30:793–803. doi:10.1177/0333102410364676
8. Diener HC, Dodick DW, Aurora SK, Turkel CC, DeGryse RE, Lipton RB, Silberstein SD, Brin MF (2010) OnabotulinumtoxinA for treatment of chronic migraine: results from the double-blind, randomized, placebo-controlled phase of the PREEMPT 2 trial. Cephalalgia 30:804–814. doi:10.1177/0333102410364677
9. Aurora SK, Winner P, Freeman MC, Spierings EL, Heiring JO, DeGryse RE, VanDenburgh AM, Nolan ME, Turkel CC (2011) OnabotulinumtoxinA for treatment of chronic migraine: pooled analyses of the 56-week PREEMPT clinical program. Headache 51:1358–1373. doi:10.1111/j.1526-4610.2011.01990.x
10. Dodick DW, Turkel CC, DeGryse RE, Aurora SK, Silberstein SD, Lipton RB, Diener HC, Brin MF (2010) OnabotulinumtoxinA for treatment of chronic migraine: pooled results from the double-blind, randomized, placebo-controlled phases of the PREEMPT clinical program. Headache 50:921–936. doi:10.1111/j.1526-4610.2010.01678.x
11. Silberstein S, Tfelt-Hansen P, Dodick DW, Limmroth V, Lipton RB, Pascual J, Wang SJ (2008) Guidelines for controlled trials of prophylactic treatment of chronic migraine in adults. Cephalalgia 28:484–495. doi:10.1111/j.1468-2982.2008.01555.x
12. Kosinski M, Bayliss MS, Bjorner JB, Ware JE Jr, Garber WH, Batenhorst A, Cady R, Dahlof CG, Dowson A, Tepper S (2003) A six-item short-form survey for measuring headache impact: the HIT-6. Qual Life Res 12:963–974
13. Yang M, Rendas-Baum R, Varon SF, Kosinski M (2011) Validation of the headache impact test (HIT-6) across episodic and chronic migraine. Cephalalgia 31:357–367. doi:10.1177/0333102410379890
14. Bayliss MS, Batenhorst A (2002) The HIT-6™: a user's guide USA. QualityMetric, Inc, Lincoln, RI
15. Lipton RB, Varon SF, Grosberg B, McAllister PJ, Freitag F, Aurora SK, Dodick DW, Silberstein SD, Diener HC, DeGryse RE, Nolan ME, Turkel CC (2011) OnabotulinumtoxinA improves quality of life and reduces impact of chronic migraine. Neurology 77:1465–1472. doi:10.1212/WNL.0b013e318232ab65
16. Silberstein SD, Dodick DW, Aurora SK, Diener HC, DeGryse RE, Lipton RB, Turkel CC (2015) Per cent of patients with chronic migraine who responded per onabotulinumtoxinA treatment cycle: PREEMPT. J Neurol Neurosurg Psychiatry 86:996–1001. doi:10.1136/jnnp-2013-307149
17. McGlothlin AE, Lewis RJ (2014) Minimal clinically important difference: defining what really matters to patients. JAMA 312:1342–1343. doi:10.1001/jama.2014.13128

# Therapeutical approaches to paroxysmal hemicrania, hemicrania continua and short lasting unilateral neuralgiform headache attacks: a critical appraisal

Carlo Baraldi[*], Lanfranco Pellesi, Simona Guerzoni, Maria Michela Cainazzo and Luigi Alberto Pini

## Abstract

**Background:** Hemicrania continua (HC), paroxysmal hemicrania (PH) and short lasting neuralgiform headache attacks (SUNCT and SUNA) are rare syndromes with a difficult therapeutic approach. The aim of this review is to summarize all articles dealing with treatments for HC, PH, SUNCT and SUNA, comparing them in terms of effectiveness and safety.

**Methods:** A survey was performed using the pubmed database for documents published from the 1st January 1989 onwards. All types of articles were considered, those ones dealing with symptomatic cases and non-English written ones were excluded.

**Results:** Indomethacin is the best treatment both for HC and PH. For the acute treatment of HC, piroxicam and celecoxib have shown good results, whilst for the prolonged treatment celecoxib, topiramate and gabapentin are good options besides indomethacin. For PH the best drug besides indomethacin is piroxicam, both for acute and prolonged treatment. For SUNCT and SUNA the most effective treatments are intravenous or subcutaneous lidocaine for the acute treatment of active phases and lamotrigine for the their prevention. Other effective therapeutic options are intravenous steroids for acute treatment and topiramate for prolonged treatment. Non-pharmacological techniques have shown good results in SUNCT and SUNA but, since they have been tried on a small number of patients, the reliability of their efficacy is poor and their safety profile mostly unknown.

**Conclusions:** Besides a great number of treatments tried, HC, PH, SUNCT and SUNA management remains difficult, according with their unknown pathogenesis and their rarity, which strongly limits the studies upon these conditions. Further studies are needed to better define the treatment of choice for these conditions.

## Background

Trigeminal autonomic cephalalgias (TACs) is a rare group of headaches characterized by unilateral attacks of severe throbbing pain, mainly localized in the orbital region, associated with unilateral cranial autonomic signs such as lacrimation, conjunctival injection, palpebral ptosis, rhinorrhoea, eyelid edema, facial sweating, facial redness and ear-fullness. The International Classification of Headache Disorders 3rd Edition beta version (ICHD-III-beta) recognizes 4 TACs: cluster headache (CH), hemicrania continua (HC), paroxysmal hemicrania (PH) and short-lasting unilateral neuralgiform headache attacks (SUNCT and SUNA) [1]. HC is characterized by a continuous background of moderate pain intensity and has only recently been classified as a TAC [2]; on the contrary, CH, PH, SUNCT and SUNA lack the history of background pain [1]. TACs rather than CH are uncommon and neglected syndromes: the annual prevalence of PH and short lasting unilateral neuralgiform headache attacks is about 0.5/1000 in the general population and is still unknown for HC [3], this facilitate their misdiagnosis, which often delays the correct treatment [4]. Treatment delay, especially in chronic forms, dramatically decreases the patients' quality of life because pain is often severe, highly-disabling and can last, even if not continuously, for many hours during the day [5]. Only a

* Correspondence: infocarlo.baraldi@gmail.com
Medical Toxicology - Headache and Drug Abuse Centre, University of Modena and Reggio Emilia, Via del Pozzo 71, 41124 Modena, Italy

few therapeutic tools are available for these conditions and this is firstly due to their infrequent diagnosis, which makes the conduction of well-prepared randomized clinical placebo-controlled trials (RCPCTs) almost impossible. The effectiveness and safety of the treatments are reported mainly in case-reports, case-series, letters to the editor and brief communications. This leads to a not-scheduled treatment for TACs and the absence of shared guidelines. Furthermore, there aren't studies clearly ranking treatments to manage TACs, nor one comparing them in terms of effectiveness and/or safety. The aim of this study is to rank all therapeutic options available in literature for HC, PH, SUNCT and SUNA treatment and to compare, when possible, their effectiveness and safety. Since there are already shared guide-lines and a large amount of reviews dealing with CH, this won't be discussed further.

## Methods
### Search strategy
A MEDLINE search using the electronic data-base pubmed has been performed to check all articles dealing with the treatment of primary HC, PH, SUNCT and SUNA form the 1st of January 1989 (the first complete year in which the first International Headache Society classification was available) onwards. All articles types were considered and non-English written ones were excluded. The research was performed using the following terms: "((paroxysmal hemicrania) AND ("1989/01/01"[Date - Publication]: "3000"[Date - Publication])) AND English[Language]" for PH, "((hemicrania continua) AND ("1989/01/01"[Date - Publication]: "3000"[Date - Publication])) AND English[Language]" for HC, "((short lasting neuralgiform headache attacks) AND ("1989/01/01"[Date - Publication]: "3000"[Date - Publication])) AND English[Language]" for SUNCT and SUNA. Short lasting unilateral neuralgiform headache attack was treated as one entity, not differentiating between short lasting neuralgiform headache attacks with conjunctival injection and tearing (SUNCT) and short lasting neuralgiform headache attacks with autonomic signs (SUNA). A few articles cited in the references of the above-mentioned ones were cited even though they were not present in pubmed, but were found in SCOPUS and EMBASE.

## Data
Altogether, 691 articles were found of which 290 articles for HC, 250 for PH and 151 for short lasting unilateral neuralgiform headache attacks. Cited articles should fulfill the ICHD-III beta guide-lines for TACs diagnosis, not deal with a symptomatic case and correctly state treatment. Reviews were considered only if new cases were included. For HC, 230 articles were excluded: 67 summarized results from other studies without adding any new case, 138 didn't deal

with HC therapy and 24 referred to symptomatic cases. For PH, 195 articles were excluded: 67 reported and summarized only the results of different works, 90 didn't consider PH therapy or described it unsatisfactorily, 29 referred to symptomatic PH and 9 didn't fulfill all ICHD-III diagnostic criteria, making a diagnosis of "probable PH". For SUNCT and SUNA 95 articles were excluded: 60 were reviews, 20 of them didn't deal with SUNCT or SUNA therapy or reported it unsatisfactorily, 11 reported symptomatic cases and 4 didn't full-filled all diagnostic criteria. Steps followed for article selection are summarized in Fig. 1. For every article, each patient was analyzed and only those treatments correctly stated in terms of regimen and response were considered. If a patient took a drug in different dosages or underwent a non-pharmacological procedure following different regimens, only the one giving the maximum effect was considered. Every patient was classified as a responder if he/she was accredited with, at least, a partial relief. Moreover, as to grade the different therapies better, pain-free patients were sub-classified as complete responders. Finally, the signaled AEs were collected. Since all these diseases are characterized by exacerbations periods in which pain attacks develops and inter-critic periods in which pain is absent (PH, SUNCT and SUNA) or slight-moderate (HC), treatments were divided in two categories: treatments used to cease attacks during exacerbations and treatments taken regularly to control pain (especially in HC), trying to prevent the incoming of new active phases. The first treatments were indicated as "acute treatments", whilst the second as "prolonged treatments". Some acute treatments in HC and PH were used also to control pain outside exacerbations and were both considered as acute and prolonged treatments.

Drug mean dosage and therapeutic standards for non-pharmacological treatments were considered and summarized, even if not statistically analyzed.

Treatments used in less than five patients or which were clearly ineffective were not pooled in the statistical analysis, even if reported. Data regarding treatments used in 5 or more patients are summarized in Table 1, those ones regarding treatments used in less than 5 patients are reported in the Additional file 1: Table S1.

### Statistical analysis
Continuous data were expressed as mean ± standard deviation. Binary variables were express as proportion and percentages. Odds and odds ratios (OR) were considered for statistical analysis. Continuous data and odds were approximated at the second decimal figure, OR and all $p$-values at the third. Statistical analysis was performed using the STATAIc 13 software. For every syndrome, the odds of responders, complete responders, AEs and AEs causing treatment reduction or discontinuation were compared based on the test of the equality of odds.

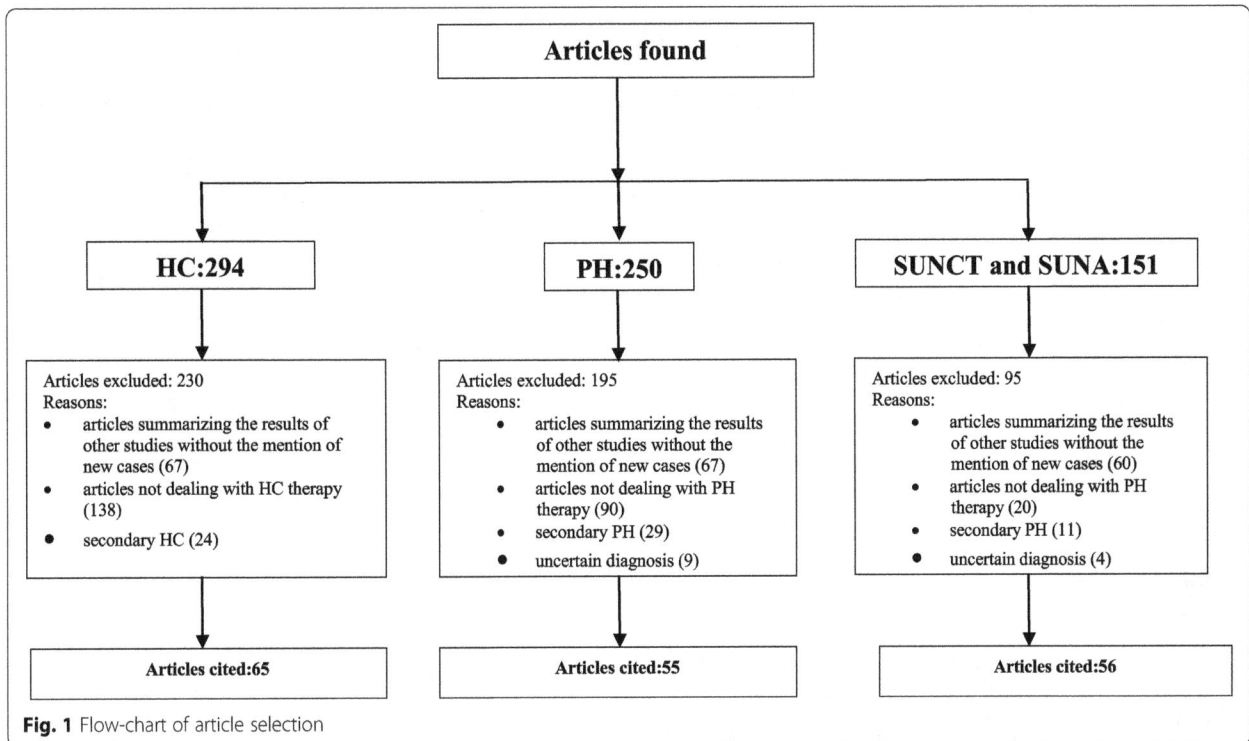

**Fig. 1** Flow-chart of article selection

## Results

### Hemicrania continua (HC)

Globally, 65 articles were considered for the statistical analysis [6–70]. Indomethacin was referred to as the most widely used treatment for HC. Melatonin was used in 17 patients, gabapentin and topiramate were utilized in 13 patients, onabotulinumtoxinA (OnabotA) in 12 patients and celecoxib in 11 patients. The other drugs were used in less than 10 patients. Supraorbital nerve blockade (SONB) was used on 17 patients, great occipital nerve blockade (GONB) on 15, occipital nerve stimulation (ONS) on 14 patients and minor occipital nerve blockade (MONB) on 6 patients.

Other drugs rather than indomethacin were used before indomethacin was given in 60% of cases, but only in the 20% of cases data were good enough to be considered (data not shown). Alternatively, since indomethacin was stopped in the 30% of cases because of its related AEs, other treatments were tried. Pharmacological treatments used in at least 5 patients, are summarized in Table 1 (section A). Statistical comparisons between the odds of responders and complete responders are summarized in Table 2 for the acute treatments and in Table 3 for the prolonged treatments. Data regarding those treatments performed in less than 5 patients are reported in Additional file 1: Table S1 (section A).

### Effectiveness

**Acute treatments** Indomethacin, supraorbital nerve blockade (SONB), great occipital nerve blockade (GONB),

celecoxib, piroxicam, minor occipital nerve blockade (MONB), oxygen, sumatriptan, methylprednisolone, ibuprofen, dorsal root ganglion blockade (DRGB), sphenopalatine ganglion blockade (SPGB) and ergotamine were the drugs considered for exacerbation management in HC.

Oxygen, minor occipital nerve blockade (MONB) and sumatriptan seemed to have no effect on HC and no responders have been registered; for this reason they weren't pooled in the statistical analysis. Ergotamine, ibuprofen, DRGB, SPGB and methylprednisolone weren't pooled in the statistical analysis because of the small number of patients treated with these. Indomethacin has a significantly higher odds of responders than celecoxib ($p < 0.001$), piroxicam ($p < 0.001$) and GONB ($p < 0.001$), but a similar proportion of responders than SONB, which reduced painful symptoms in each patient ($p = 0.541$). Indomethacin has also the highest odds of complete responders, even if compared with SONB (all $p < 0.001$). Considering other treatments rather than indomethacin, piroxicam and celecoxib haven't shown a significantly different odds of responders ($p = 0.837$) and complete responders ($p = 0.219$). Celecoxib has a higher odds of responders than GONB ($p = 0.037$) and a significantly higher odds of complete responders than GONB ($p < 0.001$) and SONB ($p = 0.028$). Finally, SONB shows a significantly higher odds of responders than GONB ($p < 0.001$), but a similar odds of pain-free patients ($p = 0.105$). All comparisons are summarized in Table 2.

**Table 1** Treatment options for HC, PH and SLUNHA used in, at least, 5 patients

| Treatment | Number of patients | Mean dosage ±SD* [range] | Route of administration | Responders proportion % [95% CI] | Complete responders proportion % [95% CI] | AE proportion % [95% CI] | AE causing the stoppage or reduction of therapy proportion % [95% CI] | References |
|---|---|---|---|---|---|---|---|---|
| Section A- Hemicrania continua | | | | | | | | |
| *Acute treatments* | | | | | | | | |
| Indomethacin | 159 | Adult: 145 ± 125 [25–325] Pediatric: 100 ± 50 [25–175] | IM 1.3% REC 0.6% OS 98.1% | 157/159 99 [97–100] | 151/159 95 [92–98] | 75/83 90 | 46/83 55 | [6–61] |
| SONB | 17 | ** | | 17/17 100 | 5/17 29 [8–50] | - | - | [62–64] |
| GONB | 15 | *** | | 6/15 40 [15–65] | 1/15 7 [0–19] | - | - | [10, 35, 43, 48, 62] |
| Celecoxib | 11 | 528 ± 241 [200–800] | OS 100% | 9/11 82 [59–100] | 8/11 73 [46–100] | - | - | [32, 49, 52, 65] |
| Piroxicam | 7 | 37 ± 10 [20–40] | OS 100% | 6/7 86 [60–100] | 5/7 71 [38–100] | - | - | [40, 66] |
| MONB | 6 | 0.5–1.5 mg/ml solution with 12μg/m andrenaline | | 0/6 0 | 0/6 0 | - | - | [62] |
| Oxygen | 13 | 8 ± 5a | INAL 100% | 0/13 0 | 0/13 0 | - | - | [39, 47] |
| Sumatriptan | 8 | 6 | SC 100% | 0/7 0 | 0/7 0 | - | - | [32, 67] |
| *Prolonged treatments* | | | | | | | | |
| Indomethacin | 159 | Adult:115 ± 100 [25–225] Pediatric:55 ± 35 [25–75]c | IM 1.3% REC 0.6% OS 98.1% | 157/159 99 [97–100] | 151/159 95 [92–98] | 75/83 90 | 46/83 55 | [6–61] |
| SONB | 17 | ** | | 17/17 100 | 5/17 29 [8–50] | - | - | [62–64] |
| Melatonin | 17 | 12 [3–30] | OS 100% | 9/17 53 [29–77] | 5/17 29 [8–50] | 6/13 45 | 3/13 23 | [13, 21, 31, 33, 37, 48] |
| GONB | 15 | *** | | 6/15 40 [15–65] | 1/15 7 [0–19] | - | - | [10, 35, 43, 48, 62] |
| ONS | 14 | **** | | 12/14 84 [68–100] | 3/14 21 [3–39] | - | - | [10, 33, 68] |
| Gabapentin | 13 | 1600 [600–3600] | OS 100% | 11/13 85 [65–100] | 6/13 46 [19–73] | 4/9 44 | 0/9 0 | [7, 21, 32, 43, 55, 69] |
| Topiramate | 13 | 133 [50–300] | OS 100% | 11/13 85 [65–100] | 8/13 62 [35–89] | 2/7 29 | 2/7 29 | [11, 24, 28, 29, 36, 38, 43, 49, 70] |

**Table 1** Treatment options for HC, PH and SLUNHA used in, at least, 5 patients (*Continued*)

| Treatment | N | Dose | Route | | | | | References |
|---|---|---|---|---|---|---|---|---|
| OnabotulinumtoxinA | 12 | 155^b [100–185] | SC 100% | 12/12 100 | 4/12 33 [6–60] | – | – | [22, 43] |
| Celecoxib | 11 | 528 ± 241 [200–800] | OS 100% | 9/11 82 [59–100] | 8/11 73 [46–100] | – | – | [32, 49, 52, 65] |
| Verapamil | 8 | 265 [120–480] | OS 100% | 3/8 38 [4–72] | 0/8 0 | 1/1 100 | 1/1 100 | [7, 21, 32, 43, 55, 69] |
| Piroxicam | 7 | 37 ± 10 [20–40] | OS 100% | 6/7 86 [60–100] | 5/7 71 [38–100] | – | – | [40, 66] |
| MONB | 6 | 0.5–1.5 mg/ml solution with 12µrg/m andrenaline | | 0/6 0 | 0/6 0 | – | – | [62] |
| **Section B- Paroxysmal hemicrania** | | | | | | | | |
| *Acute treatments* | | | | | | | | |
| Indomethacin | 168 | Adult: 97 ± 39 Pediatric: 35 ± 27 | OS 95% IM 0.6% RECTAL 4.4% | 163/168 97 [94–100] | 150/168 89 [85–94] | 42/78 54 [43–64] | 21/78 27 [17–37] | [26, 38, 53, 60, 71–118] |
| Sumatriptan | 24 | 6 | SC 100% | 5/24 21 [5–37] | 1/24 4 [0–8] | 1/1 100 | 1/1 100 | [38, 76, 84, 103, 104, 114] |
| Oxygen | 11 | 7 ± 4^a | INAL 100% | 6/18 33 [11–55] | 0/18 0 | – | – | [38, 89, 119] |
| SONB | 6 | ** | | 0/6 0 | 0/6 0 | – | – | [62] |
| GONB | 6 | ** | | 0/6 0 | 0/6 0 | – | – | [62] |
| MONB | 6 | ** | | 0/6 0 | 0/6 0 | – | – | [62] |
| Piroxicam | 5 | 36 ± 9 | OS 100% | 3/5 60 [17–100] | 2/5 40 [0–80] | – | – | [66] |
| *Prolonged treatments* | | | | | | | | |
| Indomethacin | 168 | Adult: 97 ± 39 Pediatric: 35 ± 27^c | OS 95% IM 0.6% RECTAL 4.4% | 163/168 97 [94–100] | 150/168 89 [85–94] | 42/78 54 [43–64] | 21/78 27 [17–37] | [26, 38, 53, 60, 70–118] |
| Verapamil | 30 | Adult: 248 ± 87 Pediatric: 200 ± 70 | OS 100% | 14/30 47 [26–64] | 5/30 17 [3–31] | 2/3 66 | 1/3 33 | [38, 81, 83, 87, 91, 92, 98, 101, 103, 111, 115] |
| Carbamazepine | 15 | 803 ± 275 | OS 100% | 3/15 20 [0–40] | 0/15 0 | – | – | [84, 98, 101, 107, 110, 120] |
| Topiramate | 12 | Adult: 172 ± 75 Pediatric: 48 ± 3 | OS 100% | 9/12 75 [50–99] | 5/12 42 [14–70] | 2/2 100 | 2/2 100 | [38, 75, 93, 101, 105, 109, 115] |
| SONB | 6 | ** | | 0/6 0 | 0/6 0 | – | – | [62] |
| GONB | 6 | ** | | 0/6 0 | 0/6 0 | – | – | [62] |

**Table 1** Treatment options for HC, PH and SLUNHA used in, at least, 5 patients (Continued)

| Treatment | N | Dose | Route | | | | | References |
|---|---|---|---|---|---|---|---|---|
| MONB | 6 | ** | | 0 | 0/6 0 | 0/6 0 | – | [62] |
| Piroxicam | 5 | 36 ± 9 | OS 100% | 3/5 60 [17–100] | 2/5 40 [0–80] | – | – | [66] |
| Amitriptyline | 5 | 32 ± 17 | OS 100% | 2/5 40 [0–80] | 0/5 0 | – | – | [73, 78, 91, 92] |

Section C - Short lasting unilateral neuralgiform headache attacks

*Acute treatments*

| Treatment | N | Dose | Route | | | | | References |
|---|---|---|---|---|---|---|---|---|
| Lidocaine | 36 | 1.9 [1–3.5] | IV 75% SC 25% | 34/36 94 [87–100] | 29/36 80 [67–93] | 13/36 36 [15–58] | 6/36 16 [1–31] | [124–129] |
| Prednisone | 11 | 53 [20–100] | OS 91% IV 9% | 6/11 50 [20–80] | 1/11 10 [0–28] | – | – | [124, 129–134] |
| Methylprednisolone | 7 | 193 [16–1000] | IV 57% OS 43% | 5/7 71 [38–100] | 4/7 57 [20–94] | – | – | [125, 132, 135–137] |
| Phenytoin | 5 | 270 [200–300] | OS 100% | 1/5 20 [0–55] | 0/5 [0–0] | – | – | [124, 138–141] |

*Prolonged treatments*

| Treatment | N | Dose | Route | | | | | References |
|---|---|---|---|---|---|---|---|---|
| Lamotrigine | 84 | 231 [50–900] | OS 100% | 68/84 81 [73–89] | 38/84 45 [35–55] | 32 [16–48] | 13 [12–25] | [124, 125, 127–129, 134, 139, 140, 142–155] |
| Carbamazepine | 78 | 737 [100–2000] | OS 100% | 38/78 49 [38–60] | 9/78 11 [4–18] | 50 [20–80] | 40 [10–70] | [124–127, 131–134, 137–140, 143, 146, 147, 150–152, 155–157, 159–166] |
| Indomethacin | 50 | 116 [50–225] | OS 100% | 4/50 8 [1–15] | 1/50 2 [0–4] | 50 [0–100] | – | [124, 125, 127, 129, 131, 134, 138, 139, 141, 146–148, 150, 154, 157–159, 162, 165, 167–171] |
| Gabapentin | 48 | 1581 [300–3600] | OS 100% | 28/48 59 [45–74] | 13/48 28 [15–41] | 0/8 0 | 0/8 0 | [124–127, 137, 138, 140, 141, 145, 150, 153, 167, 172, 173] |
| Topiramate | 36 | 168 [40–400] | OS 100% | 20/36 56 [39–72] | 10/36 28 [13–43] | 75 [32–100] | 2 [0–55] | [124–126, 129, 134, 135, 138, 143, 145, 148, 155] |
| VTA DBS | 9 | Amplitude: 4 mV Frequency: 185 Hz Pulse width: 60 ms | | 9/9 100 | 9/9 100 | 9/9 100 | 1/9 11 | [174] |
| GONB | 9 | Bupivacaine 12.5 every 3 months | | 5/9 55 [44–66] | 2/9 22 [33–44] | – | – | [125, 140] |

**Table 1** Treatment options for HC, PH and SLUNHA used in, at least, 5 patients (Continued)

| | | | | | | | | |
|---|---|---|---|---|---|---|---|---|
| ONS | 7 | Amplitude: 0.3–3.15 V Frequency: 60–130 Hz Pulse width: 450 ms | | 7/7 100 | 7/7 100 | 0/7 0 | 0/7 0 | [175] |
| Verapamil | 6 | 347 [240–640] | OS 100% | 2/6 33 [0–71] | 1/6 17 [0–34] | – | – | [134, 138, 139, 162, 170] |
| Valproate | 5 | 950 ± 655 [250–2000] | OS 100% | 0/5 0 | 0/5 0 | – | – | [124, 131, 139, 168] |

*For non-pharmacological procedures the method used has been reported. Drug dosages are in mg/day if not otherwise specified
**Antonaci: 0.5–1.5 mg/ml solution with 12.5 μg/m andrenaline; Guerrero 2 cm³ of 0.5% bupivacaine and 2% mepivacaine in a 1:1 ratio, Weyker 25% 0.25 ml + bupivacaine 10 mg triamcinolone
***Beams: 9 cm³ of 1% lidocaine with 40 mg triamcinolone; Garza and Guerrero: 2 cm³ of 0.5% Bupivacaine and 2% mepivacaine in a 1:1 ratio
****Burns: frequency of 60 Hz and pulse width of 250 μs for all patients; the amplitude of the bion current could be adjusted within a given range
$^a$L/min, $^b$UI; $^c$maintainance dose, unchanged for, at least, 1 month

**Table 2** comparisons between the odds of partial and complete responders for the acute treatments of HC*

| | | | | |
|---|---|---|---|---|
| | | **Responders** | | |
| **Indomethacin** | | | | |
| 0 ↑ | Celecoxib | | | |
| 0 ↑ | 1.333 [0.0902-19.692] | Piroxicam | | |
| ∞ | ∞ | ∞ | SONB | |
| 0 ↑ | 0.148 [0.019-1.179] ↑ | 9 [0.625-129.593] | ∞ ↑ | GONB |
| | | **Complete responders** | | |
| **Indomethacin** | | | | |
| 0 ↑ | Celecoxib | | | |
| 0 ↑ | 0.937 [0.107-8.217] | Piroxicam | | |
| 0 ↑ | 0.156 [0.023-1.043] ↑ | 0.167 [0.019-1.436] | SONB | |
| 0 ↑ | 0.027 [0.001-0.801] ↑ | 0.029 [0.001-1.077] ↑ | 5.833 [ 0.517-65.763] | GONB |

*Cells report the OR of responders and complete responders of the indicated treatments and the 95% CI. OR are calculated as the odds of responder/complete responders of he treatments indicated in the coloured boxes split by the odds of responders/complete responders of the column treatments. The highlighted cells indicate a p-value of the test of equality of odds lower than 0.05. Arrows indicate if the column treatment is better (↑) or worse (↓) than the coloured boxes one.

*Cells report the OR of responders and complete responders of the indicated treatments and the 95% CI. OR are calculated as the odds of responder/complete responders of he treatments indicated in the coloured boxes split by the odds of responders/complete responders of the column treatments. The highlighted cells indicate a *p*-value of the test of equality of odds lower than 0.05. Arrows indicate if the column treatment is better (↑) or worse (↓) than the coloured boxes' ones

**Prolonged treatments** Indomethacin, melatonin, gabapentin, topiramate, OnabotA, celecoxib, verapamil, piroxicam, ONS, SONB, GONB, acemethacin, amytriptiline, DRGB, SPGB, valproate, lithium, troclear injections of triamcinolone, fentanyl and tilidine are the drugs used for the treatment of HC outside exacerbations, to prevent the incoming of new active phases and control the background pain. Data regarding acemethacin, amytriptiline, DRGB, SPGB, valproate,

lithium, troclear injections of triamcinolone, fentanyl and tilidine were not pooled in the statistical analysis because of the small number of patients who tried them.

Indomethacin has a significantly higher odds of responders than all other treatments except for OnabotA (*p* = 0.723) and SONB (*p* = 0.541); moreover, it has a significantly higher odds of pain-free patients compared to the other types of treatment (all *p* < 0.001).

**Table 3** comparisons between the odds of responders and complete responders of prolonged treatments for HC*

| Indomethacin | Melatonin | Gabapentin | Topiramate | OnabotulinumtoxinA | Celecoxib | Verapamil | Piroxicam | ONS | SONB | GONB |
|---|---|---|---|---|---|---|---|---|---|---|
| | | | | **Responders** | | | | | | |
| **Indomethacin** | | | | | | | | | | |
| 0 ↑ | Melatonin | | | | | | | | | |
| 0 ↑ | 4.888 [0.715-33.433] | Gabapentin | | | | | | | | |
| 0 ↑ | 4.888 [0.715-33.433] | 1 [0.114-8.784] | Topiramate | | | | | | | |
| ∞ | ∞ ↓ | ∞ | ∞ | OnabotulinumtoxinA | | | | | | |
| 0 ↑ | 4 [0.585-27.347] | 0.818 [0.091-7.359] | 0.818 [0.091-7.359] | 0 | Celecoxib | | | | | |
| 0 ↑ | 0.533 [0.091- 3.141] | 0.109 [0.01-1.246] ↑ | 0.109 [0.01-1.246] ↑ | 0 ↑ | 7.5 [0.669-84.107] | Verapamil | | | | |
| 0 ↑ | 5.333 [0.441- 64.468] | 1.091 [0.076-15.693] | 1.091 [0.076-15.693] | 0 | 0.75 [ 0.051-11.077] | 10 [0.48-208.293] | Piroxicam | | | |
| 0 ↑ | 4.74 [0.884-25.425] ↓ | 0.97 [0.134-7.01] | 0.97 [0.134-7.01] | 0 | 1.185 [ 0.16-8.769] | 8.889 [ 1.007-78.43] ↓ | 0.889 [0.073- 10.817] | ONS | | |
| ∞ | ∞ ↓ | ∞ | ∞ | ∞ | ∞ | ∞ ↓ | ∞ | ∞ | SONB | |
| 0 ↑ | 0.593 [ 0.14-2.5] | 0.12 [ 0.015-0.98] ↑ | 0.12 [ 0.015-0.98] ↑ | 0 ↑ | 6.75 [0.848-53.738] ↑ | 1.111 [0.183-6.758] | 9 [0.625-129.593] | 0.125 [ 0.02-0.786] ↑ | 0 ↑ | GONB |
| | | | | **Complete responders** | | | | | | |
| **Indomethacin** | | | | | | | | | | |
| 0 ↑ | Melatonin | | | | | | | | | |
| 0 ↑ | 2.057 [0.433- 9.772] | Gabapentin | | | | | | | | |
| 0 ↑ | 3.84 [0.744-19.833] | 1.867 [0.373- 9.352] | Topiramate | | | | | | | |
| 0 ↑ | 1.2 [0.238-6.063] | 0.583 [0.11-3.097] | 0.313 [0.055-1.788] | OnabotulinumtoxinA | | | | | | |
| 0 ↑ | 6.4 [0.959-42.709] | 3.111 [0.503-19.227] | 1.667 [0.28-9.928] | 5.333 [ 0.729- 39.03] | Celecoxib | | | | | |
| 0 ↑ | 0 | 0 ↑ | 0 ↑ | 0 | ∞ ↑ | Verapamil | | | | |
| 0 ↑ | 6 [0.696-51.69] | 2.917 [0.363-23.405] | 1.563 [0.202-12.088] | 5 [0.53-47.222] | 1.067 [ 0.122-9.35] | ∞ ↓ | Piroxicam | | | |
| 0 ↑ | 0.64 [0.126 2.006] | 0.311 [0.061 1.604] | 0.167 [0.020 0.060] ↑ | 0.533 [0.100 2.841] | 0.1 [0.013 0.767] ↑ | ∞ | 0.107 [0.011 1.046] ↑ | ONS | | |
| 0 ↑ | 1 [0.224-4.471] | 0.486 [0.102-2.309] | 0.26 [0.050-1.345] | 0.83 [0.165-4.21] | 0.156 [0.023-1.043] ↑ | ∞ | 0.167 [0.019-1.436] | 1.563 [0.333-7.339] | SONB | |
| 0 ↑ | 0.171 [0.015-1.932] | 0.083 [0.006-1.16] ↑ | 0.044 [0.002-0.82] ↑ | 0.143 [ 0.011-1.83] | 0.028 [0.001-0.800] ↑ | ∞ | 0.29 [0.001-1.077] ↑ | 0.268 [0.024-2.932] | 0.171 [0.015- 1.933] | GONB |

*Cells report the OR of responders and complete responders of the indicated treatments and the 95% CI. OR are calculated as the odds of responder/complete responders of he treatments indicated in the coloured boxes split by the odds of responders/complete

*Cells report the OR of responders and complete responders of the indicated treatments and the 95% CI. OR are calculated as the odds of responder/complete responders of he treatments indicated in the coloured boxes split by the odds of responders/complete responders of the column treatments. The highlighted cells indicate a *p*-value of the test of equality of odds lower than 0.05. Arrows indicate if the column treatment is better (↑) or worse (↓) than the coloured boxes' ones

Considering the other types of treatment, verapamil has a lower odds of responders than gabapentin ($P = 0.03$), topiramate ($p = 0.03$), OnabotA ($p = 0.002$), ONS ($p = 0.018$) and SONB ($p < 0.001$). Verapamil has also a lower odds of complete responders than gabapentin ($p = 0.027$), topiramate ($p = 0.006$), celecoxib ($p = 0.002$) and piroxicam ($p = 0.005$). GONB has an odds of responder lower than gabapentin ($p = 0.018$), topiramate ($p = 0.018$), OnabotA ($p = 0.001$), celecoxib ($p = 0.037$), ONS ($p = 0.008$) and SONB ($p < 0.001$). Furthermore, it has a lower odds of complete responders than gabapentin ($p = 0.018$), topiramate ($p = 0.002$), celecoxib ($p < 0.001$) and piroxicam ($p = 0.002$).

Furthermore, melatonin has an odds of responders significantly lower than OnabotA ($p = 0.006$). All comparisons are summarized in Table 3.

### Safety

Considering the poor number of signaled AEs, no statistical comparisons were made between the different odds of AEs and AEs causing the discontinuation or the modification of therapy. The only mild-quality data dealing with drugs' safety profile regarded indomethacin: AEs status was clearly declared in 83 patients, 75% of whom reported an AE and 46 were forced to discontinue or reduce therapy.

### Paroxysmal hemicrania (PH)

Fifty five articles were considered for PH [26, 38, 53, 60, 62, 66, 71–123]. Indomethacin is the most used treatment (168 patients), followed by verapamil (30 patients), sumatriptan (24 patients) and oxygen (18 patients). Carbamazepine (CBZ) was tried on 15 patients, topiramate on 12 patients, amitriptyline and piroxicam on 5 patients. SONB, MONB and GONB were all used upon 6 patients. Piroxicam and amitriptyline were used upon 5 patients. All other treatments were used on less than 5 patients and were not taken into consideration for the statistical analysis. Treatments used in 5 or more patients are summarized in Table 1 (section B). Statistical comparisons of the odds of responders and complete responders for acute treatments are summarized in Table 4 whilst for the prolonged ones in Table 5. Data regarding those drugs taken by less than 5 patients are summarized in the Additional file 1: Table S1 (section B).

### Effectiveness

**Acute treatments** Indomethacin, sumatriptan, oxygen, MONB, GONB, SONB, piroxicam, rofecoxib, prednisone, valdecoxib, etoricoxib, naproxen, betamethasone, methylprednisolone, HDBS and SPGB were considered as acute treatments. The last eight were used in less than 5 patients and so weren't pooled in the statistical analysis; MONB, GONB and SONB weren't pooled in the statistical analysis either as they were clearly ineffective. Rofecoxib was not considered as it has been taken off the

International market. Indomethacin has a significantly higher odds of responders and complete responders than piroxicam, sumatriptan and oxygen (all $p < 0.001$). Moreover, piroxicam has a significantly higher odds of complete responders, both than sumatriptan ($p = 0.0187$) and oxygen ($p = 0.006$). All comparisons are reported in Table 4.

**Prolonged treatments** To prevent the recurrence of PH exacerbations 26 treatments were find out from literature. Indomethacin, verapamil, CBZ, topiramate, MONB, GONB, SONB, piroxicam and amytriptiline were those treatments used in more than 5 patients and pooled in the statistical analysis. Propranolol, acetylsalicylic acid, lithium, ergotamine, dipyrone, valproate, acetazolamide, baclofen, phenytoin, methysergide, doxepine, flunnarizine, gabapentin, bethametasone, methylprednisolone, OnabotA, hypothalamic deep brain stimulation (HDBS), sphenopalatine ganglion blockade (SPGB) were used in less than 5 patients and so weren't taken into consideration for the statistical analysis. Indomethacin has a the highest odds of responders and complete responders (all $p < 0.001$). Besides indomethacin, all other drugs show a not-significantly different odds of responders between them. Considering the complete responders, CBZ has a lower odds than piroxicam ($p = 0.012$) and topiramate ($p = 0.007$). All comparisons are reported in Table 5.

### Safety

AEs were cited in a very small number of works and many reports refers only to indomethacin; for these reasons it was not possible to make a reliable comparison between the safety profile of those drugs. Anyway, AEs were stated for 78 patients receiving indomethacin: the 54% of them suffered from an AE (mainly gastro-intestinal) and the 27% discontinued or interrupted the therapy.

### Short lasting unilateral neuralgiform headache attacks (SUNCT and SUNA)

Globally 56, studies were analyzed [124–179]. The most widely used treatment to control the excruciating and frequent attacks during active phases was lidocaine (36 patients), followed by prednisone (11 patients) and methylprednisolone (7 patients). To prevent the incoming of new active phases the most used treatments were: lamotrigine (84 patients), CBZ (78 patients), indomethacin (48 patients), gabapentin (48 patients) and topiramate (36 patients). All other treatments were used in less than 10 patients.

All these data are summarized in Table 1 (section C), data regarding statistical comparisons between the odds of responders and complete responders are summarized in Table 6 (acute treatments) and in Table 7 (prolonged treatments). Data regarding treatments used in less than 5 patients are reported in Additional file 1: Table S1 -section C.

**Table 4** statistical comparisons between the odds of responders and complete responders of acute treatments for PH*

*Short-term treatment*

| | | | |
|---|---|---|---|
| **Responders** | | | |
| Indomethacin | | | |
| **0.046 [0.006- 0.38]** ↑ | Piroxicam | | |
| **0.008 [0.001-0.063]** ↑ | 0.175 [0.019-1.588] | Sumatriptan | |
| **0.015 [0.003-0.089]** ↑ | 0.333 [0.039-2.836] | 1.9 [0.459-7.865] | Oxygen |
| **Complete responders** | | | |
| Indomethacin | | | |
| **0.08 [ 0.012-0.547]** ↑ | Piroxicam | | |
| **0.005 [ 0.001-0.089]** ↑ | **0.065 [ 0.003-1.378]** ↑ | Sumatriptan | |
| **0** ↑ | **0** ↑ | 0 | Oxygen |

*Cells report the OR of responders and complete responders of the indicated treatments and the 95% CI. OR are calculated as the odds of responder/complete responders of he treatments indicated in the coloured box split by the odds of responders/complete responders of the column treatments. The highlighted cells indicate a p-value of the test of equality of odds lower than 0.05. Arrows indicate if the column treatment is better (↑) or worse (↓) than the coloured boxes one.

*Cells report the OR of responders and complete responders of the indicated treatments and the 95% CI. OR are calculated as the odds of responder/complete responders of he treatments indicated in the coloured box split by the odds of responders/complete responders of the column treatments. The highlighted cells indicate a *p*-value of the test of equality of odds lower than 0.05. Arrows indicate if the column treatment is better (↑) or worse (↓) than the coloured boxes' ones

## Effectiveness

**Acute treatments** Lidocaine, prednisone, methylprednisolone, phenytoin, celecoxib, superior trigeminal nerve blockade (STGB) and HDBS were considered for the management of exacerbation in SUNCT and SUNA. Lidocaine was effective in the 94% of patients, of which 80% of them were completely pain-free. Lidocaine has a significantly higher odds of responders than prednisone ($p < 0.001$) and phenytoin ($p = 0.001$), but comparable to methylprednisolone ($p = 0.058$). The same trend was seen for the odds of pain-free patients: lidocaine has an odds of complete responders significantly higher than prednisone ($p = 0.002$) and phenytoin ($p < 0.001$), but comparable to methylprednisolone ($p = 0.1797$). Methylprednisolone has significantly higher odds of complete responders than phenytoin ($p = 0.0384$). All comparisons are reported in Table 6. All other treatments were used upon less than 5 patients and weren't pooled in the statistical analysis.

**Prolonged treatments** Lamotrigine, topiramate, gabapentin, verapamil, indomethacin, CBZ, GONB, ventral tegmental area deep brain stimulation, ONS, clonazepam, HDBS, OnabotA, baclofen, pregabalin, gammaknife radiosurgery of the trigeminal nerve, nifedipine, fentanyl, lithium, methysergide, zonisamide, lomerizine and STGB were those drugs used for the prevention of new active phases. The last 12 were not pooled in the statistical analysis due to the poor number of patients who tried them.

Lamotrigine has an odds of responders significantly higher than topiramate ($p = 0.004$), even if the odds of complete responders were comparable ($p = 0.074$). Lamotrigine has also a higher odds of responders ($p = 0.008$) and complete responders ($p = 0.0487$) than gabapentin and, moreover, than indomethacin, verapamil and CBZ (all *p*-value < 0.001).

Indomethacin has an odds of responders lower than topiramate, gabapentin, CBZ, VTA DBS and ONS (all

**Table 5** statistical comparisons between the odds of responders and complete responders of prolonged treatments for PH*

| | | | | | |
|---|---|---|---|---|---|
| **Responders** | | | | | |
| Indomethacin | | | | | |
| **0.046 [0.006-0.38]** ↑ | Piroxicam | | | | |
| **0.008 [0.001- 0.073]** ↑ | 0.167 [0.015-1.89] | Carbamazepine | | | |
| **0.02 [0.002-0.194]** ↑ | 0.444 [0.029-6.761] | 2.667 [0.269-26.454] | Amitriptyline | | |
| **0.092 [0.018- 0.477]** ↑ | 2 [0.199-20.146] | 1.053 [0.207-5.343] | 4.5 [0.399-50.737] | Topiramate | |
| **0.029 [ 0.006-0.11]** ↑ | 0.583 [0.082-4.159] | 3.5 [ 0.763-16.048] | 1.313 [0.186-9.298] | 0.292 [ 0.061-1.39] | Verapamil |
| **Complete Responders** | | | | | |
| Indomethacin | | | | | |
| **0.08 [ 0.012-0.547]** ↑ | Piroxicam | | | | |
| **0** ↑ | **0** ↑ | Carbamazepine | | | |
| **0** ↑ | 0 | 0 | Amitriptyline | | |
| **0.086 [ 0.023-0.325]** ↑ | 1.071 [0.12-9.586] | ∞ ↓ | ∞ | Topiramate | |
| **0.024 [0.006-0.097]** ↑ | 0.3 [0.037-2.46] | ∞ = | ∞ | 0.28 [ 0.058-1.347] | Verapamil |

*Cells report the OR of responders and complete responders of the indicated treatments and the 95% CI. OR are calculated as the odds of responder/complete responders of he treatments indicated in the coloured box split by the odds of responders/complete responders of the column treatments. The highlighted cells

*Cells report the OR of responders and complete responders of the indicated treatments and the 95% CI. OR are calculated as the odds of responder/complete responders of he treatments indicated in the coloured box split by the odds of responders/complete responders of the column treatments. The highlighted cells indicate a *p*-value of the test of equality of odds lower than 0.05. Arrows indicate if the column treatment is better (↑) or worse (↓) than the coloured boxes' ones

**Table 6** statistical comparisons between the odds of responders and complete responders of acute treatment for SUNCT and SUNA*

| Responders | | | |
|---|---|---|---|
| Lidocaine | | | |
| **0.049 [0.005-0.465] ↑** | Prednisone | | |
| 0.147 [0.015-1.466] | 3 [0.348-25.859] | Methylprednisolone | |
| **0.015 [ 0.001-0.568] ↑** | 0.3 [0.021-4.262] | 0.1 [0.004-2.757] | Phenytoin |
| **Complete Responders** | | | |
| Lidocaine | | | |
| **0.024 [0.001-0.431] ↑** | Prednisone | | |
| 0.322 [0.055-1.884] | **13.333 [ 0.619-287.219] ↓** | Methylprednisolone | |
| 0 ↑ | 0 | 0 ↑ | Phenytoin |

*Cells report the OR of responders and complete responders of the indicated treatments and the 95% CI. OR are calculated as the odds of responder/complete responders of he treatments indicated in the coloured box split by the odds of responders/complete responders of the column treatments. The highlighted cells indicate a *p*-value of the test of equality of odds lower than 0.05. Arrows indicate if the column treatment is better (↑) or worse (↓) than the coloured boxes one.

*Cells report the OR of responders and complete responders of the indicated treatments and the 95% CI. OR are calculated as the odds of responder/complete responders of he treatments indicated in the coloured box split by the odds of responders/complete responders of the column treatments. The highlighted cells indicate a *p*-value of the test of equality of odds lower than 0.05. Arrows indicate if the column treatment is better (↑) or worse (↓) than the coloured boxes' ones

*p* < 0.001). Ventral tegmental area deep brain stimulation and ONS have an odds of responders significantly higher than the ones of all other treatments despite lamotrigine (all *p*-values < 0.001).

Considering pain-free patients, indomethacin has a lower odds than lamotrigine, topiramate, gabapentin, GONB, VTA DBS and ONS (all *p*-values < 0.001). ONS has an odds of complete responders higher than all other treatments. All comparisons are reported in Table 7.

### Safety

**Acute treatments** Since the only reported AEs were for IV lidocaine, no statistical comparisons were made for short-term treatment drugs. Anyway, safety profile of IV or SC Lidocaine was stated for 36 patients, 13 of which suffered from a mild AE and 6 from an AE causing the discontinuation of therapy.

**Prolonged treatments** According with the low number of signaled AEs, verapamil and indomethacin were excluded from the statistical analysis. Lamotrigine has more AEs than gabapentin (*p* = 0.039), but no

differences were noted for the AEs causing the stop or the reduction of therapy (*p* = 0.232). No differences were found in the proportion of AEs between lamotrigine and CBZ (*p* = 0.311), but a tendency in a higher number of AEs causing the discontinuation or the modification of therapy was seen for CBZ (*p* = 0.06). Topiramate has a higher number of AEs than gabapentin (*P* = 0.002), but a similar occurrence of severe AEs. Topiramate has also the same proportion of AEs than CBZ and the same number of complete responders. Gabapentin was absolutely the safest drug, showing also a lower number of AEs than CBZ (*P* = 0.01). Because of the poor number of AEs causing the discontinuation or the modification of therapy, data regarding the comparison of their proportion between the different treatments were not shown in the previous Table.

## Discussion

### General considerations

Due to the infrequent diagnosis of these conditions, only case-reports or small case-series were found in literature and this strongly limits the reliability of the analysis. In

**Table 7** statistical comparisons between the odds of responders and complete responders of prolonged treatments for SUNCT and SUNA*

| Responders | | | | | | | | |
|---|---|---|---|---|---|---|---|---|
| Lamotrigine | | | | | | | | |
| **0.294 [0.121-0.715] ↑** | Topiramate | | | | | | | |
| **0.347 [0.152-0.79] ↑** | 1.179 [0.487-2.855] | Gabapentin | | | | | | |
| **0.118 [0.018-0.764] ↑** | 0.4 [0.062-2.582] | 0.339 [ 0.054-2.132] | Verapamil | | | | | |
| **0.021 [0.004-0.108] ↑** | **0.071 [0.017-0.298] ↑** | **0.06 [0.015-0.247] ↑** | 0.178 [0.023-1.404] | Indomethacin | | | | |
| **0.224 [0.106-0.473] ↑** | 0.76 [0.342-1.689] | 0.645 [0.308-1.35] | 1.9 [0.323-11.161] | 0 ↓ | Carbamazepine | | | |
| ∞ | 1 [0.226-4.422] | 0.848 [0.199- 3.622] | 2.5 [0.256-24.375] | 1.316 [0.325-5.32] | ∞ ↓ | GONB | | |
| ∞ | ∞ ↓ | ∞ ↓ | ∞ ↓ | ∞ ↓ | ∞ ↓ | ∞ ↓ | VTA DBS | |
| 0.294 [0.069-1.261] | ∞ ↓ | ∞ ↓ | ∞ ↓ | ∞ ↓ | ∞ ↓ | ∞ ↓ | ∞ | ONS |
| **Complete responders** | | | | | | | | |
| Lamotrigine | | | | | | | | |
| 0.466 [0.197-1.102] | Topiramate | | | | | | | |
| 0.463 [0.211-1.015] | 0.994 [0.375-2.637] | Gabapentin | | | | | | |
| 0.242 [0.026-2.24] | 0.52 [0.052-5.208] | 0.523 [0.054-5.056] | Verapamil | | | | | |
| **0.025 [0.003-0.248] ↑** | **0.054 [0.005-0.537] ↑** | **0.054 [0.006-0.514] ↑** | 0.104 [0.005-2.176] | Indomethacin | | | | |
| **0.158 [0.065-0.382] ↑** | **0.339 [0.121-0.953] ↑** | **0.341 [0.13-0.898] ↑** | 0.652 [0.067-6.326] | 6.26 [0.736- 53.141] | Carbamazepine | | | |
| 0.346[0.066-1.808] | 0.743 [0.129-4.293] | 0.747 [0.135-4.146] | 1.429 [0.09-22.582] | **13.71 [0.92-204.3487] ↓** | 2.19 [0.386- 12.436] | GONB | | |
| 0.605 [0.14-2.613] | 1.3 [0.266-6.347] | 1.308 [0.279-6.106] | 2.5 [0.169-36.882] | **24 [1.572-366.461] ↓** | 3.833 [0.784-18.778] | 0 ↑ | VTA DBS | |
| ∞ ↓ | ∞ ↓ | ∞ ↓ | ∞ ↓ | ∞ ↓ | ∞ ↓ | 0 ↑ | 1.75 [0.199- 15.37] | ONS |

*Cells report the OR of responders and complete responders of the indicated treatments and the 95% CI. OR are calculated as the odds of responder/complete responders of he treatments indicated in the coloured box split by the odds of responders/complete responders of the column treatments. The highlighted cells indicate a *p*-value of the test of equality of odds lower than 0.05. Arrows indicate if the column treatment is better (↑) or

*Cells report the OR of responders and complete responders of the indicated treatments and the 95% CI. OR are calculated as the odds of responder/complete responders of he treatments indicated in the coloured box split by the odds of responders/complete responders of the column treatments. The highlighted cells indicate a *p*-value of the test of equality of odds lower than 0.05. Arrows indicate if the column treatment is better (↑) or worse (↓) than the coloured boxes' ones many articles responders are not so well identifiable and in a very few ones the partial response was clearly described in terms of reduction of headache frequency, intensity or both, making almost impossible a comparison between the activity of different drugs on these aspects of pain. Treatment safety profile is hard to study too, primarily due to the sporadic report of AEs.

## Hemicrania continua (HC)

The first choice treatment for HC is indomethacin: for the management of recurrent exacerbations indomethacin should be the first choice drug, according with the higher effectiveness than all other treatments (see Table 2), which should be reserved to patients who don't tolerated indomethacin. SONB has a similar proportion of responders but the lower odds of pain-free patients suggest that this technique is worse and more effective in diminishing pain rather than abolishing it [180]. It should also be considered that SONB has been tested only in a smaller number of patients than indomethacin and currently the experience on the use of these techniques is scarce, both for long-term availability (mean follow-up time = 93 days-data not show) and AEs profile. Celecoxib has an odds of responders lower than indomethacin but higher than GONB and an odds of complete responders higher than GONB and SONB, so it appears a better therapeutical approach than the last two in patients who don't tolerate indomethacin. Piroxicam is comparable to celecoxib in terms of effectiveness, mirroring a similar action, as also stated by other studies [181]. GONB and MONB usefulness in relieving HC exacerbations seems to be negligible, like the usefulness of those treatments available for CH attacks, like SC sumatriptan and oxygen inhalation. This confirms that, despite the clinical over-lapping of HC and CH, the underlying pathogenetic mechanisms should be different, thus justifying a different pharmacological response [182]. HC management on long-time periods is unscheduled, but medications have been introduced trying to prevent pain recurrence. The prolonged use of drugs which were effective exacerbation control is a common practice and drugs like indomethacin, piroxicam and celecoxib are frequently used in HC patients outside active phases, even for many months: in our sample the duration of indomethacin assumption ranged between 5 and 1440 days, whereas from 18 to 540 for celecoxib. For piroxicam those data were not available, but its use for "many months" was reported in 5 patients out of 7. The stoppage of these drugs was due to AEs, mainly gastro-intestinal (GI), in the 70% of cases. The development of serious AEs is the main reason for which indomethacin, piroxicam and celecoxib should not be continued for many months outside exacerbations, even if the dose is titrated to the lowest possible or a

preventive therapy with a proton pump inhibitor is started. SONB and GONB were both used even for the prevention of HC exacerbations, but GONB seems of no effect and SONB has a low odds of pain-free patients, denoting a partial action. The incoming of GI AEs and the low effectiveness of GONB and SONB impose the use of other drugs to control pain.

Gabapentin, topiramate, melatonin and OnabotA seems to be comparable in terms of effectiveness even if, considering the $p$-values of these comparisons ($p = 0.063$), a better action for gabapentin and topiramate than melatonin should be hypothesed. ONS should be a reliable option besides pharmacological techniques, as also confirmed from a recently published statement from the European Headache Federation [183]. The usefulness of verapamil in HC is scarce, since it has a lower odds of responders than indomethacin, OnabotA, topiramate, ONS and gabapentin and an odds of complete responders lower than all other treatments, except the non-pharmacological ones and melatonin.

The question on the tolerability of these treatments remains open and the unfair data about AEs make any comparison doubtful. Anyway, from the available literature, celecoxib and piroxicam should have a similar AEs profile than indomethacin with an even higher risk of cardiovascular side-effects with celecoxib [184], but a lower risk of renal AEs according to its higher COX-2 selectivity [185]: celecoxib and other COX-2 selective NSAIDs should be avoided with cardiovascular co-morbidities, but should be chosen after indomethacin in patients with renal diseases of with gastro-intestinal co-morbidities.

## Paroxysmal hemicrania (PH)

PH is another member of the so-called indomethacin-responsive headaches [1] and, in fact, indomethacin is undoubtedly the best treatment even for this condition. The activity of other treatments is low both for the acute treatment and for the prolonged one. Piroxicam emerges as the best treatment besides indomethacin for exacerbations management, according to the higher odds of pain-free patients than oxygen and sumatriptan. The usefulness of this last two drugs is almost null and this confirms once again the differences in TACs' pathogenesis besides their clinical similarity [182]. Even when used for PH control outside active phases indomethacin is the most effective treatment. Even so, since PH is frequently chronic and indomethacin assumption for long periods of time may cause a wide range of AEs, this usually lead to the discontinuation of therapy in about 27% of cases. This imposes the use of different treatments to control the pain, but other tested drugs seems to be of little use with the most effective being rofecoxib, which has been retired from the international market because of its cardiac side-effects [186]. Piroxicam seems to be the most effective treatment other than indomethacin, even if the possibility of having GI AEs remains [187] and, like indomethacin, its use should be avoided for long periods of time. Since the hypothesized overlapping between PH and migraine pathogenesis [15], two well-known migraine prophylaxis such as topiramate and amitriptyline have been tried for PH, with comparable and moderate results. Topiramate and amitriptyline are also comparable to piroxicam and verapamil in terms of effectiveness, even though the latter shows a not-significant higher odds of responders and complete responders. CBZ usefulness seems to be low and the null number of complete responders should discourage its use for PH management.

### Short lasting unilateral neuralgiform headache attacks (SUNCT and SUNA)

To stop SUNCT and SUNA exacerbations, lidocaine (intravenously or subcutaneously) seems to be the most effective treatment and is now emerging as a novel option for chronic pain syndromes [188]. Its effectiveness is unquestionable, but paranoid idealization, depressive thoughts and cardiac arrhythmias were registered as AEs: this imposes the careful and shortest use of this drug only for the worst cases and the patient's continuous monitoring with a 12-lead ECG registration and sequential blood pressure measurements during the treatment [189]. In our sample the time of use ranged between 2 to 10 days (data not shown). Steroids represent a less effective but safer options for stopping attacks, with methylprednisolone presenting a better action than prednisone, even if not significantly. As previously discussed for lidocaine, steroids should be given intravenously for the shortest time as possible: from literature it is well-known that they can have a wide range of AEs, which can be prevented by reducing the duration of infusion to the time necessary for the ceasing of

painful exacerbations [190]. In our sample the mean time of infusion was 8 ± 4.32 days (data not shown) The usefulness of phenytoin should be considered negligible.

Lamotrigine is the best drug for the prevention of the incoming of new active phases, but seems to be more suitable in reducing attacks frequency rather than abolishing them completely: it has an odds of partial responders higher than all other drugs, but the odds of complete responders are comparable, with the exceptions of CBZ and indomethacin, which efficacy is scarce. Non-pharmacological techniques have an odds of responders comparable to lamotrigine and, moreover, ONS has even a higher odds of complete responders. Lamotrigine has also a similar AEs profile than other treatments except for gabapentin, confirming the available literature [191].

Verapamil, gabapentin and topiramate have similar effectiveness, with gabapentin showing a better AEs profile, even if the number of reported AEs is too poor to let a reliable comparison. CBZ appears less useful in treating SUNCT and SUNA than gabapentin and topiramate, according with the lower number of complete responders. Indomethacin usefulness in these conditions is sometimes reported, but should be considered as negligible: an occasional benefit of this drug in SUNCT or SUNA should rise the question of a diagnostic mistake with HC, PH or a secondary headache, imposing the reconsideration of the initial diagnosis, following scheduled diagnostic algorithms [192].

Recently, non-pharmacological techniques has gained importance in the treatment of these disorders, but the experience with these treatments is scarce and the long-term follow-up of patients is often lacking in many studies. From the available data ONS has emerged as the best technique and this result is in accordance with the findings in CH, were ONS is the only class-A evidence treatment for the American Headache Society (AHS) [193]. Moreover, even the European Headache Federation (EHF)

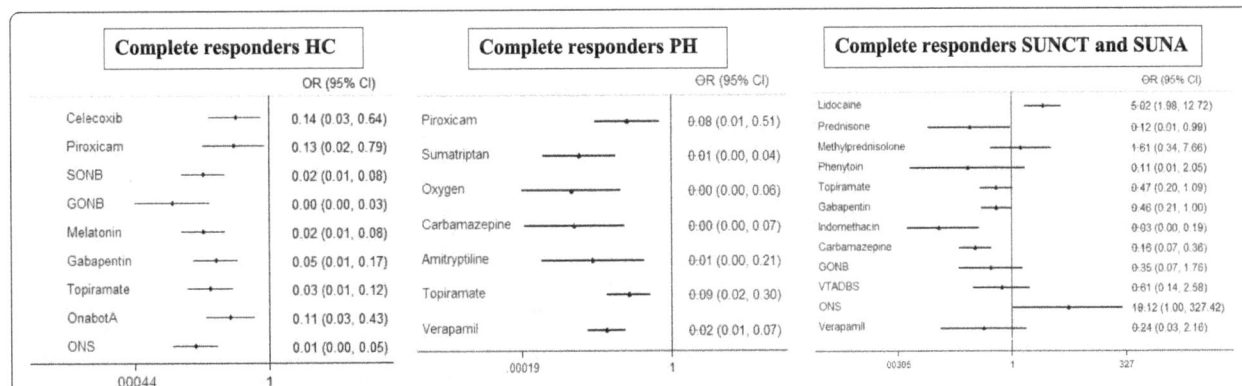

**Fig. 2** Odds ratios of complete responders. For HC and PH the referral treatment is indomethacin. For SUNCT and SUNA the referral treatment is lamotrigine. If the whole 95% CI of the OR is lower than 1, the referral treatments is better than the reported one

has confirmed the effectiveness and safety of this technique in SUNCT and SUNA, pointing out that 4 patients out of 6 analyzed were nearly pain free with mild facial paresthesia as the principal AE [183].

From the reviewed literature, ONS has demonstrated an almost complete effectiveness and a good safety profile, but it has been tried only on 7 patients. Ventral tegmental area deep brain stimulation has shown a similar effectiveness, but adverse events were reported in the 100% of cases and should be reserved to the refractory cases. Finally, GONB appears to be less effective but also safer than the previous techniques and should be considered as a reliable alternative in patients with episodic forms.

In Fig. 2 the ORs of complete responders and the relative IC95% are visually summarized for all diseases. ORs are calculated as the odds of pain-free patients for the indicated treatments split by the odds of pain-free patients for the most used treatment for every disease.

## Conclusion
PH, HC, SUNCT and SUNA represent a hard challenge for clinicians who work in headache or pain fields. Moreover, their infrequence makes difficult to study the pathogenesis of these conditions, as well as design well-done RCPCT for new drugs. From the review of the available literature indomethacin emerges as the best treatment for HC and PH, while other drugs like celecoxib, topiramate and gabapentin may be useful. SUNCT and SUNA should be managed with intravenous steroids or lidocaine in the worst cases and for short periods of time, with a subsequent change for preventive treatment to lamotrigine or ONS.

In conclusion, it should be highlighted that further studies are required to implement guidelines to treat the disease and to discover new effective and safe therapies for these conditions.

## Abbreviations
AE: Adverse event; AHS: American Headache Society; CBZ: Carbamazepine; EHF: European Headache Federation; GONB: Great occipital nerve blockade; HC: Hemicrania continua; ICHD-III-beta: International classification of headache disorders-3rd edition, beta version; IHS: International Headache Society; IV: Intravenous; MONB: Minor occipital nerve blockade; NSAIDs: Non-steroidal anti-inflammatory drugs; OnabotA: onabotulinumtoxinA; ONS: Occipital nerve stimulation; OR: Odds ratio; PH: Paroxysmal hemicrania; RCPCT: Randomized clinical placebo-controlled trials; SLUNHA: Short-lasting unilateral neuralgiform headache attacks; SON: Supra-orbital nerve; SONB: Supraorbital nerve blockade; STGB: Superior trigeminal ganglion blockade

## Authors' contributions
CB, LP, SG and MMC drafted the manuscript. CB and LAP conceived the study, participated in drafting the manuscript and made the statistical analysis. All authors read and approved the final manuscript.

## Competing interests
The authors declare that they have no competing interests.

## References
1. Headache Classification Committee of the International Headache Society (IHS) (2013) The international classification of headache disorders, 3rd edition (beta version). Cephalalgia 33:629–808
2. Vincent MB (2013) Hemicrania continua. Unquestionably a trigeminal autonomic cephalalgia. Headache 53:863–868
3. Costa A, Antonaci F, Ramusino MC, Nappi G (2015) The neuropharmacology of cluster headache and other trigeminal autonomic cephalalgias. Curr Neuropharmacol 13:304–323
4. Viana M, Tassorelli C, Allena M, Nappi G, Sjaastad O, Antonaci F (2013) Diagnostic and therapeutic errors in trigeminal autonomic cephalalgias and hemicrania continua: a systematic review. J Headache Pain 14:14
5. May A (2013) Diagnosis and clinical features of trigemino-autonomic headaches. Headache 53:1470–1478
6. Marano E, Volpe G, Della Rocca G, Di Stasio E, Bonuso S, Sorge F (1994) "Hemicrania continua": a possible case with alternating sides. Cephalalgia 14:307–308
7. Kuritzky A (1992) Indomethacin-resistant hemicrania continua. Cephalalgia 12:57–59
8. Prakash S, Brahmbhatt KJ, Chawda NT, Tandon N (2009) Hemicrania continua responsive to intravenous methylprednisolone. Headache 49:604–609
9. Moorjani BI, Rothner AD (2001) Indomethacin-responsive headaches in children and adolescents. Sem Ped Neurol 1:40–45
10. Burns B, Watkins L, Goadsby PJ (2008) Treatment of hemicrania continua by occipital nerve stimulation with a bion device: long-term follow-up of a crossover study. Lancet Neurol 7:1001–1012
11. Prakash S, Husain M, Sureka DS, Shah NP, Shah ND (2009) Is there need to search for alternatives to indomethacin for hemicrania continua? Case reports and a review. J Neurol Sci 277:187–190
12. Prakash S, Shah ND (2009) Delayed response to indomethacin in patients with hemicrania continua: real or phantom headache? Cephalalgia 30:375–379
13. Spears RC (2006) Hemicrania continua: a case in which a patient experienced complete relief on melatonin. Headache 46:515–527
14. Spitz M, Peres MFP (2004) Hemicrania continua post-partum. Cephalalgia 24:603–604
15. Terlizzi R, Cevoli S, Nicodemo M, Pierangeli G, Grimaldi D, Cortelli P (2011) A case of strictly unilateral migraine without aura transformed in an episodic hemicrania continua. Neurol Sci 32:169–170
16. Weatherall MW, Bahra A (2011) Familial hemicrania continua. Cephalalgia 31:245–249
17. Peres MFP, Stiles MA, Oshinsky M, Rozen TD (2001) Remitting form of hemicrania continua with seasonal pattern. Headache 41:592–594
18. Palmieri A, Mainardi F, Dainese F, Zanchin G (2004) Hemicrania continua evolving from migraine with aura: clinical evidence of a possible correlation between two forms of primary headache. Cephalalgia 24:1007–1008
19. Kuhn J, Kuhn KF, Cooper-Mahkorn D, Bewermeyer H (2005) Remitting form of hemicrania continua: two new cases exhibiting one unusual autonomic feature. Headache 45:751–762
20. Southerland AM, Login IS (2011) Rigorously deefined hemicrania continua presenting bilaterally. Cephalalgia 31:1490–1492
21. Rozen TD (2005) Verapamil-responsive hemicrania continua in a patient with episodic cluster headache. Cephalalgia 26:351–353
22. Miller S, Correia F, Lagrata S, Matharu MS (2015) onabotulinumtoxinA for hemicrania continua: open label experience in 9 patients. J Headache Pain 16:19
23. Baldacci F, Nuti A, Cafforio G, Lucetti C, Logi C, Cipriani G, Orlandi G, Bonuccelli U (2008) "INDOTEST" in atypical hemicrania continua. Cephalalgia 28:300–301
24. Prakash S, Rathore C (2016) Two cases of hemicrania continua-trigeminal neuralgia syndrome: expanding the spectrum of trigeminal autonomic cephalalgia-Tic (TAC-TIC) syndrome. Headache 30:1–6
25. Jurgen TP, Schulte LH, May A (2013) Indomethacin-induced de novo headache in hemicrania continua-fighting fire with fire? Cephalalgia 33:1203–1205
26. Castellanos-Pinedo F, Zurdo M, Martinez-Acebes E (2006) Hemicrania continua evolving from episodic paroxysmal hemicrania. Cephalalgia 26:1143–1145
27. Da Silva HM, Alcantara MC, Bordini CA, Speciali JG (2002) Strictly unilateral headache reminiscent of hemicrania continua resistant to indomethacin but responsive to gabapentin. Cephalagia 22:409–410

28. Spears RC (2009) Is gabapentin an effective treatment choice for hemicrania continua? J Headache Pain 10:271–275

29. Cosentino G, Fierro B, Puma AR, Talamanca S, Brighina F (2010) Different forms of trigeminal autonomic cephalalgias in the same patient: description of a case. J Headache Pain 11:281–284

30. Yablon LA, Newman LC (2010) Hemicrania continua: a second case in which the remitting form evolved from the chronic form. Headache 50:1381–1389

31. Lambru G, Castellini P, Bini A, Evangelista A, Manzoni GC, Torelli P (2008) Hemicrania continua evolving from cluster headache responsive to valproic acid. Headache 48:1374–1376

32. Allena M, Tassorelli C, Sances G, Guaschino E, Sandrini G, Nappi G, Antonaci F (2010) Is hemicrania continua a single entity of the association of two headache forms? Considerations from a case report. Headache 27:877–881

33. Androulakis XM, Krebs KA, Ashkenazi A (2016) Hemicrania continua may respond to repetitive sphenopalatine ganglion block: a case report. Headache 56:573–579

34. Cuadrado ML, Porta-Etessam J, Pareja JA, Matias-Guiu J (2009) Hemicrania continua responsive to trochlear injection of corticosteroids. Cephalalgia 30:373–374

35. Beams JL, Kline MT, Rozen TD (2015) Treatment of hemicrania continua with radiofrequency ablation and long-term follow-up. Cephalalgia 35:1208–1213

36. Brighina F, Palermo A, Cosentino G, Fierro B (2007) Prophylaxis of hemicrania continua: two new cases effectively treated with topiramate. Headache 47:441–443

37. Rozen TD (2015) How effective is melatonin as a preventive treatment for hemicrania continua? A clinic-based study. Headache 55:430–436

38. Camarda C, Camarda R, Monastero R (2008) Chronic paroxysmal hemicrania and hemicrania continua responding to topiramate: two case reports. Clin Neurol Neurosur 110:88–91

39. Cittadini E, Goadsby PJ (2010) Hemicrania continua: a clinical study of 39 patients with diagnostic implications. Brain 133:1973–1986

40. Trucco M, Antonaci F, Sandrini G (1992) Hemicrania continua: a case responsive to piroxicam-beta-cyclodextrin. Headache 32:39–40

41. Pareja JA, Sjaastad O (1996) Chronic paroxysmal hemicrania and hemicrania continua. Interval between indomethacin administration and response. Headache 36:20–23

42. Fantini J, Kosica N, Zorzon M, Belluzzo M, Granato A (2015) Hemicrania continua with visual aura successfully treated with a combination of indomethacin and topiramate. Neurol Sci 36:643–644

43. Garza I, Cutrer FM (2010) Pain relief and persistence of dysautonomic features in a patient with hemicrania continua responsive to botulinum toxin type A. Cephalalgia 30:500–503

44. Jouber J (1991) Hemicrania continua in a black patient: the importance of the non continuous stage. Headache 31:482–484

45. Rozen TD (2013) Indomethacin-responsive TACs (Paroxysmal hemicrania, hemicrania continua and LASH): further proof of a distinct spectrum of headache disorders. Headache 53:1499–1500

46. Eren O, Straube A, Schoberl F, Schankin C (2017) Hemicrania continua: beneficial effect of non-invasive vagus nerve stimulation in a patient with a contraindication for indomethacin. Headache 57:298–301

47. Goadsby PJ (2012) Trigeminal autonomic cephalalgias. Continuum Lifelong Learning Neurol 18:883–895

48. Hollingworth M, Young TM (2014) Melatonin responsive hemicrania continua in which indomethacin was associated with contralateral headache. Headache 54:916–919

49. Matharu MS, Bradbury P, Swash M (2005) Hemicrania continua: side alternation and response to topiramate. Cephalalgia 26:341–344

50. Newman LC, Spears RC, Lay CL (2004) Hemicrania continua: a third case in which attacks alternate sides. Headache 44:821–823

51. Nicpon KJ, Nicpon KW, Cicpon JJ (2010) Prophylaxis of hemicrania continua: three cases effectively treated with acemethacin. Cephalalgia 31:625–627

52. Porta-Etessam J, Cuadrado M, Rodriguez-Gomez O, Garcia-Ptacek, Valencia C (2010) Are COX-2 drugs the second line option in indomethacin responsive headaches? J Headache Pain 11:405–407

53. Prakash S, Shah ND, Bhanvadia RJ (2009) Hemicrania continua unresponsive or partial responsive to indomethacin: does it exist? A diagnostic and therapeutic dilemma. J Headache Pain 10:59–63

54. Prakash S, Rathore C, Makwana P (2015) Hemicrania continua with contralateral cranial autonomic features: a case report. J Headache Pain 16:21

55. Rajabally JA, Jacob S (2005) Hemicrania continua responsive to verapamil. Headache 45:1082–1087

56. Prakash S, Shah ND (2010) Pure menstrual hemicrania continua: does it exist? A case report. Cephalalgia 10:631–633

57. Solomon S, Newman LC (1999) Chronic daily bilateral headache responsive to indomethacin. Headache 39:754–757

58. Rozen TD (2009) Can indomethacin act as a disease modifying agent in hemicrania continua? A supportive clinical case. Headache 49:759–762

59. Young WB, Silberstein SD (1993) Hemicrania continua and symptomatic medication overuse. Headache 33:485–487

60. Goadsby PJ, Lipton RB (1997) A review of paroxysmal hemicranias, SUNCT syndrome and other short-lasting headaches with autonomic feature, including new cases. Brain 120:193–209

61. Pareja JA, Palomo T, Gorriti MA, Pareja J, Espejo J, Moron B, Trigo M (1990) Hemicrania continua. The first Spanish case: a case report. Cephalalgia 10:143–145

62. Antonaci F, Pareja JA, Caminero AB, Sjaastad O (1997) Chronic paroxysmal hemicrania and hemicrania continua: anesthetic blockades of pericranial nerves. Funct Neurol 12:11–15

63. Weyker P, Webb C, Mathew L (2012) Radiofrequency ablation of the supra-orbital nerve in the treatment algorithm of hemicrania continua. Pain Physician 15:719–724

64. Guerrero AL, Herrero-Velazquez S, Penas ML, Mulero P, Pedraza MI, Cortijo E, Fernandez R (2012) Peripheral nerve blocks: a therapeutic alternative for hemicrania continua. Cephalalgia 36:505–508

65. Peres MFP, Silberstein SD (2002) Hemicrania continua responds to cyclooxygenase-2 inhibitors. Headache 42:530–531

66. Sjaastad O, Antonaci F (1995) A piroxicam derivative partly effective in chronic paroxysmal hemicrania and hemicrania continua. Headache 35:549–550

67. Antonaci F, Pareja JA, Caminero AB, Sjaastad A (1996) Chronic paroxysmal hemicrania and hemicrania continua: lack of efficacy of sumatriptan. Headache 38:197–200

68. Schwedt TJ, Dodick DW, Hentz J, Trentman TL, Zimmerman RS (2007) Occipital nerve stimulation for chronic headache – long-term safety and efficacy. Cephalalgia 27:153–157

69. Matharu MS, Boes CJ, Goadsby PJ (2003) Management of trigeminal autonomic cephalalgias and hemicrania continua. Drugs 63:1637–1677

70. Modar K, Fayyaz A (2013) Hemicrania continua responsive to botulinum toxin type a: a case report. Headache 53:831–833

71. Micieli G, Cavallini A, Fachinetti F, Sances G, Nappi G (1989) Chronic paroxysmal hemicrania: a chronobiological study (case report). Cephalalgia 9:281–286

72. Martinez-Salio A, Porta-Etessam J, Peres-Martinez D, Balserio J, Gutierrez-Riva E (2000) Chronic paroxysmal hemicrania-TIC syndrome. Headache 40:682–685

73. Benoliel R, Sharav Y (1998) Paroxysmal hemicrania. Case studies and review of literature. Oral Surg Oral Med Oral Pathol Oral Radiol Endod 85:285–292

74. Bingel U, Weillel E (2005) An unusual indomethacin-sensitive headache: a case of bilateral episodic paroxysmal hemicrania without autonomic symptoms? Cephalalgia 25:148–150

75. Blankenburg M, Hechler T, Dubbel G, Wamsler C, Zernikow B (2009) Paroxysmal hemicrania in children—symptoms, diagnostic criteria, therapy and outcome. Cephalalgia 29:873–882

76. Antonaci F, Pareja JA, Caminero AB, Sjaastad O (1998) Chronic paroxysmal hemicrania and hemicrania continua: lack of efficacy of sumatriptan. Headache 38:197–200

77. Dodick DW (1998) Exatratrigeminal episodic paroxysmal hemicrania. Further clinical evidence of functionally relevant brain stem connections. Headache 38:794–798

78. Blau JN, Engel H (1990) Episodic paroxysmal hemicrania: a further case and review of literature. J Neurol Neurosurg Psychiatry 53:343–344

79. Boes CJ, Swanson JW, Dodick DW (1998) Chronic paroxysmal hemicrania presenting as otalgia with a sensation of external acoustic meatus obstruction: two cases and a pathophysiologic hypothesis. Headache 38:787–791

80. Mateo I, Pascual J (1999) Coexistence of chronic paroxysmal hemicrania and benign cough headache. Headache 39:437–438

81. Zidverc-Trajkovic J, Pavlovic AM, Mijajlovic M, Jovanovic Z, Sternic N, Kostic VS (2005) Cluster headache and paroxysmal hemicrania: differential diagnosis. Cephalalgia 25:244–248

82. Newman LC, Lipton RB, Solomon S (1993) Episodic paroxysmal hemicrania: 3 new cases and a review of literature. Headache 33:195–197

83. Centonze V, Bassi A, Causarano V, Dalfino L, Centonze A, Albano O (2000) Simultaneous occurrence of ipsilateral cluster headache and chronic paroxysmal hemicrania: a case report. Headache 40:54–56

84. Cohen AS, Matharu MS, Goadsby PJ (2006) Paroxysmal hemicrania in a family. Cephalalgia 26:486–488

85. Evans RW, Olesen J (2000) Remitting chronic paroxysmal hemicrania or episodic paroxysmal hemicrania? Headache 40:858–859

86. Evans RW (2007) Bilateral paroxysmal hemicrania with autonomic symptoms: the first case report. Cephalalgia 28:191–192

87. De Almeida DB, Cunali PA, Santos PL, Brioschi M, Prandini M (2004) Chronic paroxysmal hemicrania in early childhood: case report. Cephalalgia 24:608–609

88. Sarlani E, Schwartz AH, Greenspan JD, Grace EG (2003) Chronic paroxysmal hemicrania: a case report and review of literature. J Orof Pain 17:74–78

89. Cittadini E, Matharu MS, Goadsby PJ (2008) Paroxysmal hemicrania: a prospective clinical study of 31 cases. Brain 131:1142–1155

90. Fuad F, Jones NS (2002) Paroxysmal hemicrania and cluster headache: two discrete entities or is there an overlap? Clin. Otolaryngology 27:472–479

91. Warner JS, Wamil AW, McLean MJ (1994) Acetazolamide for the treatment of chronic paroxysmal hemicrania. Headache 34:597–599

92. Tehindrazanarivelo AD, Visy JM, Bousser MJ (1992) Ipsilateral cluster headache and chronic paroxysmal hemicrania: two case reports. Cephalalgia 12:318–320

93. Tarantino S, Vollono C, Capuano A, Vigevano F, Valeriani M (2011) Chronic paroxysmal hemicrania in pediatric age: report of two cases. J Headache Pain 12:263–267

94. Totczeck A, Diener HC, Gaul C (2014) Concomitant occurrence of different trigeminal autonomic cephalalgias: a case series and review of the literature. Cephalalgia 34:231–235

95. Talvik I, Peet A, Talvik T (2009) Three-year follow-up of a girl with chronic paroxysmal hemicrania. Pediatr Neurol 40:68–69

96. Siow HC (2004) Seasonal episodic paroxysmal hemicrania responding to cyclooxygenase-2 inhibitors. Cephalalgia 24:414–415

97. Pugach NL (2008) An unusual form of TAC–TAC sine autonomic phenomena. J Headache Pain 9:331–332

98. Rossi P, Di Lorenzo G, Faraoni J, Sauli E (2005) Seasonal, extratrigeminal, episodic paroxysmal hemicrania successfully treated with single suboccipital steroid injections. Eur J Neurol 12:903–906

99. Mathew NT, Kailasam J, Fischer A (2002) Responsiveness to celecoxib in chronic paroxysmal hemicrania. Neurology 55:316

100. Seidel S, Wober C (2009) Paroxysmal hemicrania with visual aura in a 17-year-old boy. Headache 49:607–609

101. Morelli N, Mancuso M, Felisati G, Lozza P, Maccaris A, Cafforio G, Gori S, Mirri L, Giudetti D (2009) Does sphenopalatine endoscopic ganglion block have an effect in paroxysmal hemicrania? A case report. Cephalalgia 30:365–367

102. Lisotto C, Maggioni F, Mainrdi F, Zanchin G (2003) Rofecoxib for the treatment of chronic paroxysmal hemicrania. Cephalalgia 23:318–320

103. Pascual J, Quijano J (1998) A case of chronic paroxysmal hemicrania responding to subcutaneous sumatriptan. J Neurol Neurosurg Psychiatry 65:407

104. Mulder LJMM, Spierings ELH (2004) Non-lateralized pain in a case of chronic paroxysmal hemicrania? Cephalalgia 24:52–54

105. Prakash S, Belani P, Susvirkar A, Trivendi A, Ahuja S, Patel A (2013) Paroxysmal hemicrania: a retrospective study of a consecutive series of 22 patients and a critical analysis of the diagnostic criteria. J Headache Pain 14:26

106. Shah ND, Prakash S (2009) Coexistence of cluster headache and paroxysmal hemicrania: does it exist? A case report and literature review. J Headache Pain 10:219–223

107. Sanahuja J, Vazquez P, Falguera M (2005) Paroxysmal hemicrania-tic syndrome responsive to acetazolamide. Cephalalgia 25:547–549

108. Muller KI, Bekkelund SI (2011) Hemicrania continua changed to chronic paroxysmal hemicrania after treatment with cyclooxygenase-2 inhibitor. Headache 51:300–305

109. Raieli V, Cicala V, Vanadia F (2015) Pediatric paroxysmal hemicrania: a case report and some clinical considerations. Neurol Sci. doi:10.1007/s10072-015-2362-3

110. Zukerman E, Peres MFP, Kaup AO, Monzillo PH, Costa AR (2000) Chronic paroxysmal hemicrania–tic syndrome. Neurology 54:1524–1526

111. Shabbir N, McAbee G (1994) Adolescent chronic paroxysmal hemicrania responsive to verapamil monotherapy. Headache 34:209–210

112. Maggioni F, Palmieri A, Viaro F, Mainardi F, Zanchin G (2007) Menstrual paroxysmal hemicrania, a possible new entity? Cephalalgia 27:1085–1087

113. Caminero AB, Pareja JA, Dobato JL (1998) Chronic paroxysmal hemicrania-TIC syndrome. Cephalalgia 18:159–161

114. Dahlof C (1993) Subcutaneous sumatriptan does not abort attacks of chronic paroxysmal hemicrania (CPH). Headache 33:201–202

115. Boes CJ, Matharu MS, Goadsby PJ (2003) The paroxysmal hemicrania-TIC syndrome. Cephalalgia 23:24–28

116. Pareja JJ, Pareja J (1992) Chronic paroxysmal hemicrania coexisting with migraine. Differential response to pharmacological treatment. Headache 32:77–78

117. Pareja JA, Caminero AB, Franco E, Casado JL, Pascual J, Sanchez del Rio M (2001) Dose, efficacy and tolerability for long-term indomethacin treatment of chronic paroxysmal hemicrania and hemicrania continua. Cephalalgia 21:906–910

118. Pareja JA (1995) Chronic paroxysmal hemicrania: dissociation of the pain and autonomic features. Headache 35:111–113

119. Boes CJ, Dodick DW (2002) Refining the clinical spectrum of chronic paroxysmal hemicrania: a review of 74 patients. Headache 42:699–708

120. Evers S, Husstedt IW (1996) Alternatives in drug treatment for chronic paroxysmal hemicrania. Headache 36:429–432

121. Kudrow DB, Kudrow L (1989) Successful aspirin prophylaxis in a child with chronic paroxysmal hemicrania. Headache 29:280–281

122. Gobel H, Heinze A, Heinze-Kuhn K, Austermann K (2001) Botulinum toxin A in the treatment of headache syndromes and pericranial pain syndromes. Pain 91:195–199

123. Walcott BP, Bamber NI, Anderson DI (2009) Successful treatment of chronic paroxysmal hemicrania with posterior hypothalamic stimulation: technical case report. Neurosurgery 5:E997

124. Matharu MS, Cohen AS, Goadsby PJ (2004) SUNCT syndrome responsive to intravenous lidocaine. Cephalalgia 24:985–992

125. Cohen AS (2007) Short-lasting neuralgiform headache attacks with conjunctival injection and tearing. Cephalalgia 27:824–832

126. Zhang Y, Zhang H, Lain YJ, Ma YQ, Xie NC, Chen X, Zhang L (2016) Botulinum toxin a for the treatment of a child with SUNCT syndrome. Pain Res Manag 2016. doi:10.1155/2016/8016065

127. Gatenbein AR, Goadsby PJ (2005) Familial SUNCT. Cephalalgia 25:457–459

128. Williams MH, Broadley SA (2008) SUNCT and SUNA: clinical features and medical treatment. J Clin Neurosci 15:526–534

129. Arroyo Martinez A, Romero Duran X, Gomez Beldarrain M, Pinedo A, Garcia-Monco JC (2010) Response to intravenous lidocaine in a patient with SUNCT syndrome. Cephalalgia 30:110–112

130. De Lourdes FM, Bruera O, Pozzo MJ, Leston J (2009) SCUNT syndrome responding absolutely to steroids in two cases with different etiologies. J Headache Pain 10:55–57

131. Sjaastad O, Saunte C, Salvesen R, Fredriksen TA, Seim A, Roe OD, Fostad K, Lobben OP, Zhao JM (1989) Shortlasting, unilateral neuralgiform headache attacks with conjunctival injection, tearing, sweating and rhinorrhea. Cephalalgia 9:147–156

132. Raimondi E, Gardella L (1998) SUNCT syndrome: two cases in Argentina. Headache 38:369–371

133. Calvo JF, Bruera OC, Lourdes-Figuerola D, Gestro D, Tinetti N, Leston JA (2004) SUNCT syndrome: clinical and 12-years follow-up case report. Cephalalgia 24:900–902

134. Rossi P, Cesarino F, Faroni J, Malpezzi MG, Sandrini G, Nappi G (2003) SUNCT syndrome successfully treated with topiramate: case reports. Cephalalgia 23:998–1000

135. Maihofner C, Speck V, Sperling W, Jeppe AG (2013) Complete remission of SUNCT syndrome by intravenous glucocorticoid treatment. Neurol Sci 34:1811–1812

136. Trauninger A, Alkonyi B, Kovacs N, Komoly S, Pfund Z (2010) Methylprednisolone therapy for short-term prevention of SUNCT syndrome. Cephalalgia 30:735–739

137. Marziniak M, Breyer R, Evers S (2009) SUNCT syndrome successfully treated with the combination of oxcarbazepine and gabapentin. Pain Med 8:1497–1500

138. Black DF, Dodick DW (2002) Two cases of medically and surgically intractable SUNCT: a reason for caution and an argument for a central mechanism. Cephalalgia 22:201–204

139. Piovesan EJ, Siow C, Kowacs PA, Werneck LC (2003) Influence of lamotrigine over the SUNCT syndrome: one patient follow-up for two years. Arq Neuropsiquiatr 61:691–694

140. Porta-Etessam J, Cuadrado ML, Galan L, Sampedro A, Valencia C (2010) Temporal response to bupivacaine bilateral great occipital nerve block in a patient with SUNCT syndrome. J Headache Pain 11:179

141. Schwaag S, Frese A, Husstedt IW, Evers S (2003) SUNCT syndrome: the first German case series. Cephalalgia 23:398–400

142. D'Andrea G, Granella F, Cadaldini M (1999) Possible usefulness of lamotrigine in the treatment of SUNCT syndrome. Neurology 53:1609

143. Antonaci F, Sances G, Loi M, Sandrini G, Dumitrache C, Cuzzoni MG (2010) SUNCT syndrome with paroxysmal mydriasis: clinical and pupillometric findings. Cephalalgia 30:987–990

144. D'Andrea G, Granella F, Ghiotto N, Nappi G (2001) Lamotrigine in the treatment of SUNCT syndrome. Neurology 57:1723–1725

145. Lambru G, Matharu M (2013) Management of trigeminal autonomic cephalalgias in children and adolescents. Curr Pain Headache Rep 17:323

146. Leone M, Rigamonti A, Usai S, D'Amico D, Grazzi L, Bussone G (2000) Two new SUNCT cases responsive to lamotrigine. Cephalalgia 20:845–847

147. Gutierrez-Garcia JM (2002) SUNCT syndrome responsive to lamotrigine. Headache 42:823–825

148. Chakravarty A, Mukherjee A (2003) SUNCT syndrome responsive to lamotrigine: documentation of the first Indian case. Cephalalgia 23:474–475

149. Malik K, Rizvi S, Vaillancourt PD (2002) The SUNCT syndrome: successfully treated with lamotrigine. Pain Med 2:167–168

150. Tan DYH, Chua ET, Ng KB, Chan KP, Thomas J (2013) Frameless linac-based stereotactic radiosurgery treatment for SUNCT syndrome targeting the trigeminal nerve and sphenopalatine ganglion. Cephalalgia 33:1132–1136

151. Paliwal VK, Singh P, Kumar A, Rahi SK, Gupta RK (2012) Short-lasting unilateral neuralgiform headache with conjunctival injection and tearing (SUNCT) with preserved refractory period: report of three cases. J Headache Pain 13:167–169

152. Martins IP, Viana P, Lobo PP (2016) Familial SUNCT in mother and son. Cephalalgia 36:993–997

153. Zabalza RJ (2012) Sustained response to botulinum toxin in SUNCT syndrome. Cephalalgia 32:869–872

154. Fantini J, Granato A, Zorzon M, Manganotti P (2016) Case report: coexistence of SUNCT and hypnic headache in the same patient. Headache 56:1503–1506

155. Cacão G, Correia Diaz F, Pereira-Monteiro J (2016) SUNCT syndrome: a cohort of 15 Portuguese patients. Cephalalgia 36:1002–1006

156. Becser N, Berky M (1995) SUNCT syndrome: a Hungarian case. Headache 35:158–160

157. Gay-Escoda C, Mayor-Subirana G, Camps-Font O, Berini-Aytes L (2015) SUNCT syndrome. Report of a case and treatment update. J Clin Exp Dent 7:342–347

158. Tada Y, Ikuta N, Negoro K (2009) Short-lasting unilateral neuralgiform headache attacks with cranial autonomic symptoms (SUNA). Inter Med 48:2141–2144

159. Pareja JA, Pareja J, Palomo T, Caballero V, Pamo M (1994) SUNCT syndrome: repetitive and overlapping attacks. Headache 34:114–116

160. Pareja JA, Sjaastad O (1994) SUNCT syndrome in the female. Headache 34:217–220

161. Cohen AS, Matharu MS, Goadsby PJ (2004) SUNCT syndrome in the elderly. Cephalalgia 24:508–509

162. Sabatovsky R, Huber M, Meuser T, Radbruch L (2001) SUNCT syndrome: a treatment option with local opioid blockade of the superior cervical ganglion? A case report. Cephalalgia 21:154–156

163. Effendi K, Jarjoura S, Mathieu D (2011) SUNCT syndrome successfully treated by gamma knife radiosurgery: case report. Cephalalgia 31:870–873

164. Bouhassira D, Attal N, Estève M, Chauvin M (1994) "SUNCT" syndrome. A case of transformation from trigeminal neuralgia? Cephalalgia 14:168–170

165. Ikawa M, Imai N, Manaka S (2010) A case of SUNCT syndrome responsive to zonisamide. Cephalalgia 31:501–503

166. Dora B (2006) SUNCT syndrome with dramatic response to oxcarbazepine. Cephalalgia 26:1171–1173

167. Hunt HC, Dodick DW, Bosch P (2002) SUNCT responsive to gabapentin. Headache 42:526–525

168. Volcy M, Tepper SJ, Rapoport AM, Sheftell FD, Bigal ME (2005) Short-lasting unilateral neuralgiform headache attacks with cranial autonomic symptoms (SUNA) – a case report. Cephalalgia 25:470–472

169. Vukovic-Cvetkovic' VV, Jensen RH (2016) A boy with bilateral SUNA: a case report. Cephalalgia. doi:10.1177/0333102416663467

170. Narbone MC, Gangemi S, Abbate M (2005) A case of SUNCT syndrome responsive to verapamil. Cephalalgia 25:476–478

171. Benoliel R, Sharav Y (1998) SUNCT syndrome. Case report and literature review. Oral Surg Oral Med Oral Palhol Oral Radiol Ended 85:158–161

172. Etemadifar M, Maghzi AH, Ghasemi M, Chitsaz A, Kaji Esfahani M (2008) Efficacy of gabapentin in the treatment of SUNCT syndrome. Cephalalgia 28:1339–1342

173. Graff-Radford SB (2000) SUNCT syndrome responsive to gabapentin (Neurontin). Cephalalgia 20:515–517

174. Miller S, Akram H, Lagrata S, Hariz M, Zrinzo L, Matharu M (2016) Ventral tegmental area deep brain stimulation in refractory short-lasting unilateral neuralgiform headache attacks. Brain 1:1–10

175. Lambru G, Shanahan P, Watkins L, Matharu MS (2014) Occipital nerve stimulation in the treatment of medically intractable SUNCT and SUNA. Pain Physician 17:29–41

176. Broggi G, Franzini A, Leone M, Bussone G (2007) Update on neurosurgical treatment of chronic trigeminal autonomic cephalalgias and atypical facial pain with deep brain stimulation of posterior hypothalamus: results and comments. Neurol Sci 28:138–145

177. Franzini A, Messina G, Cordella R, Marras C, Broggi G (2010) Deep brain stimulation of the posteromedial hypothalamus: indications, long-term results, and neurophysiological considerations. Neurosurg Focus 29:1–13

178. Lyons MK, Dodick DW, Evidente VGH (2009) Responsiveness of short-lasting unilateral neuralgiform headache with conjunctival injection and tearing to hypothalamic deppe brain stimulation. J Neurosurg 110:279–281

179. Leone M, Franzini A, D'Andrea G, Broggi G, Casucci G, Bussone G (2005) Deep brain stimulation to relieve drug-resistant SUNCT. Ann Neurol 57:924–927

180. Cuadrado ML, Aledo-Serrano Á, Navarro P, López-Ruiz P, Fernández-de-Las-Peñas C, González-Suárez I, Orviz A, Fernández-Pérez C (2016) Short-term effects of greater occipital nerve blocks in chronic migraine: a double-blind, randomised, placebo-controlled clinical trial. Cephalalgia. doi:10.1177/0333102416655159

181. Riendeau D, Charleson S, Cromlish W, Mancini JA, Wong E, Guay J (1997) Comparison of the cyclooxygenase-1 inhibitory properties of nonsteroidal anti-inflammatory drugs (NSAIDs) and selective COX-2 inhibitors, using sensitive microsomal and platelet assays. Can J Physiol Pharmacol 75:1088–1095

182. Leone M, Bussone G (2009) Pathophysiology of trigeminal autonomic cephalalgias. Lancet Neurol 8:755–764

183. Martelletti P, Jensen RH, Antal A, Arcioni R, Brighina F, de Tommaso M, Franzini A, Fontaine D, Heiland M, Jürgens TP, Leone M, Magis D, Paemeleire K, Palmisani S, Paulus W, May A, European Headache Federation (2013) Neuromodulation of chronic headaches: position statement from the European Headache Federation. J Headache Pain 14:86

184. Solomon SD, Pfeffer MA, McMurray JJ, Fowler R, Finn P, Levin B, Eagle C, Hawk E, Lechuga M, Zauber AG, Bertagnolli MM, Arber N, Wittes J, APC and PreSAP Trial Investigators (2006) Effect of celecoxib on cardiovascular events and blood pressure in two trials for the prevention of colorectal adenomas. Circulation 114:1028–1035

185. Harirforoosh S, Jamali F (2008) Renal adverse effects of nonsteroidal anti-inflammatory drugs. Expert Opin Drug Saf 8:669–681

186. Baron JA, Sandler RS, Bresalier RS, Lanas A, Morton DG, Riddell R, Iverson ER, Demets DL (2008) Cardiovascular events associated with rofecoxib: final analysis of the APPROVe trial. Lancet 372:1756–1764

187. Lipscomb GR, Wallis N, Armstrong G, Rees WDW (1998) Gastrointestinal tolerability of meloxicam and piroxicam: a double-blind placebo-controlled study. Br J Clin Pharmacol 46:133–137

188. Schwartzman RJ, Patel M, Grothusen JR, Alexander GM (2009) Efficacy of 5-day continuous lidocaine infusion for the treatment of refractory complex regional pain syndrome. Pain Med 10:401–412

189. Samarin MJ, Mohrien KM, Oliphant CS (2005) Continuous intravenous antiarrhythmic agents in the intensive care unit: strategies for safe and effective use of amiodarone, lidocaine, and procainamide. Crit Care Nurs Q 38:329–344

190. Prakash S, Shah ND (2010) Post-infectious new daily persistent headache may respond to intravenous methylprednisolone. J Headache Pain 11(1):59–66. doi:10.1007/s10194-009-0171-x

191. French JA, Gazzola DM (2011) New generation antiepileptic drugs: what do they offer in terms of improved tolerability and safety? Ther Adv Drug Saf 2: 141–158

192. Mitsikostas DD, Ashina M, Craven A, Diener HC, Goadsby PJ, Ferrari MD, Lampl C, Paemeleire K, Pascual J, Siva A, Olesen J, Osipova V, Martelletti P, EHF committee (2015) European Headache Federation consensus on technical investigation for primary headache disorders. J Headache Pain 17: 5. doi:10.1186/s10194-016-0596-y

193. Robbins MS, Starling AJ, Pringsheim TM, Becker WJ, Schwedt TJ (2016) Treatment of cluster headache: the American Headache Society evidence-based guidelines. Headache 56:1093–1106

# Treatment of disabling headache with greater occipital nerve injections in a large population of childhood and adolescent patients

Francesca Puledda[1]* [iD], Peter J. Goadsby[1] and Prab Prabhakar[2]

## Abstract

**Background:** Pediatric headache disorders can be extremely disabling, with marked reduction in the quality of life of children and their carers. Evidenced-based options for the treatment of primary headache disorders with preventive medication is limited and clinical outcomes are often unsatisfactory. Greater occipital nerve injections represent a rapid and well-tolerated therapeutic option, which is widely used in clinical practice in adults, and has previously shown a good outcome in a pediatric population.

**Methods:** This service evaluation reviewed greater occipital nerve injections performed unilaterally with 30 mg 1% lidocaine and 40 mg methylprednisolone, to treat disabling headache disorders in children and adolescents.

**Results:** We analyzed a total of 159 patients who received 380 injections. Of the population, 79% had chronic migraine, 14% new daily persistent headache, 4% a trigeminal autonomic cephalalgia, 3% secondary headache and one patient had chronic tension-type headache. An improvement after injection was seen in 66% ($n = 105$) of subjects, lasting on average $9 \pm 4$ weeks. Improvement was seen in 68% of patients with chronic migraine, 67% with a trigeminal autonomic cephalalgia and 59% with new daily persistent headache. Side effects were reported in 8% and were mild and transient. Older age, female gender, chronic migraine, increased number of past preventive use, medication overuse and developing side effects were all associated with an increased likelihood of positive treatment outcome.

**Conclusions:** This large single centre service evaluation confirms that unilateral injection of the greater occipital nerve is a safe, rapid-onset and effective treatment strategy in disabling headache disorders in children, with a range of diagnoses and severity of the condition, and with minimal side effects.

**Keywords:** Pediatric headache, Greater occipital nerve injection, Chronic migraine, Trigeminal autonomic cephalalgia, Cluster headache, New daily persistent headache

## Background

Headache is the most common manifestation of pain in childhood and can severely impact the health, functional status and quality of life of pediatric patients [1]. In particular, headache disorders with high frequency of attacks in children and adolescents can be extremely disabling. The one-year prevalence of migraine in children between the ages of 5 and 15 years ranges around 10% depending on the study [2], while chronic migraine affects between 0.8% and 1.7% of adolescents [3] and up to 1.7% of subjects in pediatric age groups [4]. The prevalence is up to three times higher in females [5, 6]. When primary headache disorders manifest daily they may be misdiagnosed and very often present co-morbidities such as anxiety, mood disorders, sleep issues and other pain syndromes [7], which require themselves to be addressed.

For all these reasons, early management of disabling headache as early in its course as possible is highly

---

* Correspondence: Francesca.puledda@kcl.ac.uk
[1]Headache Group, Department of Basic and Clinical Neuroscience, King's College London, and NIHR-Wellcome Trust King's Clinical Research Facility, Wellcome Foundation Building, King's College Hospital, London SE5 9PJ, UK

desirable and should involve several strategies, including prevention. In this context, therapy can be extremely challenging, with physicians often facing difficulty in finding rapid and sustained treatment options with a demonstrated efficacy and tolerability in the pediatric population. Recent evidence confirms this, showing that common preventive treatments used in adult migraineurs may not be as effective in pediatric patients [8].

Infiltration of the area around the greater occipital nerve with a mixture of local anesthetic and corticosteroids is a well-established therapy for primary headache prevention in adults [9, 10] that has been recently reported in children to have excellent results [11]. Greater occipital nerve (GON) injections have shown to provide a quick onset of therapeutic response, which is also sustained [12], while avoiding the common side effects of classic migraine preventives or more invasive treatments [13]. The mechanism of action is linked to the anatomical overlap between spinal afferents providing sensory innervation from the C2 occipital region and trigeminal afferents at the trigeminocervical complex, a complex brain area involved in the pathophysiology of primary headache disorders [14].

Our objective was to determine the efficacy and safety of greater occipital nerve injections in a large population of paediatric headache patients.

## Methods
### Study population and design
We performed a service evaluation of the Specialist Headache Centre at Great Ormond Street Hospital for Children and required no Research Ethics Committee approval (http://www.hra-decisiontools.org.uk/research/). A retrospective chart review was performed on all letters and clinical correspondence for patients who received a greater occipital nerve injection between 2009 and 2016. The population comprised children and adolescents seen within the Headache Centre by authors (PP and PJG), always in the presence of either a parent or guardian. Whenever possible, patient histories were taken directly from the children themselves. Headache diagnoses were defined according to ICHD-III-beta [15].

### Data collection
Retrospective data abstraction was performed by one of the authors (FP). For each patient who received a GON injection, information on age (measured as a continuous variable), gender, headache diagnosis, date of first visit, time from first visit to injection, site of injection, past and current medication, effects of injection and eventual follow-up treatment was collected using a standardized pro forma.

### Greater occipital nerve injections
Infiltrations of the region of the greater occipital nerve were always performed unilaterally and consisted of 30 mg 1% lidocaine and 40 mg methylprednisolone acetate. The clinician palpated over the greater occipital nerves and injected the side that was most tender. GON injection was administered 1–2 cm below the midpoint between the occipital tubercle and mastoid process in all patients. The injection site was then massaged to spread the solution.

For the purpose of data collection, we included both first time and repeat injections. The primary outcome of 'improvement' from the injection was defined as either a significant, more than one third, decrease in headache frequency or intensity or by a documented headache improvement in the clinical notes.

### Data analysis
All data was tabulated in Excel and analysed using IBM SPSS Statistics 22. $P < 0.05$ was considered significant. Descriptive analysis of numeric variables was performed using measures of central tendency and dispersion. For categorical variables, distribution was described as percentages. Differences in frequencies were examined using Chi-square analysis. A binary logistic regression analysis was performed in order to determine the effect of several predictor variables on the dichotomous primary outcome measure of improvement.

## Results
Two hundred and five patients received at least one greater occipital nerve block, for a total of 458 injections. All patients who were offered an injection had a disabling headache condition.

### Clinical phenotype
Follow-up data for the first injection was available for 78% of patients ($n = 159$), who had a total 380 injections. Of these, 159 patients with follow-up, 79% ($n = 126$) had chronic migraine, 15% ($n = 24$) with aura, 14% ($n = 22$) new daily persistent headache (NDPH), 4% ($n = 6$) a trigeminal autonomic cephalalgia (TAC), 3% ($n = 4$) a form of secondary headache and one patient had chronic tension-type headache. Demographic characteristics of the population are summarized in Table 1.

Medication overuse was present in 23% ($n = 36$) of subjects.

The mean age was $15 \pm 2$ with a range between 8 and 18 years. $n = 12$ subjects fell within the 8–12 age range, $n = 78$ in the 13–15 range and $n = 69$ in the 16–18 range.

Female to male ratio was 2.2:1 Mean number of headache years was $4 \pm 3$ and on average patients had tried at least two previous preventives with a range between 0 and 5.

**Table 1** Demographic characteristics of 159 patients treated with greater occipital nerve injection

| | | |
|---|---|---|
| Total patients | $n = 159$ | |
| Mean age (years ± SD; range) | 15 ± 2; | range 8–18 years |
| Female: male (n:n); % | 108:50; | 68% - 32% |
| Headache diagnosis (n; %) | | |
| Chronic migraine without aura (CM) | 102 | 64% |
| Chronic migraine with aura (CMwA) | 24 | 15% |
| *Total chronic migraine* | 126 | 79% |
| NDPH | 22 | 14% |
| CH | 3 | 2% |
| HC | 1 | 0.6% |
| SUNCT/SUNA | 2 | 1% |
| *Total TAC* | 6 | 4% |
| TTH | 1 | 0.6% |
| Secondary HA | 4 | 3% |
| Years of headache to 1st injection (years ± SD; range) | 4.5 ± 3.2; | range 0–12 years |
| Past medication (mean ± SD) | 2.1 ± 1.5 | range 0–5 |
| Patients on preventive medication at time of injection (n) | 115 | |
| Diagnosis of medication overuse at time of injection (n; %) | 36; | 23% |

## Efficacy

A benefit from the GON injection was seen in 66% ($n = 105$) of subjects and this was significant respect to the number of patients who had no effect ($p < 0.001$; see Table 2). The mean duration of improvement was 9 ± 4 weeks with a minimum of 3 weeks (in $n = 5$ patients); the remaining one-hundred patients had an improvement which lasted for more than 3 weeks.

Improvement was seen in 68% of the chronic migraine population ($n = 85$) and 59% ($n = 13$) in the NDPH subgroup. Four of the six patients (67%) with trigeminal autonomic cephalalgias had benefit from the injection. We performed a Chi-square analysis to find differences in frequencies between headache diagnosis and the primary outcome measure; having excluded tension-type headache and secondary headache cases for low numbers, there was no significant difference in improvement between migraine, NDPH and trigeminal autonomic cephalalgias. Sustained headache freedom of more than 3 weeks was seen in 17 patients, of which the majority had chronic migraine.

A total of ninety-nine patients received subsequent injections, and fifty-one of these went on to have more than two. These were given at variable intervals, with a minimum twelve-week gap in between injections. Of patients who had subsequent injections $n = 15$ were headache free and $n = 67$ had a general benefit after treatment.

## Side effects

Side effects were reported in thirteen patients: eleven subjects had a headache worsening, however in five of these a beneficial effect followed after a maximum ten-day interval. One patient reported soreness at the site of injection and one had an allergic reaction, possibly to the sedative that had to be used during the procedure.

## Modelling

A binary logistic regression model was created in order to examine the effect of age, gender, medication overuse, headache diagnosis and frequency, years of disease, number of past preventives used and presence of side effects, on the primary outcome measure of improvement for the first GON injection. Results of the regression analysis are shown in Table 3. In summary, no specific variable was responsible for significantly predicting a positive outcome, although a diagnosis of migraine and a trigeminal autonomic cephalalgia increased the odds of having an improvement from the injection by 4 and 3 times, respectively. Each increase in age by year made the odds of improvement 1.2 times more likely (95% CI 0.8–1.8) as well as each increase in discreet number of past medications used and being a female. Having a diagnosis of medication overuse and having developed side effects to the injection were also associated with an increase likelihood of having an improvement after the treatment. The predictor variables inserted in the model were subsequently removed one at a time, causing no significant change in results and therefore allowing to exclude any confounding effect of single variables on the model.

## Discussion

Disabling headaches can be extremely challenging for both patients and clinicians [1], especially given that the

**Table 2** Effects of first greater occipital nerve injection in 159 chronic headache patients with available follow-up

| Improvement from injection | $n = 105\ P < 0.001$ | 66% |
|---|---|---|
| Duration of improvement (weeks) | $9.3 \pm 4.3$ | |
| Benefit per HA diagnosis (n; %) | | |
| CM | 70 | 69% |
| CMwA | 15 | 63% |
| Total migraine | 85 | 68% |
| NDPH | 13 | 59% |
| CH | 3 | 100% |
| HC | 0 | 0% |
| SUNCT/SUNA | 1 | 50% |
| Total TAC | 4 | 67% |
| TTH | 1 | 100% |
| Secondary HA | 2 | 50% |
| Sustained HA freedom (>3 weeks) | 17 | 16% |
| CM | 11 | 16% |
| CMwA | 2 (one brainstem) | 13% |
| Total migraine | 13 | 10% of total migraine |
| NDPH | 2 | 15%, 9% of total NDPH |
| CH | 1 | 33% |
| SUNCT | 1 | 100% |
| Total TAC | 2 | 33% of total TAC |
| Side effects | 13 | 8% |
| Worsened HA int/freq for up to 5 weeks | 6 (with no improvement) | |
| Worsened HA int/freq for up to 10 days | 5 (with improvement) | |
| Soreness | 1 | |
| Reaction to sedative | 1 | |

armamentarium of available strategies presents several caveats, making adherence to treatment generally quite low [16]. Our service evaluation suggests greater occipital nerve injections can be useful across a range of primary headache disorders, offering an effective, low-risk procedure.

The majority of patients improved after the first GON injection. This is in accordance with previous observations in adults [12] and children [11]. Interestingly, our study found no significant difference with regards to response to treatment in different headache phenotypes,

**Table 3** Results of binary logistic regression analysis for likelihood of improvement from greater occipital nerve injection. Variables in italics were associated with negative beta values and therefore a decreased likelihood of the outcome

| Predictor Variable | p value | Odds ratio | 95% Confidence Interval |
|---|---|---|---|
| Age (measured in years) | 0.38 | 1.2 | 0.8–1.8 |
| Gender (female) | 0.74 | 1.2 | 0.4–3.6 |
| Chronic migraine diagnosis | 0.32 | 4.0 | 0.3–62.2 |
| TAC diagnosis | 0.45 | 3.0 | 0.2–50.6 |
| Medication overuse | 0.89 | 1.1 | 0.4–3.1 |
| Headache frequency (days) | 0.47 | 1.0 | 0.9–1.1 |
| Years of headache | 0.58 | 1.0 | 0.8–1.1 |
| Number of past preventives | 0.46 | 1.2 | 0.8–1.6 |
| Time from diagnosis to injection (weeks) | 0.18 | 1.0 | 0.9–1.0 |
| Side effects | 0.53 | 1.8 | 0.3–11.0 |

even if we observed an increased likelihood of response in migraineurs and patients with TACs. It must be noted however that the number trigeminal autonomic cephalalgia patients was quite low ($n$ = 6). It is noteworthy that the clinical trial literature for GON injections is stronger in cluster headache [10, 17] than migraine [18]. Our results are quite encouraging, as it shows that GON injections can be used to treat a variety of complex headache problems regardless of the underlying diagnosis.

Reported studies have shown a great variability exists with regards to clinical practice and approach to this technique [19, 20], and more effort needs to be expended to standardize the general procedure, as well as in obtaining data from controlled trials in different population groups. Even though GON injections have been used for several years in headache practice [21] and other paediatric conditions [22], generally the paediatric headache literature is quite limited, with only one systematic study being performed recently in a North-American headache centre [11]. To the best of our knowledge, this is the first large survey on the practice of greater occipital nerve injections in a European paediatric population.

Treatment response was generally prolonged with 16% of patients remaining headache free for more than 3 weeks. This, even if not comparable with that of regular pharmacological preventives, represents a positive result especially considering that GON injections are a one-off intervention. In this context their use as a transitional therapy can be encouraging for patients. Unfortunately, data on onset of effect from the procedure was not available for all patients, therefore we cannot comment on time of therapeutic response, even though past studies have shown this to be quite rapid [11].

GON infiltrations showed a very high tolerability in our population, with the most common side effect being an initial worsening of the pre-existing headache condition, which lasted up to 5 weeks in the worst case. However, almost half of patients who experienced this side effect subsequently responded to treatment with a significant improvement.

A repeat injection was performed in more than half the patients who had an initial improvement, a large majority of which continued to report a benefit from treatment.

Results from binary logistic regression analysis suggested no significant effect of several clinical parameters in predicting a positive outcome to treatment, although certain conditions, such as chronic migraine, were linked to an increased likelihood of developing an effect from the injection. This result, however, does not exclude that an effective response could be achieved in new daily persistent headache - the second most common chronic headache diagnosis in our population - or other headache phenotypes, as seen by the Chi-square sub analysis.

It is interesting to note that conditions normally associated with a more severe clinical picture, such as an increased number of headache preventive medications used in the past and a diagnosis of medication overuse, not only did not predict a poorer response to treatment but on the contrary were linked with a higher likelihood of improvement. This is also true for the developing of injection side effects, such as a worsening of headache conditions, which in almost half the cases showed to revert to a substantial improvement after a few days. It is therefore possible to infer that greater occipital nerve injections are a valid therapeutic approach even in refractory headache patients who would normally be bound to fail normal preventives [23]; patients should also be informed that side effects are not to be considered as a marker of poor outcome. Finally, our data showed that older children and female patients are generally more likely to have a response to treatment and this is in line with previous studies.

## Limitations

An important limitation of this study is that being compiled from an open label series, a placebo effect cannot be excluded. It is worth noting this is a relatively invasive procedure and the proportion of patients showing a placebo response in headache studies is well established [24]. However, the large number of patients analysed does offer insight on the advantages of this treatment with respect to more classic preventive therapies. In the future, research should focus on performing large randomized controlled studies in paediatric subjects to establish how objectively effective this approach may be.

## Conclusions

Greater occipital nerve injections are a safe, effective and useful strategy for disabling primary headache disorders in children. They appear especially beneficial in patients with migraine and trigeminal autonomic cephalalgias, although phenotypical diagnosis is not an apparent limitation to its effect. Presence of side effects and refractory headache does not predict poor treatment outcome. In the clinical approach to the treatment of chronic primary headache disorders in a paediatric setting, GON injections should be considered as first line management alongside the classic medications, which are often more side-effect prone.

**Abbreviations**
CH: Cluster headache; CM: Chronic migraine without aura; CMwA: Chronic migraine with aura; GON: Greater occipital nerve; HA: Headache; HC: Hemicrania continua; ICHD-III-beta: International classification of headache disorders 3 beta; NDPH: New Daily Persistent Headache; SUNA: Short-lasting unilateral neuralgiform headache attacks with cranial autonomic symptoms; SUNCT: Short lasting unilateral neuralgiform headache

attacks with conjunctival injection and tearing; TAC: Trigeminal autonomic cephalalgia; TTH: Tension-type headache

## Acknowledgements

The authors would like to acknowledge all patients who were seen at the Specialist Headache Centre at Great Ormond Street Hospital for Children over the years.

## Financial disclosures

FP has no disclosures.

PJG has no disclosures relevant to this work. They reports grants and personal fees from Allergan, Amgen, and Eli-Lilly and Company; and personal fees from Akita Biomedical, Alder Biopharmaceuticals, Avanir Pharma, Cipla Ltd., Dr. Reddy's Laboratories, eNeura, Electrocore LLC, Novartis, Pfizer Inc., Quest Diagnostics, Scion, Teva Pharmaceuticals, Trigemina Inc., Scion; and personal fees from MedicoLegal work, Journal Watch, Up-to-Date, Massachusetts Medical Society, Oxford University Press; and in addition, Dr. Goadsby has a patent Magnetic stimulation for headache assigned to eNeura.

PP has no disclosures relevant to this work. Over the last 5 years he has advised, lectured in meetings sponsored by, received honorarium in association with the following commercial organisations - Amgen, Bristol Myers Squibb (BMS), Merck Sharpe and Dohme (MSD), Janssen India, Allergan and Novartis.

## Authors' contributions

FP reviewed all letters, collated and analysed the data and wrote the first draft of the manuscript. PP and PJG saw the patients, wrote the clinical letters, reviewed the data and edited the manuscript. PP performed all GON injections. All authors read and approved the final manuscript.

## Competing interests

The authors declare that they have no competing interests for this work.

## Author details

[1]Headache Group, Department of Basic and Clinical Neuroscience, King's College London, and NIHR-Wellcome Trust King's Clinical Research Facility, Wellcome Foundation Building, King's College Hospital, London SE5 9PJ, UK. [2]Department of Paediatric Neurology, Great Ormond Hospital for Children NHS Foundation Trust, London, UK.

## References

1. Kernick D, Campbell J (2009) Measuring the impact of headache in children: a critical review of the literature. Cephalalgia 29(1):3–16
2. Abu-Arafeh I, Razak S, Sivaraman B, Graham C (2010) Prevalence of headache and migraine in children and adolescents: a systematic review of population-based studies. Dev Med Child Neurol 52(12):1088–1097
3. Lipton RB, Manack A, Ricci JA, Chee E, Turkel CC, Winner P (2011) Prevalence and burden of chronic migraine in adolescents: results of the chronic daily headache in adolescents study (C-dAS). Headache 51(5):693–706
4. Wober-Bingol C (2013) Epidemiology of migraine and headache in children and adolescents. Curr Pain Headache Rep 17(6):341
5. Arruda MA, Guidetti V, Galli F, Albuquerque RC, Bigal ME (2010) Frequent headaches in the preadolescent pediatric population: a population-based study. Neurology 74(11):903–908
6. Wang SJ, Fuh JL, Lu SR, Juang KD (2006) Chronic daily headache in adolescents: prevalence, impact, and medication overuse. Neurology 66(2): 193–197
7. Seshia SS (2012) Chronic daily headache in children and adolescents. Curr Pain Headache Rep 16(1):60–72
8. Powers SW, Coffey CS, Chamberlin LA, Ecklund DJ, Klingner EA, Yankey JW et al (2017) Trial of Amitriptyline, Topiramate, and placebo for Pediatric migraine. N Engl J Med 376(2):115–124
9. Inan LE, Inan N, Karadas O, Gul HL, Erdemoglu AK, Turkel Y et al (2015) Greater occipital nerve blockade for the treatment of chronic migraine: a randomized, multicenter, double-blind, and placebo-controlled study. Acta Neurol Scand 132(4):270–277
10. Ambrosini A, Vandenheede M, Rossi P, Aloj F, Sauli E, Pierelli F et al (2005) Suboccipital injection with a mixture of rapid- and long-acting steroids in cluster headache: a double-blind placebo-controlled study. Pain 118(1–2): 92–96
11. Gelfand AA, Reider AC, Goadsby PJ (2014) Outcomes of greater occipital nerve injections in pediatric patients with chronic primary headache disorders. Pediatr Neurol 50(2):135–139
12. Afridi SK, Shields KG, Bhola R, Goadsby PJ (2006) Greater occipital nerve injection in primary headache syndromes–prolonged effects from a single injection. Pain 122(1–2):126–129
13. Martelletti P, Giamberardino MA, Mitsikostas DD (2016) Greater occipital nerve as target for refractory chronic headaches: from corticosteroid block to invasive neurostimulation and back. Expert Rev Neurother 16(8):865–866
14. Goadsby PJ, Holland PR, Martins-Oliveira M, Hoffmann J, Schankin C, Akerman S (2017) Pathophysiology of migraine- a disorder of sensory processing. Physiol Rev 97:553–622
15. Headache Classification Committee of the International Headache Society (IHS) (2013) The international classification of headache disorders, 3rd edition (beta version). Cephalalgia 33(9):629–808
16. Evans RW, Linde M (2009) Expert opinion: adherence to prophylactic migraine medication. Headache 49(7):1054–1058
17. Leroux E, Valade D, Taifas I, Vicaut E, Chagnon M, Roos C et al (2011) Suboccipital steroid injections for transitional treatment of patients with more than two cluster headache attacks per day: a randomised, double-blind, placebo-controlled trial. Lancet Neurol 10(10):891–897
18. Dilli E, Halker R, Vargas B, Hentz J, Radam T, Rogers R et al (2015) Occipital nerve block for the short-term preventive treatment of migraine: a randomized, double-blinded, placebo-controlled study. Cephalalgia 35(11): 959–968
19. Szperka CL, Gelfand AA, Hershey AD (2016) Patterns of use of peripheral nerve blocks and trigger point injections for Pediatric headache: results of a survey of the American headache society Pediatric and adolescent section. Headache 56(10):1597–1607
20. Blumenfeld A, Ashkenazi A, Grosberg B, Napchan U, Narouze S, Nett B et al (2010) Patterns of use of peripheral nerve blocks and trigger point injections among headache practitioners in the USA: results of the American headache society interventional procedure survey (AHS-IPS). Headache 50(6):937–942
21. Anthony M (1992) Headache and the greater occipital nerve. Clin Neurol Neurosurg 94(4):297–301
22. Johr M (2015) Regional anaesthesia in neonates, infants and children: an educational review. Eur J Anaesthesiol 32(5):289–297
23. Schulman E (2013) Refractory migraine - a review. Headache 53(4):599–613
24. Macedo A, Banos JE, Farre M (2008) Placebo response in the prophylaxis of migraine: a meta-analysis. Eur J Pain 12(1):68–75

# 19

# OnabotulinumtoxinA in the treatment of refractory chronic cluster headache

Christian Lampl[1]* (iD), Mirjam Rudolph[1] and Elisabeth Bräutigam[2]

## Abstract

**Background:** Cluster headache (CH) is a clinically well-defined primary headache disorder, approximately 20% of cluster headache sufferers experience recurrent attacks without periods of significant remission. For the treatment of chronic cluster headache (CCH) only limited therapeutic options are available.

**Methods:** A potential refractory CCH patient group was identified according to the clinical definition of rCCH based on the consensus statement of the European Headache Federation (EHF). Treatment with OnabotulinumtoxinA (BoNT-A; Botox®, 150 Allergan IU) was done according to the PREEMPT study protocol. A standardized headache diary was used for recording frequency, duration of attacks and pain intensity. To assess personal burden the HIT-6 and the Hospital Anxiety and Depression scale was used. Primary outcome measure was a > 50% reduction in headache minutes.

**Results:** Seventeen male patients suffering from rCCH, aged $32 \pm 11$ (mean ± SD) years, presenting a mean disease duration of 6.6 years completed the study of 28 weeks. The cut-off point of > 50% reduction in headache minutes as positive result was reached in 58.8%, 29.4% experienced an improvement of 30–50%. Mean frequency of headache days dropped from 28.2 to 11.8 days at week 24 ($p = 0.0001$; 95% CI -21.33 to − 11.61;). Intensity of remaining attacks was also reduced significantly. Headache disability scores showed a trend to improvement after BoNT-A.

**Conclusions:** Encouraging results for the treatment with BoNT-A in rCCH patients were observed in our study population.

**Keywords:** Headache, Cluster headache, Refractoriness, Onabotulinumtoxin a, Prophylactic treatment

## Background

Cluster headache (CH) is a clinically well-defined primary headache disorder occurring in both episodic and chronic forms. Chronic cluster headache (CCH) is a rare condition - approximately 20% of cluster headache sufferers experience recurrent attacks without periods of significant remission [1]. CCH may be unremitting from onset or evolve from episodic CH [2]. The evolution to CCH has been reported to occur in 3.8% to 12.9% of episodic CH sufferers [3]. According to the IHS classification ICHD-3rd version [4] CCH fulfils criteria for episodic cluster headache with attacks recurring without a remission period or with remissions lasting < 3 month for at least one year. For the treatment of CCH only limited therapeutic options are available so far. CCH sufferers often overuse symptomatic medications to treat CH attacks and may develop medication overuse headache (MOH) in addition. To avoid this risk it is worth noting that the preventive treatment of CCH is essential. The decision about how to treat is largely based on clinical experience. For those with CCH preventive treatments are used for an indefinite period of time at least until the patient has been in remission without attacks for 6 months. It is often used in conjunction with a transitional agent and in combinations. Preventive medication should be preferably used as monotherapy but combinations of suggested preventive treatments are recommended especially if one preventive treatment decreases the attack frequency but does not control the situation satisfactorily, upon the physician's decision [5].

Botulinum Neurotoxin Type A (OnabotulinumtoxinA; BoNT-A) is well established in the treatment of chronic

---

* Correspondence: christian.lampl@ordensklinikum.at
[1]Headache Medical Center, Ordensklinikum Linz Barmherzige Schwestern, Linz, Austria

migraine (for review [6]). The intention of this study was to evaluate the efficacy and tolerability of BoNT-A as add-on therapy in refractory CCH (rCCH) patients.

## Methods

Potential rCCH patients were identified from the database of our headache medical centre and from the registry of Linde Austria. The clinical definition of rCCH was based on the consensus statement of the European Headache Federation (EHF) [5]. This study was performed as an open label, non-randomised, single-centre study. Patients between 18 and 60 years of age were included. Exclusion criteria were those for BoNT-A therapy (e.g., generalised muscle weakness, myasthenia gravis, gravidity or known antibodies against botulinum toxin), symptomatic CCH and patients with occipital nerve stimulation (ONS) in situ. After a detailed elucidation of the procedure, injection sites, possible side effects and communication about the off label use of BoNT-A eligible patients undersigned informed consent. BoNT-A (Botox®, 150 Allergan IU) was used according to the Phase 3 REsearch Evaluating Migraine Prophylaxis Therapy (PREEMPT) [7, 8] study protocol (Fig. 1). A standardized headache diary was used including frequency (days/month), duration of attacks (min/attacks/day) and pain intensity (numeric rating scale, NRS). Pain duration was measured with a stop-watch (either commercial one or with mobile phone stop-watch). To assess personal burden patients were asked to fill out the six-item Headache Impact Test (HIT-6) and the Hospital Anxiety and Depression scale (HADS). The HIT 6 was designed to provide a global measure of adverse headache impact [9, 10] and was developed for use in screening and monitoring patients with headaches in both clinical practice and clinical research. The HADS [11] consists of two subscales: HADS-Anxiety (HADS-A) and

HADS-Depression (HADS-D) - each of seven items. In response to each item, participants report their subjective experience at the end of week 4 (baseline), week 12 and week 24, rating it 0–3 (3 indicating maximum symptom severity). The sum of each subscale has a potential range of 0–21. As recommended in the original description [11] we took a threshold of 11 on the respective subscale to indicate caseness for anxiety or depression.

Observational period was 28 weeks, 4 weeks pre-treatment (baseline) and 24 weeks treatment phase. Headache frequency and duration was recorded per day and added at the end of each 4 weeks period (baseline; mean of each 4 weeks period at week 12 and mean of each 4 weeks period at week 24 of the treatment phase). 150 Allergan IU was injected in week 1 after baseline and in week 12. BoNT-A was given as add-on therapy, prior acute and prophylactic treatment was allowed to continue. Any change in medication was recorded. Mean and median values of baseline and week 24 were compared using Wilcoxon Signed Ranks tests and a statistically significant result set at the 95% level ($p = 0.05$). Statistical Package for Social Studies (SPSS) version 17.0 (Aug 23, 2008) (SPSS Inc., Chicago, IL) was used to analyse our data. The study got approval by the local ethic committee (EK 4217; EudraCT No: 2017–003873-33). Primary endpoints were the change in headache days, change in headache minutes comparing baseline and week 24, with a cut-off point of 50% or greater improvement. Secondary outcomes were achieving a 30% to 50% improvement in headache minutes, change in pain intensity of the attacks, change in HIT6 and HADS scores and change in daily analgesics and prophylactic treatment.

## Results

In total 27 patients (21 from the Linde data base, 6 from our headache center; f:m/5:16) were identified. Twentyone

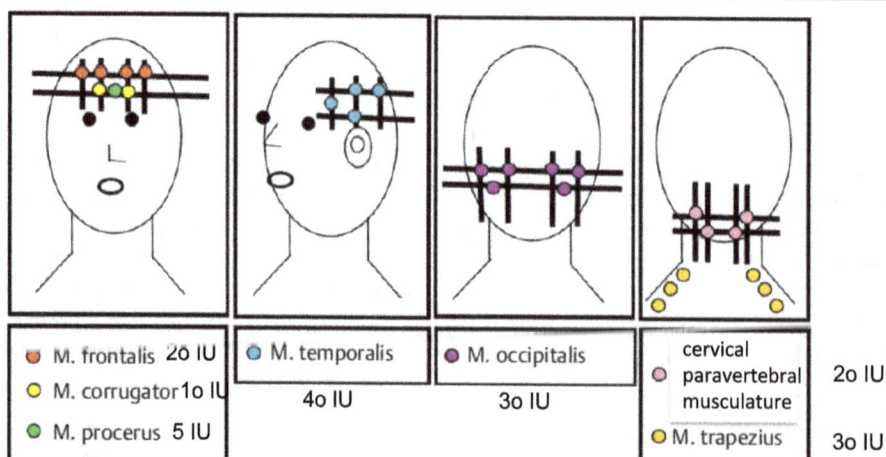

**Fig. 1** Injection procedure of OnabotulinumtoxinA according to the PREEMPT study protocol

patients were contacted, all of them agreed to participate. Due to the exclusion criteria 19 male patients with rCCH, aged 32 ± 11 (mean ± SD) years, with a mean disease duration of 6.6 years were enrolled in the study and received initial treatment with BoNT-A. Two patients had to be excluded because of missing data according to the study protocol. Table 1 shows which treatment and which dose was tested before the patients were classified as rCCH. The results of BoNT-A treatment are summarized in Table 2. The cut-off point of > 50% as positive result was reached in 10/17 patients (58.8%). Three patients experienced total cessation of attacks within the study period; five patients (29.4%) achieved a 30–50% reduction of attack minutes. In 2 patients no improvement was observed. Mean frequency of headache days dropped significantly to – 16 days ($p = 0.0001$; 95%CI -21.33 to – 11.61;). Mean headache minutes decreased to – 1.329 (p = 0.0001; 95% CI -1.778.82 to – 878.24). Intensity of remaining attacks was also reduced significantly. The mean primary pain score at subjects' referral was 7.80 ± 1.25. It dropped to a mean of 3.85 ± 1.11 ($p = 0.0038$; 95% CI -6.85 to – 0.1). Percentage of pain score reduction did not correlate with the subjects' duration of illness (correlation coefficient = 0.113, $p = 0.756$). Headache disability scores showed a trend to improvement after BoNT-A (Table 3), HIT-6 showed a mean change of – 12.7 points ($p = 0.021$; 95% CI -21,3 to – 1.8), HADS-A a mean

change of – 2.2 ($p = 0.078$; 95% CI -6.1 to – 0.1); HADS-D a mean change of – 3.2 ($p = 0.063$; 95% CI -8.2 to – 0.1). Adverse events were reported in 7 patients: Four observed an eyebrow ptosis, 3 patients mentioned a transient worsening in headache before improvement. All adverse events were rated as mild by patients and transient in nature. Preventive medication could be stopped in 6 patients (4 with topiramate, 2 with verapamil). In 4 patients dosage of verapamil could be bisected, 2 patients had no prophylactic treatment at baseline and 5 patients recorded no change in their prophylactic medication.

## Discussion

BoNT-A was highly effective in rCCH in 10/17 patients. Three "super-responders" were identified as well as a median reduction in headache minutes of 62% in all patients. Nine patients (52.9%) reported a > 70% improvement in headache minutes. Clinically significant improvements were also seen in both HIT-6 and HADS scores. Our patients tried at least 3 preventive medications in recommended dosage and had suffered from CCH for a mean of 6.6 years at the time of BoNT-A treatment. This refractory nature of the group means that it is doubtful that our observations are due to spontaneous remission.

The efficacy of BoNT-A as CCH prophylaxis has so far been studied only in single case reports [12–14] and

**Table 1** Demographic details, medication used to manage CCH before enrolment in the study

| patients ID | triptans | oxygen | mid analgesics | Verapamil (mg) | | Lithium (mg)* | | Propranolol (mg)* | | Amitriptyline (mg)* | | Topiramate (mg)* | | Corticosteroids (mg)** |
|---|---|---|---|---|---|---|---|---|---|---|---|---|---|---|
| | | | | hd | ld | hd | ld | hd | ld | hd | ld | hd | ld | |
| 1 | ✓ | 12 l | ✓ | 480 | 480 | X | X | 120 | 80 | X | X | 200 | 200 | 25 |
| 2 | ✓ | 15 l | ✓ | 480 | 480 | 450 | X | 120 | 80 | ? | 10 | 100 | 100 | X |
| 3 | ✓ | 15 l | ✓ | 600 | 480 | 450 | X | 120 | X | X | X | 200 | 200 | X |
| 4 | ✓ | 15 l | ✓ | 600 | 240 | X | X | 120 | X | 75 | 75 | 100 | X | X |
| 5 | ✓ | 12 l | ✓ | 720 | 480 | X | X | 80 | 40 | X | X | 100 | X | 75 |
| 6 | ✓ | 12 l | ✓ | 240 | 240 | 900 | 450 | 240 | X | 25 | 25 | X | X | 10 |
| 7 | ✓ | 12 l | ✓ | 840 | 480 | X | 240 | X | X | 10 | X | 100 | 100 | 50 |
| 8 | ✓ | 10 l | ✓ | 480 | 480 | X | X | 40 | X | X | X | 100 | 100 | X |
| 9 | ✓ | 12 l | ✓ | 600 | X | 450 | X | 80 | X | ? | X | 100 | X | 50 |
| 10 | ✓ | 15 l | ✓ | 240 | 240 | 450 | X | 120 | X | 25 | X | X | X | 50 |
| 11 | ✓ | 15 l | ✓ | 480 | 240 | 450 | 450 | X | X | X | X | 100 | 100 | X |
| 12 | ✓ | 15 l | ✓ | 480 | 480 | X | X | 120 | X | X | X | 100 | 100 | 50 |
| 13 | ✓ | 15 l | ✓ | 600 | 600 | X | X | 40 | X | X | X | 200 | 200 | 25 |
| 14 | ✓ | 15 l | ✓ | 600 | X | 450 | X | X | X | ? | X | 150 | X | X |
| 15 | ✓ | 12 l | ✓ | 600 | 480 | 450 | X | X | X | X | X | 200 | 200 | X |
| 16 | ✓ | 15 l | ✓ | 240 | 240 | 450 | 450 | X | X | X | X | 100 | 100 | 25 |
| 17 | ✓ | 10 l | ✓ | 720 | X | 450 | X | ? | X | X | X | 200 | 200 | X |

l = litre; hd = highest dosage used; ld = last dosage used before enrolled in the study; mg = milligram; ✓□ = used; X = not used;? = not known; ** no longer than 1 month

**Table 2** Demographic details, headache scores pre- and post- treatment with OnabotulinumtoxinA

| patients ID | duration/y | baseline | | treatment phase | | | | improvement %[b] | patient subjective estimate of response %[b] |
|---|---|---|---|---|---|---|---|---|---|
| | | frequency d/mo | duration min | week 12 | | week 24 | | | |
| | | | | frequency d/mo[a] | sum of min/ bout[a] | frequency d/mo[a] | sum of min bout[a] | | |
| 1 | 7 | 30 | 2.250 | 17 | 1.755 | 14 | 1.320 | 41.3 | 50 |
| 2 | 4 | 25 | 1.632 | 8 | 337 | 0 | 0 | 100 | 90–100 |
| 3 | 3 | 28 | 1.328 | 11 | 472 | 7 | 221 | 83.3 | 60–70 |
| 4 | 5 | 29 | 2.598 | 0 | 0 | 0 | 0 | 100 | 100 |
| 5 | 5 | 30 | 3.148 | 12 | 1.065 | 8 | 531 | 83.1 | 75 |
| 6 | 5 | 30 | 1.912 | 8 | 867 | 5 | 312 | 83,6 | 70 |
| 7 | 9 | 28 | 2.491 | 12 | 1.289 | 7 | 1.333 | 46.4 | 50 |
| 8 | 7 | 30 | 1.870 | 8 | 473 | 6 | 328 | 82.4 | 70–80 |
| 9 | 7 | 25 | 1.140 | 13 | 833 | 11 | 618 | 45.8 | 50 |
| 10 | 4 | 27 | 3.456 | 14 | 2.855 | 12 | 1.565 | 54.7 | 50 |
| 11 | 3 | 30 | 1.080 | 30 | 1.418 | 30 | 1.377 | 0 | 0 |
| 12 | 3 | 30 | 3.020 | 16 | 1.844 | 14 | 813 | 73 | 50 |
| 13 | 3 | 30 | 2.280 | 29 | 2.065 | 30 | 2.555 | 0 | 0 |
| 14 | 6 | 28 | 1.680 | 0 | 0 | 0 | 0 | 100 | 100 |
| 15 | 4 | 27 | 2.479 | 18 | 1.349 | 22 | 1.662 | 32,9 | 20–30 |
| 16 | 2 | 30 | 3.040 | 17 | 1.364 | 14 | 839 | 72.4 | 50–70 |
| 17 | 5 | 23 | 1.855 | 21 | 989 | 20 | 1.200 | 35,3 | 20 |
| Mean | 5 | 28.2 | 2.192 | 13.8 | 1.117 | 11.8 | 863 | 62 | |
| median | 5 | 29 | 2.250 | 13.5 | 1.065 | 11 | 813 | 62 | |
| (range) | (2–9) | (23–30) | (1.080–3.148) | (0–30) | (0–2.855) | (0–30) | (0–2.555) | (0–100) | |

pre = before treatment (=baseline), y = year; mo = month, w = week, d = day, min = minutes; [a] = mean of every 4 weeks over past 12 weeks; [b]= baseline vs week 24

in one open trial with a group of 12 CH patients following a standardised injection scheme [15], but not the PREEMPT study protocol. Using 50 IU of BoNT-A the German study group observed a reduction of attack frequency in 25% (3/12) of all study patients and in 33% (3/9) of patients with CCH. Interestingly they observed a better approach in the majority of patients who suffered from CCH for a shorter period (1.5–2 years) than patients with a longer duration of CCH (3–12 years). That could not be observed in our study population. Although the aetiology and pathophysiology of CH is still not completely understood we do have evidence from PET studies [16, 17], voxel-based morphometry [18] and stereotactic hypothalamic deep brain stimulation [19, 20], that a dysfunction of the ipsilateral posterior hypothalamus may cause a secondary activation of the trigemino-autonomic brainstem pathways [21]. This activation leads to the release of calcitonin gene-related peptide (CGRP) a potent vasodilator and neurotransmitter [22]. The activation of the trigeminal system during CH attack is indicated by the elevation of CGRP plasma levels in the external jugular vein [23]. CGRP plasma levels are also elevated interictally in episodic CH patients in the bout compared to outside the bout [23]. The question now is how BoNT-A interferes with the pathophysiology of CCH and whether it is responsible for the positive effects observed in our study. BoNT-A inhibits the release of CGRP from peripheral trigeminal neurons and consequently reduces the CGRP-mediated trigeminal sensitization in migraine [24, 25]. Furthermore, it was suggested that BoNT-A exhibits its actions in pain and migraine by reaching dural trigeminal afferents [26, 27]. Due to the ability of BoNT-A to undergo retrograde axonal transport to the CNS [28] neurotransmitters like Substance P [29] or CGRP [30] might be modulated not only locally at the injection site but also at anatomically connected sites in the trigeminal terminals.

The effects of BoNT-A in the cranial dura could be reconstructed as follows [31]: after peripheral injection BoNT-A is taken up by sensory nerve endings and axonally transported to trigeminal ganglion. After transcytosis the toxin reaches dural nerve endings containing CGRP, suppresses the CGRP-mediated sensitization of the trigeminovascular system, resulting

**Table 3** Headache-associated disability scores pre- and post- treatment with OnabotulinumtoxinA

| patients ID | HIT- 6 (36–76) | | | HADS - A (0–21) | | | HADS - D (0–21) | | |
|---|---|---|---|---|---|---|---|---|---|
| | pre | w 24 | change in score | pre | w 24 | change in score | pre | w 24 | change in score |
| 1 | 70 | 50 | 20 | 18 | 15 | 3 | 8 | 6 | 2 |
| 2 | 58 | 36 | 22 | 15 | 9 | 6 | 12 | 8 | 4 |
| 3 | 67 | 47 | 20 | 17 | 15 | 2 | 15 | 12 | 3 |
| 4 | 76 | 42 | 34 | 15 | 6 | 9 | 6 | 3 | 3 |
| 5 | 78 | 58 | 20 | 15 | 12 | 3 | 9 | 4 | 5 |
| 6 | 58 | 52 | 6 | 11 | 8 | 3 | 10 | 3 | 7 |
| 7 | 63 | 58 | 5 | 13 | 11 | 2 | 10 | 7 | 3 |
| 8 | 63 | 42 | 21 | 13 | 12 | 1 | 8 | 2 | 6 |
| 9 | 57 | 42 | 13 | 12 | 11 | 1 | 12 | 11 | 1 |
| 10 | 78 | 68 | 10 | 11 | 12 | -1 | 11 | 9 | 2 |
| 11 | 65 | 68 | −3 | 13 | 15 | −2 | 14 | 15 | −1 |
| 12 | 68 | 57 | 11 | 11 | 12 | −1 | 11 | 5 | 6 |
| 13 | 65 | 65 | 0 | 18 | 21 | −3 | 16 | 16 | 0 |
| 14 | 56 | 36 | 20 | 12 | 6 | 6 | 4 | 0 | 4 |
| 15 | 53 | 57 | −4 | 14 | 12 | 2 | 15 | 12 | 3 |
| 16 | 68 | 54 | 14 | 14 | 9 | 5 | 12 | 9 | 3 |
| 17 | 76 | 72 | 4 | 12 | 11 | 1 | 14 | 11 | 3 |
| Mean (95% CI) | 65.8 | 53.1 | −12.7 (−21.3; −1.8) | 13.8 | 11.6 | −2.2 (−6.1; −0.1) | 11.0 | 7.8 | −3.2 (−8.2; −0.1) |
| median (range) | 65 (53–78) | 54 (36–72) | 13 (− 3–34) | 13 (11–18) | 12 (6–21) | 2 (− 2–9) | 11 (6–16) | 8 (0–16) | 3 (− 1–7) |

pre = before treatment (=baseline), w = week; HIT-6 = Headache Impact Test, HADS=Hospital Anxiety and Depression Scale, A = anxiety, D = depression

in reduction in local neurogenic inflammation. At present this seems to be the most convincing hypothesis of the action of BoNT-A in migraine and CH. Moreover modulation of neurotransmitter release at higher order neurons could contribute to pain attenuation as brain Gamma-aminobutyric acid (GABA) concentration may be correlated to migraine intensity [32]. This could also be a mechanism in cluster headache patients to modulate pain intensity.

Although we observed encouraging results for the treatment with BoNT-A in rCCH patients, major limitations of this study arise from its open design and the small patient number. Previous studies of BoNT-A have also reported a significant placebo response; therefore we cannot exclude this as a potential confounding factor in our outcomes as well as effects of concomitant preventive therapy. However, the good response rates and consistent efficacy of repeated BoNT-A application in our study population with an extraordinary pain condition suggest that the response to BoNT-A in this series entirely cannot be attributed to a placebo response. Further multicentre studies with higher patient numbers will be needed to further clarify if BoNT-A is effective in the prophylactic treatment of rCCH. As the syndrome is quite rare, it is still essential to collect and publish large case series regarding clinical manifestations and treatment options.

## Conclusions

Our data suggest that the injection of BoNT-A could be beneficial as add-on therapy in patients with otherwise rCCH. However, these preliminary results has to be confirmed in double-blind, randomised, controlled studies. Especially patient characteristics that predict benefit from BoNT-A treatment should be identified. In our experience it is essential to use the PREEMPT study protocol for the injection procedure.

### Abbreviations
BoNT-A: OnabotulinumtoxinA; CCH: Chronic Cluster Headache; CGRP: Calcitonin gene-related peptide; CH: Cluster Headache; GABA: Gamma-aminobutyric acid; HADS: Hospital Anxiety and Depression scale; HIT-6: Headache Impact Test; ICHD: International Classification of Headache Disorders; IU: International Units; MOH: Medication Overuse Headache; NRS: Numeric Rating Scale; PREEMPT: Phase 3 REsearch Evaluating Migraine Prophylaxis Therapy –; rCCH: Refractory Chronic Cluster Headache; SPSS: Statistical Package for Social Studies

### Authors' contributions
CL and MR conceived the idea for this analysis, made possible by the design of the original questionnaire, which had been led by CL and MR. Both contributed to data acquisition. CL, MR and EB performed analysis and data interpretation. CL drafted the article with input from MR and EB. All authors reviewed and approved the final manuscript.

## Authors' information
No relevant information about the authors that may aid the reader's interpretation of the article, and understand the standpoint of the authors.

## Competing interests
The authors declare that they have no competing interests.

## Author details
[1]Headache Medical Center, Ordensklinikum Linz Barmherzige Schwestern, Linz, Austria. [2]Headache Medical Center, Department of Radio-Oncology, Ordensklinikum Linz Barmherzige Schwestern, Linz, Austria.

## References
1. Bahra A, May A, Goadsby PJ (2002) Cluster headache: a prospective clinical study with diagnostic implications. Neurology 58:354–361
2. Pearce JM (1993) Natural history of cluster headache. Headache 33:235–236
3. Manzoni GC, Micieli G, Granella F, Tassorelli C, Zanferrari C, Cavallini A (1991) 189 patients. Cephalalgia 11:169–174
4. Headache Classification Committee of the International Headache Society (IHS) (2018) The international classification of headache disorders, 3rd edition. Cephalalgia 38:1–211
5. Mitsikostas DD, Edvinsson L, Jensen RH, Katsarava Z, Lampl C, Negro A, Osipova V, Paemeleire K, Siva A, Valade D, Martelletti P (2014) Refractory chronic cluster headache: a consensus statement on clinical definition from the European headache federation. J Headache Pain 27(15):79
6. Frampton JE, Silberstein S (2018) OnabotulinumtoxinA: a review in the prevention of chronic migraine. Drugs 78:589–600
7. Aurora SK, Dodick DW, Turkel CC, RE DG, Silberstein SD, Lipton RB, Diener HC, Brin MF (2010) PREEMPT 1 Chronic Migraine Study Group (2010) Onabotulinumtoxin a for treatment of chronic migraine: results from the double-blind, randomized, placebo-controlled phase of the PREEMPT 1 trial. Cephalalgia 30:793–803
8. Diener HC, Dodick DW, Aurora SK, Turkel CC, RE DG, Lipton RB, Silberstein SD, Brin MF (2010) PREEMPT 2 Chronic Migraine Study Group (2010) Onabotulinumtoxin a for treatment of chronic migraine: results from the double-blind, randomized, placebo-controlled phase of the PREEMPT 2 trial. Cephalalgia 30:804–814
9. Ware JE Jr, Bjorner JB, Kosinski M (2000) Practical implications of item response theory and computerized adaptive testing: a brief summary of ongoing studies of widely used headache impact scales. Med Care 38: 73–82
10. Kosinski M, Bayliss MS, Bjorner JB, Ware JE Jr, Garber WH, Batenhorst A, Cady R, Dahlöf CG, Dowson A, Tepper S (2003) A six-item short-form survey for measuring headache impact: the HIT-6. Qual Life Res 12:963–974
11. Zigmond AS, Snaith RP (1983) The hospital anxiety and depression scale. Acta Psychiatr Scand 67:361–370
12. Robbins L (2001) Botulinum toxin a (Botox) for cluster headache: 6 cases. Cephalalgia 21:499–500
13. Freund BJ, Schwartz M (2000) The use of botulinum toxin-a in the treatment of refractory cluster headache: case reports. Cephalalgia 20: 325–331
14. Smuts JA, Barnard PWA (2000) Botulinum toxin type a in the treatment of headache syndromes: a clinical report on 79 patients. Cephalalgia 20:332
15. Sostak P, Krause P, Förderreuther S, Reinisch V, Straube A (2007) Botulinum toxin type-a therapy in cluster headache: an open study. J Headache Pain 8: 236–241
16. Sprenger T, Valet M, Hammes M, Erhard P, Berthele A, Conrad B, Tolle TR (2004) Hypothalamic activation in trigeminal autonomic cephalgia: functional imaging of an atypical case. Cephalalgia 24:753–757
17. May A, Bahra A, Buchel C, Frackowiak RS, Goadsby PJ (1998) Hypothalamic activation in cluster headache attacks. Lancet 352:275–278
18. Hardebo JE (1994) How cluster headache is explained as an intracavernous inflammatory process lesioning sympathetic fibers. Headache 34:125–131
19. Franzini A, Ferroli P, Leone M, Broggi G (2003) Stimulation of the posterior hypothalamus for treatment of chronic intractable cluster headaches: first reported series. Neurosurgery 52:1095 1099
20. Leone M, Franzini A, Broggi G, Bussone G (2003) Hypothalamic deep brain stimulation for intractable chronic cluster headache: a 3-year followup. Neurol Sci 24(2):143–145
21. Malick A, Strassman RM, Burstein R (2000) Trigeminohypothalamic and reticulohypothalamic tract neurons in the upper cervical spinal cord and caudal medulla of the rat. J Neurophysiol 84:2078–2112
22. Zagami AS, Goadsby PJ, Edvinsson L (1990) Stimulation of the superior sagittal sinus in the cat causes release of vasoactive peptides. Neuropeptides 16:69–75
23. Goadsby PJ, Edvinsson L (1994) Human in vivo evidence for trigeminovascular activation in cluster headache. Neuropeptide changes and effects of acute attacks therapies. Brain 117:427–434
24. Fanciullacci M, Alessandri M, Sicuteri R, Marabini S (1997) Responsiveness of the trigeminovascular system to nitroglycerine in cluster headache patients. Brain 120:283–288
25. Cernuda-Morollón E, Martínez-Camblor P, Ramón C, Larrosa D, Serrano-Pertierra E, Pascual J (2014) CGRP and VIP levels as predictors of efficacy of onabotulinumtoxin type a in chronic migraine. Headache 54:987–995
26. Matak I, Lacković Z (2014) Botulinum toxin a, brain and pain. Prog Neurobiol 119–120:39–59
27. Ramachandran R, Yaksh TL (2014) Therapeutic use of botulinum toxin in migraine: mechanisms of action. Br J Pharmacol 171:4177–4192
28. Huang P, Khan I, Suhail M, Malkmus S, Yaksh T (2011) Spinal botulinum neurotoxin B: effects on afferent transmitter release and nociceptive processing. PLoS One 6:e19126
29. Chien C, Lee H, Wu C, Li P (2012) Inhibitory effect of botulinum toxin type a on the NANC system in rat respiratory models of neurogenic inflammation. Arch Biochem Biophys 524:106–113
30. Hou YP, Zhang YP, Song YF, Zhu CM, Wang YC, Xie GL (2007) Botulinum toxin type a inhibits rat pyloric myoelectrical activity and substance P release in vivo. Can J Physiol Pharmacol 85:209–214
31. Lacković Z, Filipović B, Matak I, Helyes Z (2016) Activity of botulinum toxin type a in cranial dura: implications for treatment of migraine and other headaches. Br J Pharmacol 173:279–291
32. Wiegand H, Erdmann G, Wellhoner HH (1976) 125I-labelled botulinum a neurotoxin: pharmacokinetics in cats after intramuscular injection. Naunyn Schmiedeberg's Arch Pharmacol 292:161–165

# 20

# Oxygen treatment for cluster headache attacks at different flow rates

Thijs H. T. Dirkx* ⓘ, Danielle Y. P. Haane and Peter J. Koehler

## Abstract

**Background:** Cluster headache attacks can, in many patients, be successfully treated with oxygen via a non-rebreather mask. In previous studies oxygen at flow rates of both 7 L/min and 12 L/min was shown to be effective. The aim of this study was to compare the effect of 100% oxygen at different flow rates for the treatment of cluster headache attacks.

**Methods:** In a double-blind, randomized, crossover study, oxygen naïve cluster headache patients, treated attacks with oxygen at 7 and 12 L/min. The primary outcome measure was the percentage of attacks after which patients (treating at least 2 attacks/day) were painfree after 15 min, in the first two days of the study. Secondary outcome measures were percentage of successfully treated attacks, percentage of attacks after which patients were painfree, drop in VAS score and patient preference in all treatment periods (14 days).

**Results:** Ninety-eight patients were enrolled, 70 provided valid data, 56 used both flow rates. These 56 patients recorded 604 attacks, eligible for the primary analysis. An exploratory analysis was conducted using all eligible attacks of 70 patients who provided valid data. We could only include 5 patients, treating 27 attacks on the first two days of the study, for our primary outcome, which did not show a significant difference ($p = 0.180$). Patients tended to prefer 12 L/min ($p = 0.005$). Contradicting this result, more patients were painfree using 7 L/min ($p = 0.039$). There were no differences in side effects or in our other secondary outcome measures. The exploratory analysis showed an odds ratio of being painfree using 12 L/min of 0.73 (95% CI 0.52–1.02) compared to 7 L/min ($p = 0.061$) as scored on a 5-point scale. The average drop in score on this 5-point scale, however, was equal between groups. Also slightly more patients noticed, no or not much, relief on 7 L/min, and found 12 L/min to be effective in all their attacks.

**Conclusion:** There is lack of evidence to support differences in the effect of oxygen at a flow rate of 12 L/min compared to 7 L/min. More patients were painfree using 7 L/min, but our other outcome measures did not confirm a difference in effect between flow rates. As most patients prefer 12 L/min and treatments were equally safe, this could be used in all patients. It might be more cost-effective, however, to start with 7 L/min and, if ineffective, to switch to 12 L/min.

**Keywords:** Cluster headache, Oxygen, Acute treatment, Randomized controlled trial

* Correspondence: thijsdirkx@hotmail.com
Department of Neurology, Zuyderland Medical Center Heerlen, PO Box 4446,
6401, CX, Heerlen, The Netherlands

## Background

Cluster headache (CH) attacks can, in many patients, be successfully treated with oxygen via a non-rebreather mask [1–4]. A study by Kudrow (1981) ($N = 52$) demonstrated that 75% of patients treated with oxygen at a flow rate of 7 L/min have adequate or complete relief, in at least 7 out of 10 attacks [1]. In a second study by Kudrow ($N = 50$), oxygen at 7 L/min was effective in 82%, compared to 70% with ergotamine [1]. In a small study by Fogan (1985) ($N = 19$) oxygen at a flow rate of 6 L/min was shown to be more effective than room air [2]. The endpoint was a mean relief score (0 = no relief to 3 = complete relief). The average relief score for all oxygen-treated patients was 1.93, compared to 0.77 for room air.

The usual oxygen flow rate applied has remained 7 L/min until the study by Cohen (2009) ($N = 76$) showed that treatment with oxygen at a flow rate of 12 L/min was effective as well [3]. The CH attacks stopped, or adequate relief was obtained, within 15 min of oxygen usage in 78%, compared to 20% using room air. In this study the primary endpoint was to render the patient painfree or have adequate relief while treating a single attack. As this endpoint is very different from the one used by Kudrow and Fogan [1, 2], these studies are difficult to compare. A beneficial effect of oxygen at 14–15 L/min in patients not responding to 7–10 L/min has been described in a small case series of 3 patients [5].

A controlled study to compare different oxygen flow rates has not been conducted. The use of oxygen at a flow rate of 12 L/min without proper evidence of its superiority to 7 L/min seems inefficient, considering the additional costs of production and delivery. In the present study we compared treatment of CH attacks with 100% oxygen via a non-rebreather mask at different flow rates, 7 L/min vs. 12 L/min. We hypothesized that oxygen at a higher flow rate (12 L/min) might be more effective for the treatment of cluster headache attacks.

## Methods

### Study design

The study was designed as a double-blind, randomized, crossover study, in which patients used 100% oxygen at a flow rate of 7 L/min and 12 L/min.

The study was approved by the Medical Ethics Board of Zuyderland Medical Center Heerlen, the Netherlands. The study was registered with the European Union Clinical Trials Register (nr. 2012–003648-59) and the Dutch Trial Register (NTR3801). Written informed consent was obtained from all patients. The authors had full access to all data.

All newly diagnosed CH patients and known CH patients aged 18–65, who were naïve to oxygen treatment could be included in the study. Exclusion criteria were previous oxygen usage, pregnancy or lactation, chronic obstructive pulmonary disease, other primary or secondary headache diagnoses or other distracting painful conditions, which could interfere with the patient's pain perception, incapacitation to understand and sign informed consent, and other contraindication for oxygen therapy as determined by the patient's physician. If patients with secondary CH were included before imaging was conducted, they were excluded afterwards, when they were diagnosed as a secondary CH.

Patients were included with the aid of an oxygen supplier in the Netherlands. All patients were diagnosed with cluster headache by their treating neurologist, according to the ICHD-2 criteria. If the treating neurologist chose to start oxygen treatment and the patient was interested in the study, we were informed by the oxygen supplier. Patients were then contacted by us to give further details. After informed consent participants were randomized. Randomization was conducted via a random-number generator and we used a blocked-randomization design. An independent investigator kept the randomization key, which was only shared with the researchers when performing the final analysis. An oxygen tank was delivered to all patients with two covered valves, labeled valve A and valve B. Both oxygen valves were modified, so that it was not possible to change the flow rate and the flow rate itself was not visible either. One valve was set at a flow rate of 7 L/min, the other at 12 L/min. Patients as well as investigators were blinded for the flow rates. Patients were randomized into 4 groups: AB ABBA, BA ABBA, AB BAAB and BA BAAB. The first two treatment periods lasted only 1 day. Each of the other treatment periods lasted for 3 days.

As an example, the AB ABBA-scheme meant: use of valve A on day 1, B on day 2, A on days 3–5, B on days 6–8 and on days 9–11 and A on days 12–14. The treatment periods were independent of the number of attacks that occurred during each period. After completing the study, patients continued the treatment with oxygen in concordance with the dosage prescribed by their own neurologist. All patients used the same type of non-rebreather mask with a reservoir (Salter Labs E-8140).

At the start of the study patients were asked to fill in a questionnaire about characteristics of their CH attacks, medication usage (preventive medication and previously used acute treatments), and other patient characteristics. During the treatment period patients were asked to fill in a diary, in which they described, for each attack, the time until the start of oxygen treatment, pain scores before and following treatment, how long the oxygen treatment lasted, and any side effects using valve A or B. Following the 14-day study period or at the end of the cluster period, patients were asked to fill in a final questionnaire. This included questions about whether or not they had noticed any difference between flow rate A and B and if so, what that difference was and which flow rate they thought was most effective.

Patients were instructed to start treatment as soon as possible after onset of the CH attack. They had to continue oxygen treatment until the CH attack had ended or for at least 15 min. After 15 min patients were allowed to use rescue medication, usually a sumatriptan injection or nasal spray. If patients already used preventive medication (usually verapamil) at the start of the study, they were allowed to continue this medication. In order not to affect the evaluation of the primary endpoint, patients were not allowed to change the dosage or start new preventive medication until after the first 2 days of the study.

### Endpoints

The main endpoint of the study was the percentage of attacks, in which a painfree state was achieved after 15 min of treatment with oxygen, in at least 2 attacks/day on the first 2 days. Patients were asked to rate their pain before and after 15 min of oxygen treatment on a 5-point scale: 0 for pain free, 1 for mild pain, 2 for moderate pain, 3 for severe pain, 4 for very severe pain.

The secondary endpoints were, percentage of attacks treated successfully (defined as drop in VAS score of over 50%), percentage of attacks after which patients were painfree, absolute drop in VAS-score, and the patient preference to the flow rates of 7 or 12 L/min in all treatment periods. Patient preference was visualised on a 11-point scale using score – 5 for maximal preference to flow rate A and + 5 for maximal preference to flow rate B. Moreover, they were asked to choose either A, B or equal.

Attacks treated with oxygen that occurred within 12 h of other attack treatment (usually triptans) were excluded from all analysis, as these results might be confounded by the ongoing effect of that treatment. Attacks occurring within 3 h of oxygen treatment were excluded as well, as pain scores might be less reliable, when measured shortly after a previous attack.

### Sample size calculation

As studies comparing the effect of oxygen at 7 or 12 L/min have not been conducted, we did not have reliable data for conducting a sample size calculation. Therefore, we looked at the average drop in VAS score using different flow rates in our prospective study on oxygen treatment and CH [6]. Based on these results we would need to study 100 pairs of subjects or 100 subjects in a crossover design to be able to reject a null hypothesis that the response difference is zero with a probability (power) of 0.8. The type I error probability associated with the test of this null hypothesis is 0.05. It is important to note that these data do not represent our primary endpoint, but one of our secondary endpoints. Furthermore, these

data were obtained in a small population and patients were not randomized between the two different flow rates. We decided to include 110 patients. This number allowed for a drop-out rate of 9.1%.

### Statistics

It was not necessary that patients completed the entire crossover design as described in the protocol, but patients could be included in the analysis if they treated attacks with both flow rates. If patients dropped out before using both treatments, or if all attacks using one flow rate had to be excluded, they were not included in the primary and secondary endpoints. As our data were not normally distributed, we had to apply non-parametric tests.

For patient preference we used a One Sample Wilcoxon Signed Rank Test and Chi square test. We calculated the percentage of successfully treated attacks, the percentage of attacks after which patients were painfree, and the average drop in VAS score, for each flow rate in every individual patient. Additionally we calculated the average drop in score on the 5-point scale. For these outcome measures we used a test for paired samples, the Wilcoxon Signed Ranks Test. To test if there was a difference between randomization groups, we used the Kruskal-Wallis Test.

We conducted an additional exploratory analysis, in which all eligible treated attacks were included. As this analysis included patients, who used only one flow rate, we used statistical tests for unpaired data. The odds ratio of treating an attack successfully or being painfree after an attack was calculated using the Chi square test and the Fisher's exact test. We used a independent samples T-test for the drop in VAS-score and drop in score on the 5 point-scale.

All statistical tests were 2-tailed and the significance threshold was set at 0.05. All statistical analyses were performed using SPSS.

### Results

In total we included 98 patients, from 28 Dutch centers, between March 2013 and October 2016. The initial goal was to include 110 patients. Patient recruitement, however, was slower than expected and we had to stop inclusion before reaching our goal.

Out of 98 patients, 28 had to be excluded (Fig. 1). We did not receive adequate data (questionnaires and diary) of most of these patients. We were not always able to identify the reasons for not participating in the study, but the most common reason was that cluster headache attacks did not occur anymore (end of the cluster period). There were 2 cases of secondary CH (1 intracerebral arteriovenous malformation located just cranial to the tectum and 1 pituary tumour). Of the 70 patients who provided adequate data, 56 patients used both

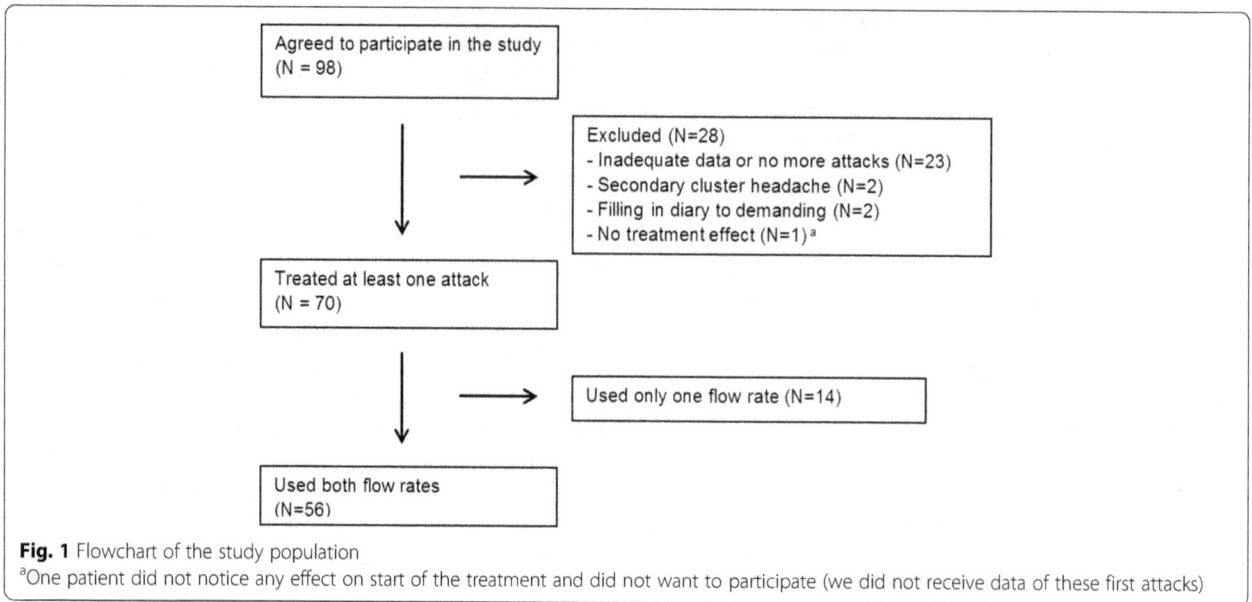

**Fig. 1** Flowchart of the study population

aOne patient did not notice any effect on start of the treatment and did not want to participate (we did not receive data of these first attacks)

treatments. Table 1 shows the baseline characteristics of these 56 patients. These patients treated a total of 680 attacks, of which 76 attacks had to be excluded, leaving 604 attacks for the analysis.

Because most patients were recently diagnosed with CH, and often were experiencing their first cluster period, it was not always possible to differentiate between chronic or episodic CH. Of 31 patients who answered this question, 67.7% reported having episodic CH. Five patients had an average attack duration of longer than 180 min and 3 patients had less than one attack in 2 days. As all of the patients, who did not fulfil the duration or frequency criterium, had individual attacks that met the ICHD-2 criteria [7] and otherwise had typical symptoms apart from frequency or duration, the most likely diagnosis remained CH. As reported in a previous study, these patients were not excluded from the analysis [8]. All patients had at least one autonomic symptom or reported restlessness during attacks.

**Table 1** Baseline data. $N = 56$

| Gender | 61.1% male - 38.9% female |
|---|---|
| Age (median – range) | 43.0 (20–76) |
| Current or past smoker | 74.1% (50% current - 24.1% past) |
| Painfree periods (episodic) (N = 31) | 67.7% |
| Pain between attacks | 50.9% |
| Attack duration untreated (median-range) | 60 min (9–330) |
| Attack frequency (median-range) | 2 attacks per day (0.1–8) |
| Verapamil usage | 55.4% |

### Side effects

No serious side effects were reported in either treatment group and there was no significant difference in the occurrence of these side effects between treatment groups (Table 2). All patients were able to continue treatment despite of these side effects.

### Primary outcome measure

Only 5 patients met the inclusion criteria for our primary outcome measure; two treated attacks on each of the first 2 days. These patients treated a total of 27 attacks on the first 2 days. No significant difference was found in the percentage of attacks after which patients were painfree between 7 and 12 L/min ($p = 0.180$) (Table 3).

Looking at the individual attacks, the odds ratio (Fisher's exact test) for being painfree after 15 min of treatment was 3.75 (95% CI 0.58–24.28), favouring 12 L/min ($p = 0.209$). However, as numbers were so small, there was clearly inadequate power.

### Secondary outcome measures

The percentage of attacks treated successfully and absolute drop in VAS-score showed no significant difference between both treatment groups (Table 3). Patient's preference at the end of the study, expressed on a scale of 0–10, showed a median score of 3.5 (favouring 12 L/min). This was statistically significant ($p = 0.005$). Twenty-four out of 49 patients chose 12 L/min over 7 L/min, compared to 11 patients who preferred 7 L/min ($p = 0.059$). Contradicting this result, a higher percentage of attacks after which patients were painfree, as scored on a 5-point scale, was found in the 7 L/min group. This was statistically

**Table 2** Side effects

| Side effects | 7 L / min (n) | 12 L /min (n) |
|---|---|---|
| Lightheadedness | 10 | 11 |
| Dry mouth | 5 | 6 |
| Tired after treatment | 2 | 2 |
| Difficulty breathing[a] | 2 | 1 |
| Nasal congestion | 1 | 1 |
| Coughing | 1 | 1 |
| Difficulty sleeping after treatment | 0 | 2 |
| Nausea | 1 | 1 |
| Hoarse voice | 0 | 1 |
| Tingling | 1 | 0 |
| Burning eyes | 1 | 0 |
| Cold feeling | 1 | 0 |
| Blurry vision | 0 | 1 |

[a]Severity not specified, both patients were able to continue treatment

significant ($p = 0.039$). The average drop in score on this 5-point scale was equal between groups.

### Missing data

Ten patients used both treatments but did not answer the question considering preferred valve. There were no significant differences in these 10 patients on other outcome measures.

Fourteen patients only used one treatment; 6 used 12 L/min and 8 used 7 L/min. We conducted an exploratory analysis, in which all eligible attacks in 70 patients were included. Seven hundred ten attacks were reported, of which 78 had to be excluded, leaving 632 attacks for the analysis. Table 4 gives an overview of all attacks included in this analysis. No significant differences were found between groups. However, the likelihood of being painfree was lower using 12 L/min, OR 0.73 (95% CI 0.52–1.02), which was nearly statistically significant ($p = 0.061$). The average drop on the 5-point scale was equal between groups.

### Randomization effect

No significant differences were found between randomization groups on success or painfree percentages and patient preference. Considering the drop in VAS score, randomization group 4 showed a larger drop in VAS score using 12 L/min compared to group 3, which showed a larger drop in VAS score of 7 L/min. This showed statistical significance. On all other outcome measures, group 3 and 4 were equal to the other groups.

### Discussion

Our primary outcome did not show a significant difference between 7 L/min and 12 L/min. As this was based on a small number of patients, we feel that this result is of little clinical significance. The results of our secondary outcome measures are somewhat conflicting. More patients seem to be painfree using 7 L/min, although the

**Table 3** Results primary and secondary endpoints

| | Included (N) | Results (Median+IQR[a]) | P-value |
|---|---|---|---|
| % Painfree after treatment (first 2 days) | 5 | 7 L/min: 0 (0–37.50) | 0.180[b] |
| | | 12 L/min: 0 (0–83.50) | |
| Drop in VAS score | 56 | 7 L/min: 4.09 (2.67–5.48) | 0.243[b] |
| | | 12 L/min: 4.33 (2.71–5.41) | |
| % Successfully treated attacks | 56 | 7 L/min: 92.86 (45.10–100) | 0.505[b] |
| | | 12 L/min: 84.52 (33.33–100) | |
| Patients preference (0–10) | 46 | 3.50 (0.50–5.50) | 0.005[c] |
|   0 favouring 12 L/min | | | |
|   10 favouring 7 L/min | | | |
| Patients preference | 49 | 7 L/min: N = 11 | 0.059[d] |
|   7 L/min - 12 L/min - equal | | 12 L/min: N = 24 | |
| | | Equal: N = 14 | |
| % Painfree after treatment (all attack periods) | 55 | 7 L/min: 28.57 (0–66.67) | 0.039[b] |
| | | 12 L/min: 0 (0–50.00) | |
| Drop on 5-point scale | 55 | 7 L/min: 1.50 (1–2) | 0.475[b] |
| | | 12 L/min 1.50 (1–2) | |

[a]Median + interquartile range (25–75)
[b]Wilcoxon Signed Ranks Test
[c]One sample Wilcoxon Signed Rank Test
[d]Chi square test

**Table 4** Overview of all attacks treated in 70 patients

|  | 7 L/min | 12 L/min | Odds ratio (95% confidence interval) | P-value |
|---|---|---|---|---|
| Patients | 64 | 62 |  |  |
| Total number of attacks treated | 344 | 366 |  |  |
| Attacks excluded[a] | 37 (10.8%) | 41 (11.2%) |  |  |
| Attacks included in analysis | 307 | 325 |  |  |
| Attacks / patient (range) | 4.80 (1–19) | 5.24 (1–17) |  |  |
| Successfully treated | 211 (68.7%) | 219 (67.4%) | 0.94 (0.67–1.31) | 0.717[c] |
| Drop in VAS score (Mean – SD) | 4.23 SD 2.06 | 4.28 SD 1.75 |  | 0.734[d] |
| Painfree after treatment[b] | 109 (36.2%) | 93 (29.2%) | 0.73 (0.52–1.02) | 0.061[c] |
| Drop on 5-point scale (Mean – SD)[b] | 1.61 SD 0.77 | 1.63 SD 0.66 |  | 0.683[d] |

[a]Attacks were excluded because of occurrence within 3 h of previous oxygen treatment or within 12 h of other attack treatment
[b]No data available of 6 attacks treated with both 7 L/min and 12 L/min
[c]Chi square test
[d]Independent samples T-test

absolute differences are small (29.2 vs 36.2%). We could not confirm this trend in our other outcome measures and contradicting these results, patients tended to favour 12 L/min.

The average drop in score on the 5- point scale was equal between groups. This suggests that the average response, besides the patients being painfree, was worse in the 7 L/min group. This explanation was supported by some of the questions on our final questionnaire. Figure 2 shows that slightly more patients had no or not much relief on 7 L/min. Figure 3 shows that slightly more patients found 12 L/min to be effective in all attacks. This might explain the preference for 12 L/min. These results, combined with our other outcome measures, suggest that although more patients were painfree using 7 L/min, this is insufficient to state that 7 L/min is the more effective treatment.

Patient preference scored by patients from 0 (favouring 12 L/min) to 10 (favouring 7 L/min), shows a considerable number scoring lower than 1.0 (13/46), and only 1 patient scoring higher than 9.0. Besides this difference the results are almost normally distributed. This could be interpreted in a way that there seems to be a subgroup of patients, who absolutely favours 12 L/min, while in the rest of the population there does not seem to be a difference between both treatment groups. We wondered if we could identify this population of patients having an absolute preference for 12 L/min. As a considerable number of patients experienced their first attack period, we could not always differentiate between episodic or chronic CH. Five out of 9 patients in the 12 L/min preference group, compared to only 4 out of 20 in the no-preference group had chronic CH. The Chi square test did not show statistical significance, possibly due to low power, but this might be an interesting trend.

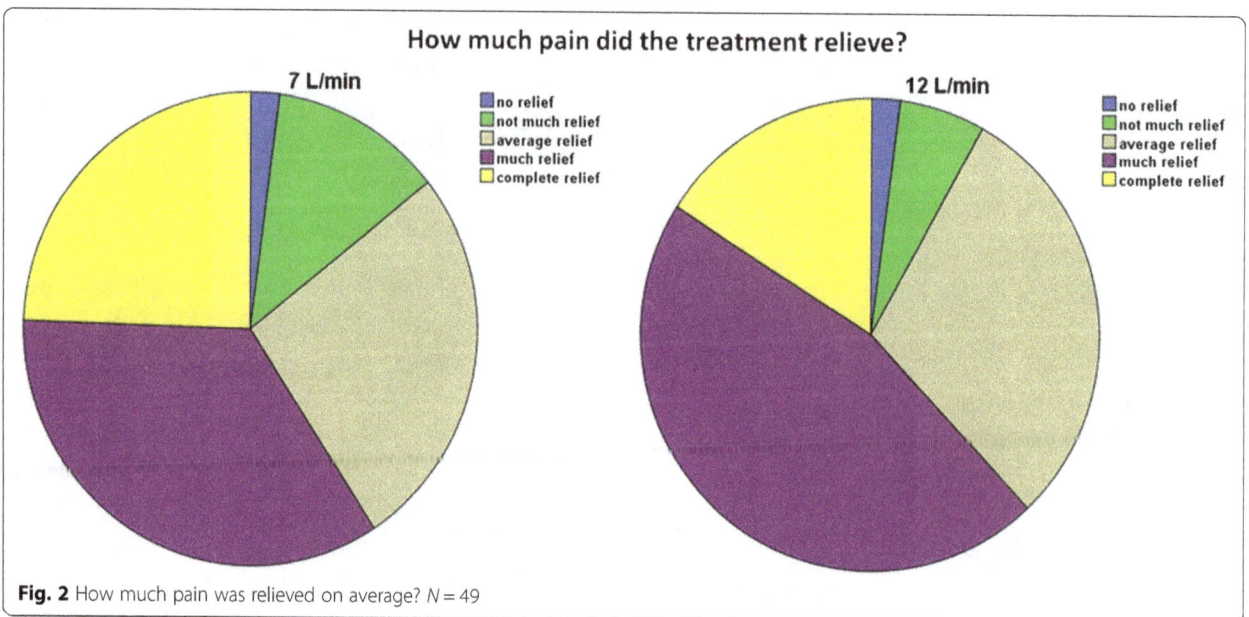

**Fig. 2** How much pain was relieved on average? N = 49

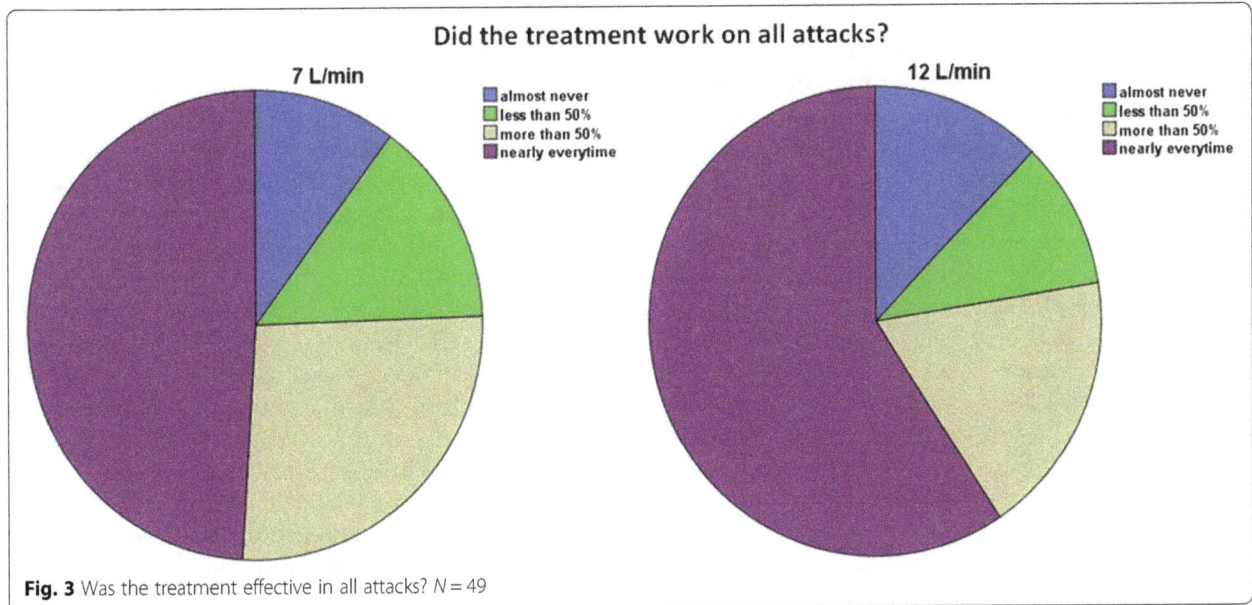

**Fig. 3** Was the treatment effective in all attacks? $N = 49$

No significant differences were found between episodic or chronic CH on our other secondary outcome measures. The use of verapamil was not related with a preference for one of the two flow rates. We also screened for gender, age, smoking, attack characteristics and specific autonomic symptoms or restlessness, but no significanct between group differences were found.

The most common side effect of oxygen usage was lightheadedness. This was equally found in both flow rates. Patients were instructed to breathe normally while using the oxygen. However, some patients might have been hyperventilating, which could have caused this lightheadedness.

No other controlled trials compared different oxygen flow rates for CH attacks. In previous studies oxygen at both 7 L/min and 12 L/min was shown to be effective [1, 3]. As these studies used different outcome measures they are difficult to compare. As our study did not show any difference in the occurrence of side effects between groups, we can state that there is no consistent difference in treatment effect and safety between oxygen at a flow rate of 7 and 12 L/min. An interpretation of our results may be to treat all patients with 12 L/min, as the only disadvantage would be the higher production and delivery costs. An alternative would be to treat people with 7 L/min, and if this is not successful, or not sufficiently satisfying, use 12 L/min instead, as is often current practice today.

**Methodological considerations**

A crossover design was used in previous studies on oxygen treatment and CH [1–3, 9]. We chose this type of design as new or oxygen naïve CH patients are not easily recruited.

An important benefit of a crossover design is that each patient receives both treatments. This eliminates confounders caused by different treatment groups and results in a smaller sample size necessary to detect a significant treatment effect. An important disadvantage of crossover designs is the potential carry over effect. As oxygen is assumed to have a very short washout period, a crossover design is suitable for a trial with oxygen treatment.

Randomization groups were not equally distributed due to drop-out and we found a significant difference in drop in VAS score between groups 3 and 4. We do not have a good explanation, why results in these groups were different, however, as group 4 was the smallest ($n = 11$) and there was a wide variation between results, this might well be a sampling error. The way the randomization scheme was built, makes it less likely that there is a significant carry over effect. More specifically, group 3 and 4 only differed on the first 2 days.

Our aim was to include 110 patients, but we were only able to include 98. Patient recruitment was slower than expected, and due to the long duration of the study, we had to stop recruitment before including 110 patients. We chose to allow for an estimated drop-out rate of 9.1%. In retrospect, this should have been considerably higher. There was a large group of patients, who agreed to participate, but eventually did not. As most patients were recently diagnosed with CH and it often takes some time before the diagnosis is made, several patients would be near the end of their cluster period at the time of inclusion. As in most of these cases, we did not receive the first questionnaire with baseline characteristics, we are not sure if this may have resulted in a bias, but there is no reason to assume this.

Fourteen patients only used one flow rate. As these were nearly equally distributed between flow rates and treatment results were not significantly different in these patients, we have no reason to assume selective drop-out. Furthermore, the exploratory analysis, including all eligible treated attacks, showed similar results.

The reason for our primary outcome was that we would find a difference before verapamil was started or the dosage increased. It did not seem ethical to exclude patients from prophylactic treatment during the 14 days of the trial. We could only include 5 patients for analysis of our primary outcome measure. There were more patients who had over 2 attacks a day on average. However, as patients mostly started oxygen treatment immediately after they received there tanks at home, day 1 of the study often started halfway through the day. As attacks often occured at night this resulted in relatively few attacks being registered on the first day. Furthermore we had to exclude attacks in some patients. In retrospect the primary outcome measure should have been chosen differently. However, we do think that our secondary outcome measures are adequately chosen. These outcome measures reflect the results of a large number of attacks and we did not find a confounding effect of verapamil usage on our results.

In our study, patients were not treated clinically and we had to rely on data delivered in a diary and questionnaires. Depending on the way patients interpreted questions and scores this may have created a bias in results. However, it is unlikely that this would create a specific bias favouring one of the two treatment methods. Patients had to note the date and timing of each attack and what valve they used. We contacted patients before the start of the study and one week after the start of the study to make sure all data was correctly noted. If there were inconsistencies, these attacks were excluded. We checked whether oxygen was used in each case (by checking the oxygen tanks), but we were unable to check if both valves had been used. This made it difficult to detect a possible violation of protocol. The blind was not broken for any patient during the study.

### Future studies
Ideally another study with more power should be conducted to see if oxygen at a flow rate of 12 L/min is consistently preferred by patients and if subgroups can be found. It is, however, difficult to recruit oxygen naïve cluster headache patients. It remains unclear which outcome measure is the most appropriate for a trial on the treatment of cluster headache.

### Conclusion
Patients preferred the treatment with oxygen at a flow rate of 12 L/min compared to 7 L/min. We did not find a

significant difference in drop in VAS score or successfully treated attacks, but more patients were painfree after using 7 L/min. The preference for 12 L/min might be explained by the fact that there were more patients in which treatment with 12 L/min was effective in all attacks, and less patients in which treatment was ineffective. These results suggest, that although more patients were painfree using 7 L/min, this is insufficient to state that 7 L/min is the more effective treatment. We suggest there is a subgroup of patients, who benefit from using the higher flow rate. In this study we were unable to further define this subgroup, possibly due to small sample sizes. As no difference in side effects were found, the usage of oxygen at a flow rate of 12 L/min is at least equally safe as 7 L/min and could be used in all patients. From an economic perspective it might be more cost-effective to start treatment with 7 L/min and if ineffective to switch to 12 L/min. This, however, remains open for debate.

#### Abbreviations
CH: Cluster headache; CI: Confidence interval; IQR: Interquartile range; OR: Odds ratio

#### Acknowledgements
We thank Tiny Simons (Zuyderland medical center), Alexandra Plaum and Jerome Oude Nijhuis (Maastricht University medical center) for assistance with the gathering of data and contacting participants, prof. Michel Ferrari and dr. Joost Haan (Leiden University Medical Center) for assistance with the design of the study and dr. Anke Linssen (Zuyderland medical center) for assistance with the statistical analysis. Special thanks to Westfalen medical BV for providing the blinded oxygen valves.

#### Funding
This research received no specific grant from any funding agency in the public, commercial, or not-for-profit sectors.

#### Authors' contributions
TD Acquisition of data, statistical analysis and interpretation of data, preparation of the manuscript. DH Study concept and design, acquisition of data, critical review of the manuscript. PK Study concept and design, acquisition of data, preparation of the manuscript, study supervision, critical review of the manuscript. All authors read and approved the final manuscript.

#### Competing interests
The authors declare that they have no competing interests.

#### References
1. Kudrow L (1981) Response of cluster headache attacks to oxygen inhalation. Headache 21:1–4
2. Fogan L (1985) Treatment of cluster headache. A double-blind comparison of oxygen v air inhalation. Arch Neurol 42:362–363
3. Cohen AS, Burns B, Goadsby PJ (2009) High-flow oxygen for treatment of cluster headache. JAMA 302:2451–2457
4. Bennett MH, French C, Schnabel A et al (2015) Normobaric and hyperbaric oxygen therapy for the treatment and prevention of migraine and cluster headache. Database Syst Rev 28(12). https://doi.org/10.1002/14651858. CD005219.pub3
5. Rozen TD (2004) High oxygen flow rates for cluster headache. Neurology 63:593

6. Haane DY, De Ceuster LM, Geerlings RP et al (2013) Cluster headache and oxygen: is it possible to predict which patients will be relieved? A prospective cross-sectional correlation study. J Neurol 260:2596–2605
7. Headache Classification Committee of the International Headache Society (2004) The international classification of headache disorders, 2nd edn. Cephalalgia 24(Suppl 1):9–160
8. Van Vliet JA, Eekers PJ, Haan J et al (2016) Evaluating the IHS criteria for cluster headache --a comparison between patients meeting all criteria and patients failing one criterion. Cephalalgia 26:241–245
9. Petersen AS, Barloese MC, Lund NL et al (2017) Oxygen therapy for cluster headache. A mask comparison trial. A single-blinded, placebo-controlled, crossover study. Cephalalgia 37:214–224

# Evaluation of ADMA-DDAH-NOS axis in specific brain areas following nitroglycerin administration: study in an animal model of migraine

Rosaria Greco[1*], Andrea Ferrigno[2†], Chiara Demartini[1†], Annamaria Zanaboni[1,3], Antonina Stefania Mangione[1], Fabio Blandini[4], Giuseppe Nappi[1], Mariapia Vairetti[2] and Cristina Tassorelli[1,3]

### Abstract

**Background:** Nitric oxide (NO) is known to play a key role in migraine pathogenesis, but modulation of NO synthesis has failed so far to show efficacy in migraine treatment. Asymmetric dimethylarginine (ADMA) is a NO synthase (NOS) inhibitor, whose levels are regulated by dimethylarginine dimethylaminohydrolase (DDAH). Systemic administration of nitroglycerin (or glyceryl trinitrate, GTN) is a NO donor that consistently induces spontaneous-like headache attacks in migraneurs. GTN administration induces an increase in neuronal NOS (nNOS) that is simultaneous with a hyperalgesic condition. GTN administration has been used for years as an experimental animal model of migraine. In order to gain further insights in the precise mechanisms involved in the relationships between NO synthesis and migraine, we analyzed changes induced by GTN administration in ADMA levels, DDHA-1 mRNA expression and the expression of neuronal and endothelial NOS (nNOS and eNOS) in the brain. We also evaluated ADMA levels in the serum.

**Methods:** Male Sprague–Dawley rats were injected with GTN (10 mg/kg, i.p.) or vehicle and sacrificed 4 h later. Brain areas known to be activated by GTN administration were dissected out and utilized for the evaluation of nNOS and eNOS expression by means of western blotting. Cerebral and serum ADMA levels were measured by means of ELISA immunoassay. Cerebral DDAH-1 mRNA expression was measured by means of RT-PCR. Comparisons between experimental groups were performed using the Mann Whitney test.

**Results:** ADMA levels and nNOS expression increased in the hypothalamus and medulla following GTN administration. Conversely, a significant decrease in DDAH-1 mRNA expression was observed in the same areas. By contrast, no significant change was reported in eNOS expression. GTN administration did not induce any significant change in serum levels of ADMA.

**Conclusion:** The present data suggest that ADMA accumulates in the brain after GTN administration *via* the inhibition of DDAH-1. This latter may represent a compensatory response to the excessive local availability of NO, released directly by GTN or synthetized by nNOS. These findings prompt an additional mediator (ADMA) in the modulation of NO axis following GTN administration and offer new insights in the pathophysiology of migraine.

**Keywords:** Nitroglycerin; Migraine; Rat brain; nNOS; eNOS; ADMA; DDAH

* Correspondence: rosaria.greco@mondino.it
†Equal contributors
[1]Laboratory of Neurophysiology of Integrative Autonomic Systems, Headache Science Centre, "C. Mondino" National Neurological Institute, Pavia, Italy
Full list of author information is available at the end of the article

## Background

Nitric oxide (NO) may function as a signaling molecule in controlling neuronal activity and plays an important role in governing sensory inputs during migraine [1]. Endogenous NO is produced by the constitutive isoforms of NO synthase, endothelial nitric oxide synthase (eNOS) and neuronal nitric oxide synthase (nNOS). Asymmetric dimethylarginine (ADMA), a major endogenous inhibitor of NOS, inhibits NO production *in vivo* and *in vitro* [2, 3]. Besides ADMA, two other forms of methylated arginine — which can be considered arginine analogues — have been identified in eukaryotes: *NG*-monomethyl-l-arginine (l-NMMA), and ω-*NG,N'G*-symmetric dimethylarginine (SDMA) [4]. All three methylated arginines (ADMA, l-NMMA and SDMA) are inhibitors of arginine transport at superphysiological concentrations, while the physiological relevance of this inhibition remains unclear [5, 6]. Circulating ADMA is present at higher concentrations than l-NMMA and is often considered to be the principal inhibitor of NOS activity [2]. Most of ADMA is degraded by dimethylarginine dimethylaminohydrolase (DDAH), which hydrolyzes ADMA to L-citrulline and dimethylamine [7]. Therefore, this enzymatic pathway is a potential endogenous mechanism for the regulation of NO production by competitive inhibition. ADMA has been associated to cardiovascular risk [7, 8] as it seems involved in the development and progression of cardiovascular disease, *via* the inhibition of eNOS activity and increased production of superoxides [9]. However, high levels of ADMA and increased DDAH-1 expression have been detected in the brain, and spinal cord, thus suggesting a possible role for the ADMA-DDAH pathway in the modulation of neuronal activity [10–12]. This hypothesis seems even more compelling when considering that DDAH-1 co-localizes with nNOS [11]. Increased ADMA levels seem to induce endothelial dysfunction and oxidative stress [9, 12], two potential factors involved in migraine pathogenesis [13, 14]. Available data on ADMA plasma levels and migraine have yielded inconclusive findings so far [15–17] and there is no information on ADMA/DDAH pathway in animal models of migraine.

Exogenous NO, released by nitroglycerin (or glyceryl trinitrate, GTN), induces migraine-like headache in predisposed subjects and it has been used as a human [18, 19] and animal model for the study of migraine [20–22]. GTN also activates the NO synthetic pathway in humans and rats [23, 24].

In order to gain new insights in ADMA-DDAH-NO axis in migraine pain, in this study we investigated changes in brain and serum ADMA levels, together with nNOS and eNOS expression and DDHA-1 expression in discrete areas of the rat brain following GTN administration.

## Methods

Male Sprague–Dawley rats were injected with GTN (10 mg/kg, i.p.) or vehicle and sacrificed 4 h after the injection. The principles of the Helsinki declaration and IASP's guidelines for pain research in animal were rigorously applied [25]. Animals were housed in plastic boxes in groups of 2 with water and food available *ad libitum* and kept on a 12:12 h light–dark cycle. A total of 28 animals were used for the experiments and all procedures were in accordance with the European Convention for Care and Use of Laboratory Animals and were approved by the local animal ethic committee of the University of Pavia (Document n. 2, 2012). GTN [Bioindustria L.I.M. Novi Ligure (AL), Italy] was prepared from a stock solution of 5.0 mg/1.5 mL dissolved in 27 % alcohol and 73 % propylene glycol. For the injections, GTN was further diluted in saline (0.9 % NaCl) to reach the final concentration of propylene glycol (PG) 16 % and alcohol 6 % and administered at a dose of 10 mg/kg. A solution of saline (0.9 % NaCl), PG 16 % and alcohol 6 % was used as vehicle (CT group).

On the basis of the distribution of the nuclei that are known to be activated by GTN and involved in migraine pain, the following discrete brain areas were dissected out 4 h after GTN or vehicle administration and used for analysis: medulla-pons, containing nucleus trigeminalis caudalis (NTC), nucleus tractus solitarius and area postrema; mesencephalon, containing ventrolateral column of the periaqueductal grey and parabrachial nucleus, and hypothalamus, containing the paraventricular and supraoptic nuclei of the hypothalamus.

### Western blotting

Rats ($N = 6$ per experimental group) were perfused transcardially with 250 ml cold saline, 4 h after GTN or vehicle administration. Brains were immediately removed and chopped into parts; brain areas of interest were dissected out and used for the preparation of total extracts. The samples were homogenized on ice with a homogenizer in at least 5 volumes of modified RIPA buffer (Tris 50 mM, pH 7.4, NaCl 150 mM, EDTA 1 mM, SDS 0,2 %) supplemented with cocktail inhibitors protease. Then, they were incubated on ice for 20 min. The tissue lysate was centrifuged at $10,000 \times g$ for 45 min at 4 °C and supernatants stored at –80 °C. Protein assay was performed by bicinchoninic acid (BCA) method. A 20 μg of protein were submitted to SDS-poliacrylamide gels 10 % and transferred onto a PVDF membrane (Amersham Biosciences). After blocking with 5 % dry milk, the blots were probed overnight at 4 C° with rabbit polyclonal anti-nNOS serum (1:1000; Cayman Chemical) or anti-eNOS serum (1:1000; Santa Cruz Bioctenology) and then probed for 1 h with an anti-rabbit horseradish peroxidase coupled secondary antibody (1:10000; Amersham Biosciences). An enhanced chemiluminescence system (ECL Advance; Amersham Biosciences) was used for visualization. Membranes were also probed with a rabbit polyclonal anti-β actin antibody (1:1000; Santa Cruz Biotechnology) as a housekeeping protein.

For semiquantitative analysis, a Bio-Rad GS800 densitometer was used. NOS expression was evaluated in each sample by dividing the optical density of the NOS band by the intensity of the optical density of the band corresponding to the housekeeping protein. The specificity of the antibodies was confirmed by immunoprecipitation with a specific blocking peptide.

### Enzyme-linked immunosorbant assays (ELISA)

Rats ($N = 8$ per experimental group) were injected with GTN (10 mg/kg i.p.) or vehicle and then killed with a lethal dose of anaesthetic 4 h after treatment. Their brains were immediately chopped into parts; brain areas of interest were dissected out and frozen at $-80\ °C$ until further processing.

Blood was drawn from the vena cava and centrifuged at 3000 g for 10 min at 4 °C.

ADMA levels (ng/mg proteins or nmol/ml) were quantified by ELISA kit (Antibodies Online) according to the manufacturer's instructions.

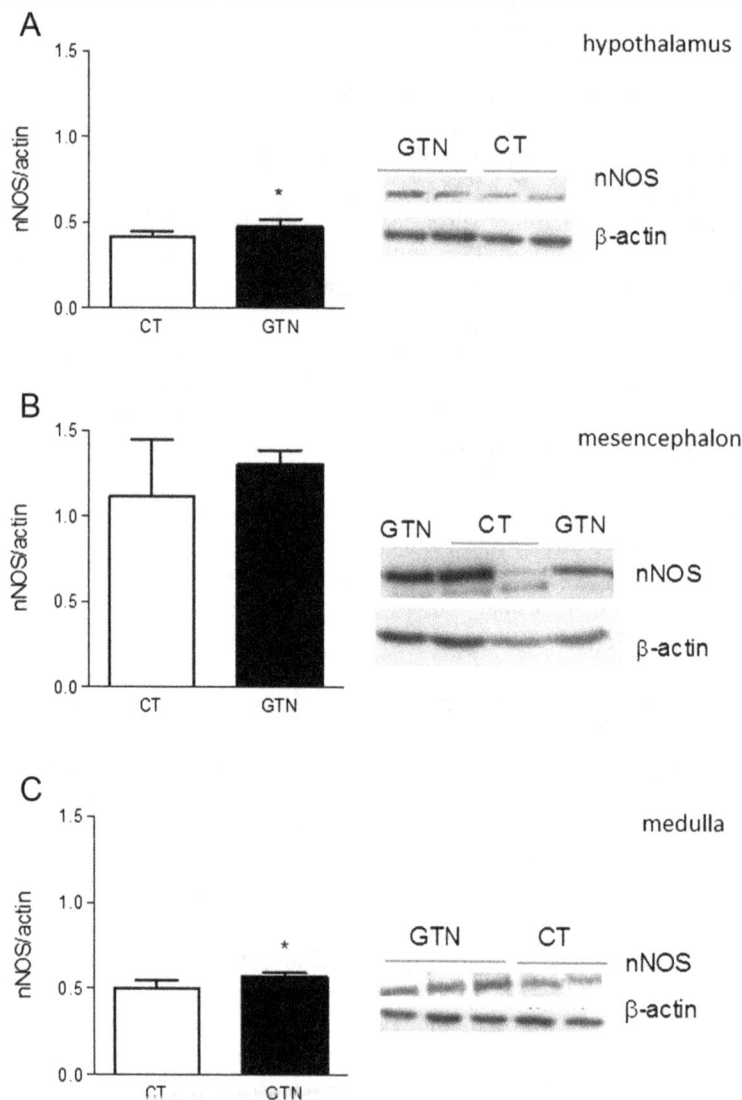

**Fig. 1** nNOS expression in homogenates of hypothalamus (**a**), mesencephalon (**b**) and medulla (**c**) of rats injected with glyceryl trinitrate (GTN) or vehicle (CT). The histograms illustrate the densitometric analysis representing expression levels of nNOS (155KDa), evaluated as the ratio vs β-actin (39 kDa). The latter protein was used as a housekeeping protein on the same membrane previously incubated with nNOS. nNOS expression was evaluated after 4 h of GTN or vehicle injection. In the right of each panel are illustrated representative western blots of nNOS protein. Data are expressed as mean ± SD. Mann Whitney test, *$p < 0.05$ vs vehicle (CT)

## Real-time polymerase chain reaction

Rats ($N = 6$ per experimental group) were injected with GTN (10 mg/kg i.p.) or vehicle and then killed with a lethal dose of anaesthetic 4 h after treatment. Their brains were immediately chopped into parts and frozen at −80 °C until further processing.

DDAH-1 mRNA expression was analyzed by a real-time polymerase chain reaction (RT-PCR) and total RNA was isolated from the cerebral samples with Trizol reagent in accordance with the method of Chomczynski and Mackey [26]. RNA was quantified by measuring the absorbance at 260/280 nm. cDNA was generated using the iScript cDNA Synthesis kit (Bio-Rad) following the supplier's instructions. Gene expression was analyzed using the Fast Eva Green supermix (Bio-Rad). As regards housekeeping, gene glyceraldehyde 3-phosphate dehydrogenase (GAPDH) was used. The expression of the housekeeping gene remained constant in all the experimental groups considered. The amplification was performed through two-step cycling (95–60 °C) for 45 cycles in a light Cycler 480 Instrument RT-PCR Detection System (Roche) following the supplier's instructions. All samples were assayed in

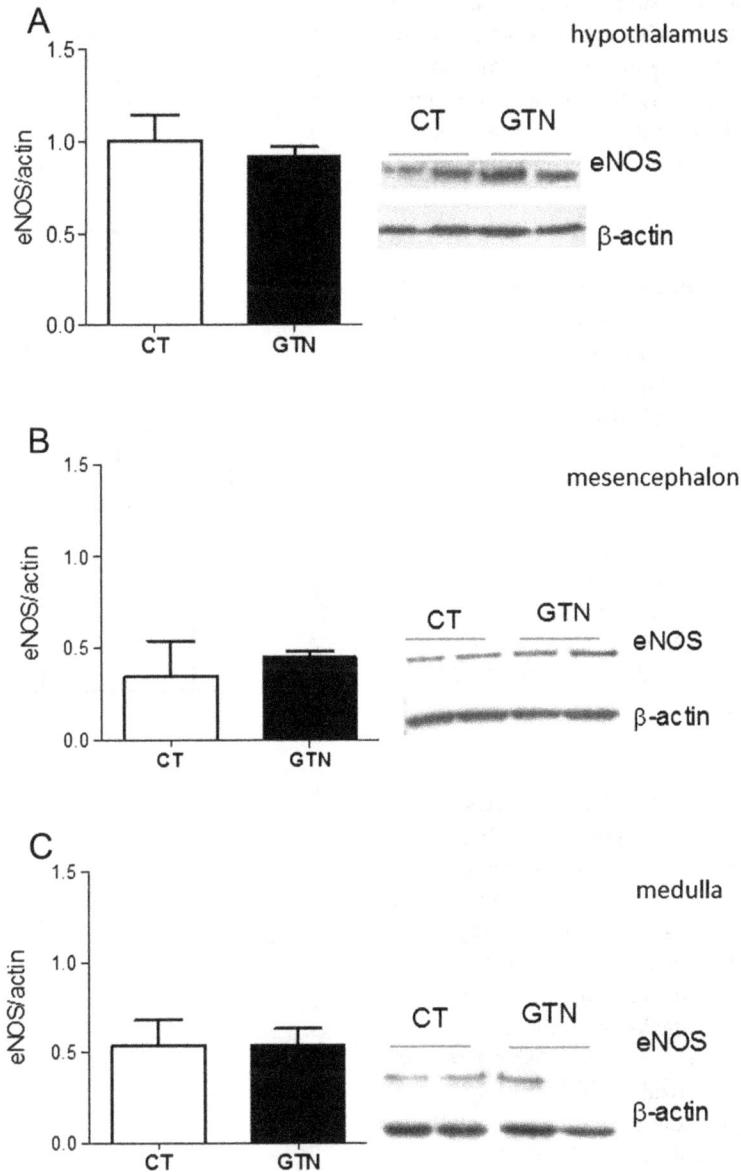

**Fig. 2** eNOS expression in homogenates of hypothalamus (**a**), mesencephalon (**b**) and medulla (**c**) of rats injected with glyceryl trinitrate (GTN) or vehicle (CT). The histograms illustrate the densitometric analysis representing expression levels of eNOS (130KDa) as ratio vs β-actin (39 kDa). The latter protein was used as a housekeeping protein on the same membrane previously incubated with eNOS. In the right of each panel are illustrated representative western blots of eNOS protein. eNOS expression was evaluated after 4 h of GTN or vehicle injection. Data are expressed as mean ± SD. Mann Whitney test, *$p < 0.05$ vs vehicle (CT)

triplicate. Gene expression was calculated using the ΔCt method.

## Statistical evaluation

Data are expressed as mean ± SD. Comparisons between groups (GTN and CT) were performed using the Mann Whitney test. The minimum level of statistical significance was set at $p < 0.05$.

## Results

### nNOS and eNOS expression

Western blotting analyses using the anti-nNOS antibody revealed the presence of one band at 155 KDa. In the GTN Group, the intensity of this band was significantly increased in the hypothalamus and medulla, when compared to the control group (Fig. 1). By contrast, no change in eNOS expression (135KDa) was detected in any of the cerebral areas under evaluation after GTN administration (Fig. 2).

### AMDA levels

ADMA levels were significantly increased in the hypothalamus and medulla of GTN treated rats, when compared to CT group. Conversely, we did not detect any significant differences in mesencephalon (Fig. 3). No significant difference was observed in serum ADMA concentrations between GTN and CT groups (Fig. 4).

### DDAH-1mRNA expression

DDAH-1 mRNA expression was significantly decreased in the hypothalamus and in the medulla of rats treated with GTN when compared to CT group. No significant difference in DDAH-1 mRNA expression was found in the mesencephalon of rats treated with GTN when compared to CT group (Fig. 5).

## Discussion

Strong evidence supports the idea that NO plays a pivotal role in the pathogenesis of migraine [27, 28], a disorder characterized by pain sensitization associated with cranial vascular changes [29–31], but mechanisms and modalities of NO activity are still largely unknown. Systemic GTN activates neuronal groups in selected areas of the rat brain involved in nociception [21, 32, 33] and induces spontaneous-like attacks in migraineurs via multimodal mechanisms that include GTN- induced vasodilation, peripheral sensitization induced by the increased availability of NO at the trigeminovascular level, and possibly also central sensitization [34–37].

GTN administration induces an increase in nNOS that is simultaneous with a hyperalgesic condition and neuronal activation in brain areas involved in migraine pain [38, 39], thus suggesting that NOS inhibition may be a potential therapeutic target for migraine. Experimental

and clinical studies suggest that NOS inhibition influences the activation of the trigeminal vascular system and that nonselective NOS inhibition is associated to antimigraine activity [40, 41]. Clinical application of non selelctive NOS inhibition is however hindered by the

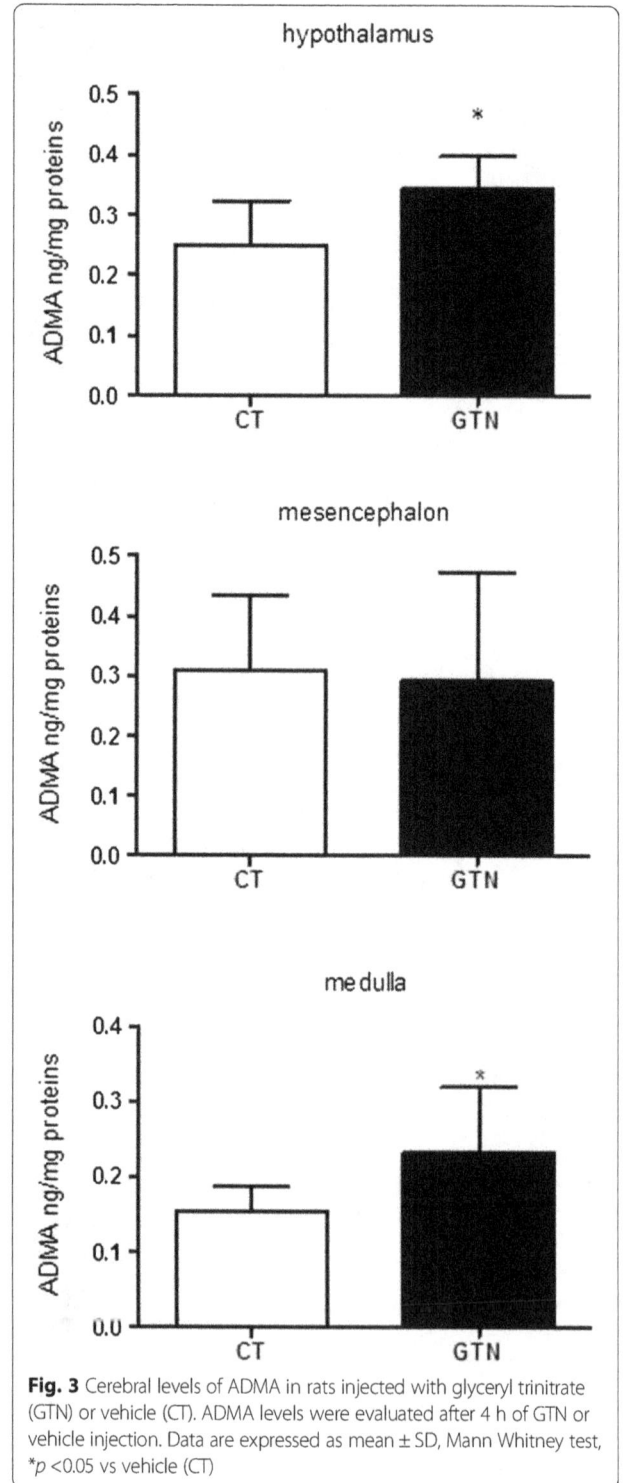

**Fig. 3** Cerebral levels of ADMA in rats injected with glyceryl trinitrate (GTN) or vehicle (CT). ADMA levels were evaluated after 4 h of GTN or vehicle injection. Data are expressed as mean ± SD, Mann Whitney test, *$p$ <0.05 vs vehicle (CT)

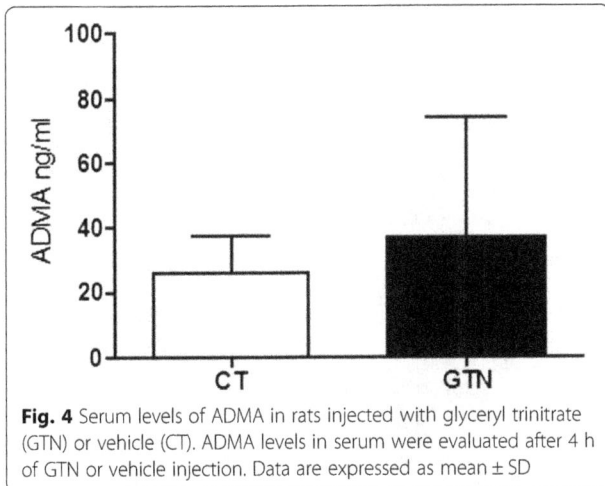

**Fig. 4** Serum levels of ADMA in rats injected with glyceryl trinitrate (GTN) or vehicle (CT). ADMA levels in serum were evaluated after 4 h of GTN or vehicle injection. Data are expressed as mean ± SD

cardiovascular effects, *i.e.,* increase of mean arterial pressure and a decrease of heart rate for its pharmacokinetic profile [41].

ADMA, is a methylated arginine found in plasma, urine and different tissues [2], which is released when methylated proteins are degraded into their amino acid components during hydrolytic protein turnover [8]. ADMA blocks NO synthesis and can induce endothelial dysfunction, both *in vivo* and *in vitro* [2, 3], and cause oxidative stress [42], two potential factors involved in migraine pathogenesis [13, 14]. DDAH regulates ADMA levels and NO signalling *in vivo* and ADMA/DDAH system is considered as a novel pathway for modulating NO production [43]. DDAH-1 predominates in tissues that express nNOS, whereas DDAH-2 predominates in tissues expressing eNOS [44]. Since large amounts of ADMA and DDAH-1 have been detected in the brain and spinal cord, probably ADMA/DDAH-1 pathway may have a role also in neuronal, inflammatory and other non-cardiovascular pathologies, as migraine pain, where NO has pivotal role [15]. Uzar *et al.,* [15] found elevated plasma levels of ADMA and NO in migraine patients as compared to control subjects, suggesting that an increase in ADMA levels in migraine might represent a compensatory mechanism for blocking NO production and NO-induced excessive vasodilatation [15]. However, differences in ADMA and NO levels when comparing ictal and interictal levels in migraineurs yielded inconclusive findings [15–17]. To the best of our knowledge, no information is available on cerebral ADMA and DDAH-1 expression in experimental animal models of migraine.

In this study, we evaluated the simultaneous changes in ADMA levels and DDAH-1 mRNA expression in brain areas in an animal model specific for migraine in order to evaluate whether ADMA-DDAH-pathway may be involved in migraine. We also evaluated nNOS and eNOS expression in the same brain areas, and ADMA levels

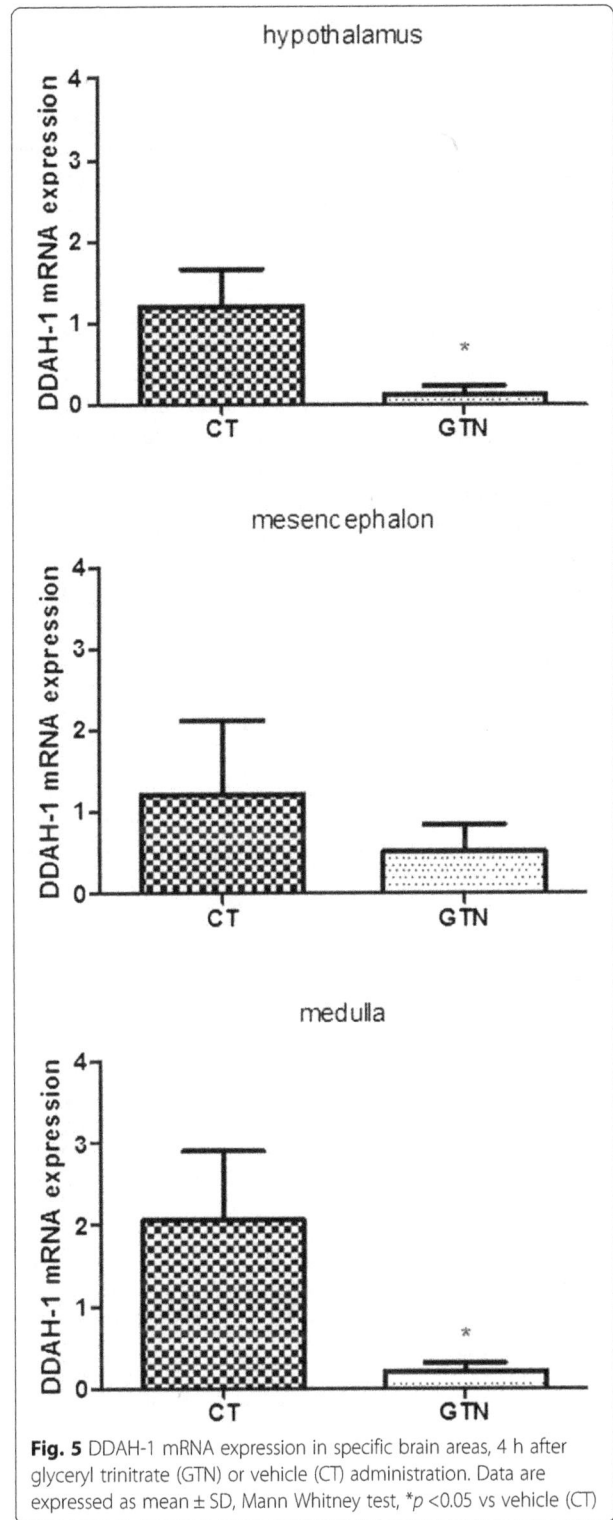

**Fig. 5** DDAH-1 mRNA expression in specific brain areas, 4 h after glyceryl trinitrate (GTN) or vehicle (CT) administration. Data are expressed as mean ± SD, Mann Whitney test, *$p < 0.05$ vs vehicle (CT)

in the venous blood, drawn from the vena cava. Our findings show that AMDA levels significantly increased in the hypothalamus and medulla 4 h after GTN administration, the timing where we observe neuronal activation and hyperlagesia. This increase was associated to the inhibition of DDAH-1 expression and to the increase in nNOS expression in the same areas. eNOS expression instead was not affected. Taken together, these results suggest that the increase in brain NO availability, secondary to GTN exposure [45], may have interfered with DDAH-1 expression, possibly *via* S-nitrosylation of DDAH-1 active site [46, 47]. Indeed, deletion of DDAH-1 gene, or the inhibition of its transcription, is associated with an increase of ADMA levels [48]. Alternatively, DDAH-1 expression may have been inhibited *via* GTN-induced oxidative stress [49] or GTN-induced activation of inflammatory pathway [50, 51]. Previous reports have indeed shown that DDAH activity and protein expression may be markedly reduced during oxidative stress and/or inflammation [52–54].

Circulating levels of ADMA were not affected by GTN treatment to suggest that GTN interferes with DDAH-1 expression only at cerebral level, but not at peripheral level such as the liver, where high net hepatic uptake of ADMA occurs [55]. In agreement with a selective 'neuronal' activity of AMDA in this experimental paradigm is the absence of changes observed in eNOS.

## Conclusions

The present data suggest that ADMA accumulates in the brain after GTN administration *via* the inhibition of DDAH-1. This latter may represent a compensatory response to the excessive local availability of NO, released directly by GTN or synthetized by nNOS. These findings prompt an additional mediator (ADMA) in the modulation of NO axis following GTN administration and offer new insights in the pathophysiology of migraine.

### Abbreviations
GTN: Nitroglycerin or Glyceryl trinitrate; ADMA: Asymmetric dimethylarginine; NO: Nitric oxide, nNOS, neuronal nitric oxide synthase; eNOS: endothelial nitric oxide synthase; NMMA: NG-monomethyl-l-arginine (l-); SDMA: ω NG,N' G-symmetric dimethylarginine; DDAH: dimethylarginine dimethylaminohydrolase.

### Competing interests
The authors declare that they have no competing interests.

### Authors' contributions
RG instructed the experiments, AF, CD and AZ performed the experiments. RG analysed the data and drafted the manuscript. CT revised the manuscript. All authors contributed to the idea of the study, and read and approved the final manuscript.

### Acknowledgements
This study was supported by a grant from the Italian Ministry of Health to "C. Mondino" National Neurological Institute (Ricerca Corrente 2011).

### Author details
[1]Laboratory of Neurophysiology of Integrative Autonomic Systems, Headache Science Centre, "C. Mondino" National Neurological Institute, Pavia, Italy. [2]Department of Internal Medicine and Therapeutics, Pharmacology and Toxicology Unit, University of Pavia, Pavia, Italy. [3]Department of Brain and Behavioural Sciences, University of Pavia, Pavia, Italy. [4]Laboratory of Functional Neurochemistry, Center for Research in Neurodegenerative Diseases, "C. Mondino" National Neurological Institute, Pavia, Italy.

### References
1. Olesen J, Thomsen LL, Lassen LH, Olesen IJ (1995) The nitric oxide hypothesis of migraine and other vascular headaches. Cephalalgia 15(2):94–100
2. Vallance P, Leone A, Calver A, Collier J, Moncada S (1992) Accumulation of an endogenous inhibitor of nitric oxide synthesis in chronic renal failure. Lancet 339:572–575
3. MacAllister RJ, Whitley GS, Vallance P (1994) Effects of guanidino and uremic compounds on nitric oxide pathways. Kidney Int 45(3):737–742
4. Kakimoto Y, Akazawa S (1970) Isolation and identification of NG, NG-and NG, N'G-dimethyl-arginine, Nε-mono-, di-, and trimethyllysine, and glucosylgalactosyl- and alactosyl-δ-hydroxylysine from human urine. J Biol Chem 245:575–578
5. Closs EI, Basha FZ, Habermeier A, Forstermann U (1997) Interference of l arginine analogues with l arginine transport mediated by the y + carrier hCAT 2B. Nitric Oxide 1:65–73
6. Tsikas D, Boger RH, Sandmann J, Bode-Boger SM, Frolich JC (2000) Endogenous nitric oxide synthase inhibitors are responsible for the l arginine paradox. FEBS Lett 478:1–3
7. Vallance P, Leiper J (2004) Cardiovascular biology of the asymmetric dimethylarginine: dimethylarginine dimethylaminohydrolase pathway. Arterioscler Thromb Vasc Biol 24(6):1023–1030
8. Böger RH (2003) The emerging role of ADMA as a novel cardiovascular risk factor. Cardiovasc Res 59:824–833
9. Pou S, Keaton L, Surichamorn W, Rosen GM (1999) Mechanism of superoxide generation by neuronal nitric-oxide synthase. J Biol Chem 274(14):9573–9580
10. Selley ML (2004) Homocysteine increases the production of asymmetric dimethylarginine in cultured neurons. J Neurosci Res 77(1):90–93
11. D'Mello R, Sand C, Pezet S, Leiper JM, Gaurilcikaite E, McMahon SB, Dickenson AH, Nandi M (2015) Dimethylarginine dimethylaminohydrolase-1 is involved in spinal nociceptive plasticity. Pain [Epub ahead of print]
12. Luo Y, Yue W, Quan X, Wang Y, Zhao B, Lu Z (2015) Asymmetric dimethylarginine exacerbates Aβ-induced toxicity and oxidative stress in human cell and Caenorhabditis elegans models of Alzheimer disease. Free Radic Biol Med 79:117–126
13. Yilmaz G, Sürer H, Inan LE, Coskun O, Yücel D (2007) Increased nitrosative and oxidative stress in platelets of migraine patients. Tohoku J Exp Med 211(1):23–30
14. Rajan R, Khurana D, Lal V (2014) Interictal cerebral and systemic endothelial dysfunction in patients with migraine: a case–control study. J Neurol Neurosurg Psychiatry. doi:10.1136/jnnp-2014-309571
15. Uzar E, Evliyaoglu O, Toprak G, Acar A, Yucel Y, Calisir T, Cevik MU, Tasdemir N (2011) Increased asymmetric dimethylarginine and nitric oxide levels in patients with migraine. J Headache Pain 12(2):239–243
16. Guldiken B, Demir M, Guldiken S, Turgut N, Ozkan H, Kabayel L, Tugrul A (2009) Asymmetric dimethylarginine and nitric oxide levels in migraine during the interictal period. J Clin Neurosci 16(5):672–674
17. Gruber HJ, Bernecker C, Lechner A, Weiss S, Wallner-Blazek M, Meinitzer A, Höbarth G, Renner W, Fauler G, Horejsi R, Fazekas F, Truschnig-Wilders M (2009) Increased nitric oxide stress is associated with migraine. Cephalalgia 30:486–492
18. Ashina M, Simonsen H, Bendtsen L, Jensen R, Olesen J (2004) Glyceryl trinitrate may trigger endogenous nitric oxide production in patients with chronic tension-type headache. Cephalalgia 24(11):967–972
19. Ashina M, Tfelt-Hansen P, Dalgaard P, Olesen J (2011) Lack of correlation between vasodilatation and pharmacologically induced immediate headache in healthy subjects. Cephalalgia 31(6):683–690
20. Buzzi MG, Tassorelli C (2010) Experimental models of migraine. Handb Clin Neurol 97:109–123
21. Greco R, Mangione AS, Sandrini G, Maccarrone M, Nappi G, Tassorelli C (2011) Effects of anandamide in migraine: data from an animal model. J Headache Pain 12(2):177–183
22. Greco R, Bandiera T, Mangione A, Demartini C, Siani F, Nappi G, Sandrini G, Guijarro A, Armirotti A, Piomelli D, Tassorelli C (2015) Effects of peripheral FAAH blockade on NTG-induced hyperalgesia-evaluation of URB937 in an animal model of migraine. Cephalalgia [Epub ahead of print]

23. Sarchielli P, Alberti A, Codini M, Floridi A, Gallai V (2000) Nitric oxide metabolites, prostaglandins and trigeminal vasoactive peptides in internal jugular vein blood during spontaneous migraine attacks. Cephalalgia 20:907–918

24. Reuter U, Bolay H, Jansen-Olesen I, Chiarugi A, Sanchez del Rio M, Letourneau R, Theoharides C, Waeber C, Moskowitz MA (2001) Delayed inflammation in rat meninges: implications for migraine pathophysiology. Brain 124(Pt 12):2490–2502

25. Zimmerman M (1983) Ethical guidelines for investigations of experimental pain in conscious animals. Pain 16:109–110

26. Chomczynski P, Mackey K (1995) Substitution of chloroform by bromo-chloropropane in the single-step method of RNA isolation. Anal Biochem 225(1):163–164

27. Olesen J, Jansen-Olesen I (2000) Nitric oxide mechanisms in migraine. Pathol Biol (Paris) 48(7):648–657

28. Thomsen LL, Olesen J (1997) A pivotal role of nitric oxide in migraine pain. Ann N Y Acad Sci 835:363–372

29. Burstein R (2001) Deconstructing migraine headache into peripheral and central sensitization. Pain 89(2–3):107–110

30. May A, Goadsby PJ (1999) The trigeminovascular system in humans: pathophysiologic implications for primary headache syndromes of the neural influences on the cerebral circulation. J Cereb Blood Flow Metab 19(2):115–127

31. Moskowitz MA, Macfarlane R (1993) Neurovascular and molecular mechanisms in migraine headaches. Cerebrovasc Brain Metab Rev 5(3):159–177

32. Tassorelli C, Joseph SA, Nappi G (1999) Reciprocal circuits involved in nitroglycerin-induced neuronal activation of autonomic regions and pain pathways: a double immunolabeling and tract-tracing study. Brain Res 842(2):294–310

33. Tassorelli C, Greco R, Morocutti A, Costa A, Nappi G (2001) Nitric oxide-induced neuronal activation in the central nervous system as an animal model of migraine: mechanisms and mediators. Funct Neurol 16(4 Suppl):69–76

34. Sances G, Tassorelli C, Pucci E, Ghiotto N, Sandrini G, Nappi G (2004) Reliability of the nitroglycerin provocative test in the diagnosis of neurovascular headaches. Cephalalgia 24(2):110–119

35. Thomsen LL, Kruuse C, Iversen HK, Olesen J (1994) A nitric oxide donor (nitroglycerin) triggers genuine migraine attacks. Eur J Neurol 1(1):73–80

36. de Tommaso M, Libro G, Guido M, Difruscolo O, Losito L, Sardaro M, Cerbo R (2004) Nitroglycerin induces migraine headache and central sensitization phenomena in patients with migraine without aura: a study of laser evoked potentials. Neurosci Lett 363(3):272–275

37. Tuka B, Helyes Z, Markovics A, Bagoly T, Németh J, Márk L, Brubel R, Reglődi D, Párdutz A, Szolcsányi J, Vécsei L, Tajti J (2012) Peripheral and central alterations of pituitary adenylate cyclase activating polypeptide-like immunoreactivity in the rat in response to activation of the trigeminovascular system. Peptides 33(2):307–316

38. Pardutz A, Szatmári E, Vecsei L, Schoenen J (2004) Nitroglycerin-induced nNOS increase in rat trigeminal nucleus caudalis is inhibited by systemic administration of lysine acetylsalicylate but not of sumatriptan. Cephalalgia 24(6):439–445

39. Ramachandran R, Bhatt DK, Ploug KB, Hay-Schmidt A, Jansen-Olesen I, Gupta S, Olesen J (2014) Nitric oxide synthase, calcitonin gene-related peptide and NK-1 receptor mechanisms are involved in GTN-induced neuronal activation. Cephalalgia 34(2):136–147

40. Barbanti P, Egeo G, Aurilia C, Fofi L, Della-Morte D (2014) Drugs targeting nitric oxide synthase for migraine treatment. Expert Opin Investig Drugs 23(8):1141–1148

41. Lassen LH, Ashina M, Christiansen I, Ulrich V, Grover R, Donaldson J, Olesen J (1998) Nitric oxide synthase inhibition: a new principle in the treatment of migraine attacks. Cephalalgia 18(1):27–32

42. Teerlink T, Luo Z, Palm F, Wilcox CS (2009) Cellular ADMA: regulation and action. Pharmacol Res 60(6):448–460

43. Jiang DJ, Jia SJ, Dai Z, Li YJ (2006) Asymmetric dimethylarginine induces apoptosis via p38 MAPK/caspase-3-dependent signaling pathway in endothelial cells. J Mol Cell Cardiol 40(4):529–539

44. Leiper JM, Santa Maria J, Chubb A, MacAllister RJ, Charles IG, Whitley GS, Vallance P (1999) Identification of two human dimethylarginine dimethylaminohydrolases with distinct tissue distributions and homology with microbial arginine deiminases. Biochem J 343:209–214

45. Ma SX, Ignarro LJ, Byrns R, Li XY (1999) Increased nitric oxide concentrations in posterior hypothalamus and central sympathetic function on nitrate tolerance following subcutaneous nitroglycerin. Nitric Oxide 3(2):153–161

46. Leiper J, Murray-Rust J, McDonald N, Vallance P (2002) S-nitrosylation of dimethylarginine dimethylaminohydrolase regulates enzyme activity: further interactions between nitric oxide synthase and dimethylarginine dimethylaminohydrolase. Proc Natl Acad Sci U S A 99(21):13527–13532

47. Stamler JS (2008) Nitroglycerin-mediated S-nitrosylation of proteins: a field comes full cycle. Circ Res 103(6):557–559

48. Davids M, Richir MC, Visser M, Ellger B, van den Berghe G, van Leeuwen PA, Teerlink T (2012) Role of dimethylarginine dimethylaminohydrolase activity in regulation of tissue and plasma concentrations of asymmetric dimethylarginine in an animal model of prolonged critical illness. Metabolism 61(4):482–490

49. Nazıroğlu M, Çelik Ö, Uğuz AC, Bütün A (2015) Protective effects of riboflavin and selenium on brain microsomal Ca2 + −ATPase and oxidative damage caused by glyceryl trinitrate in a rat headache model. Biol Trace Elem Res 164(1):72–79

50. Greco R, Tassorelli C, Cappelletti D, Sandrini G, Nappi G (2005) Activation of the transcription factor NF-kappaB in the nucleus trigeminalis caudalis in an animal model of migraine. Neurotoxicology 26(5):795–800

51. Yin Z, Fang Y, Ren L, Wang X, Zhang A, Lin J, Li X (2009) Atorvastatin attenuates NF-kappaB activation in trigeminal nucleus caudalis in a rat model of migraine. Neurosci Lett 465(1):61–65

52. Pope AJ, Druhan L, Guzman JE, Forbes SP, Murugesan V, Lu D, Xia Y, Chicoine LG, Parinandi NL, Cardounel AJ (2007) Role of DDAH-1 in lipid peroxidation product-mediated inhibition of endothelial NO generation. Am J Physiol Cell Physiol 293(5):C1679–C1686

53. Yang TL, Chen MF, Luo BL, Xie QY, Jiang JL, Li YJ (2005) Fenofibrate decreases asymmetric dimethylarginine level in cultured endothelial cells by inhibiting NF-kappaB activity. Naunyn Schmiedebergs Arch Pharmacol 371(5):401–407

54. Tain YL, Kao YH, Hsieh CS, Chen CC, Sheen JM, Lin IC, Huang LT (2010) Melatonin blocks oxidative stress-induced increased asymmetric dimethylarginine. Free Radic Biol Med 49(6):1088–1098

55. Nijveldt RJ, Siroen MP, Teerlink T, van Leeuwen PA (2004) Elimination of asymmetric dimethylarginine by the kidney and the liver: a link to the development of multiple organ failure? J Nutr 134(10 Suppl):2848S–2852S

# Single-pulse transcranial magnetic stimulation (sTMS) for the acute treatment of migraine: evaluation of outcome data for the UK post market pilot program

Ria Bhola[1], Evelyn Kinsella[1], Nicola Giffin[2], Sue Lipscombe[3], Fayyaz Ahmed[4], Mark Weatherall[5] and Peter J Goadsby[6,7*]

## Abstract

**Background:** Single pulse transcranial magnetic stimulation (sTMS) is a novel treatment for acute migraine. Previous randomised controlled data demonstrated that sTMS is effective and well tolerated in the treatment of migraine with aura. The aim of the programme reported here was to evaluate patient responses in the setting of routine clinical practice.

**Methods:** Migraine patients with and without aura treating with sTMS had an initial review ($n = 426$) and training call, and then participated in telephone surveys at week six ($n = 331$) and week 12 during a 3-month treatment period ($n = 190$).

**Results:** Of patients surveyed with 3 month data (n = 190; episodic, $n = 59$; chronic, $n = 131$), 62 % reported pain relief, finding the device effective at reducing or alleviating migraine pain; in addition there was relief reported of associated features: nausea- 52 %; photophobia- 55 %; and phonophobia- 53 %. At 3 months there was a reduction in monthly headache days for episodic migraine, from 12 (median, 8–13 IQ range) to 9 (4–12) and for chronic migraine, a reduction from 24 (median, 16–30 IQ range) to 16 (10–30). There were no serious or unanticipated adverse events.

**Conclusion:** sTMS may be a valuable addition to options for the treatment of both episodic and chronic migraine.

## Background

Migraine is the most common cause of disability due to a neurological disorder [1] on a worldwide basis [2]. Migraine can be ameliorated in some patients by life-style advice, and when troublesome, requires treatment of both attacks and strategies to reduce attack frequency with preventives [3]. While much has been determined about the biology of migraine in recent times [4], and the future is promising [5], much needs to be done for the burden on patients and society that migraine brings. A particular issue in migraine is that of side effects, such as weight gain with many preventives [6], or

vascular issues with acute attack therapies [7], or both, are driving a need for new effective and well tolerated treatments.

Transcranial magnetic stimulation (TMS) was first described in 1985 [8] and followed seminal work by Merton, Morton and Marsden [9] who had used electrical stimulation of the cortex to dissect questions around the cortical influence on motor reflexes [9–11], and had found the stimulus painful to subjects. sTMS is a non-invasive, safe and painless method of activating the human motor cortex [12]. TMS is based on the principle of electromagnetic induction. A pulse of current passes through a coil located within the device and when the device is placed over a person's head for a very short duration, it aims to depolarise neurons rapidly within a target area [13]. Given early suggestions of an effect of sTMS in migraine with aura [14], single pulse TMS was

---

* Correspondence: peter.goadsby@kcl.ac.uk
[6]Headache Group, Basic & Clinical Neuroscience, King's College London, London, UK
[7]NIHR-Wellcome Trust Clinical Research Facility, King's College Hospital, London SE5 9PJ, UK
Full list of author information is available at the end of the article

studied in cortical spreading depression (CSD) in rat [15], as CSD in rat is considered an excellent model of human aura [16]. sTMS inhibits CSD in rat and cat [15]. It has no effect on nociceptive trigeminocervical neurons [17], while it certainly inhibits nociceptive trigeminothalamic neurons [18, 19].

sTMS has been shown to be effective in acute migraine treatment in patients with migraine with aura in a sham-controlled study [20]. Moreover, it is well accepted to be safe [21]. The device is CE-marked in Europe, so it can be used in clinical practice. The SpringTMS device was introduced to open clinical practice through the post-market pilot program in the UK and migraine patients, both with and without aura, were selected for this treatment. The aim of this program was to assess the impact of sTMS on migraine symptoms and treatment during an initial 3 month treatment period: assessing the effect on pain severity, associated migraine symptoms, attack duration and acute medication use. Patients prescribed treatment from December 2012, were also asked to provide data on disability (HIT-6). We report on the treatment outcomes over a 3 year period, having presented interim outcomes previously in an abbreviated form [22].

## Methods

Twenty specialist headache clinics in the UK participated in the post market pilot program, which commenced in June 2011 following receipt of the CE mark for the SpringTMS device. Five centres, the authors of this report, contributed all but 60 patients.

The headache specialists selected patients in the clinic who had previously found acute medications intolerable ($n = 89$), ineffective or inadequately effective ($n = 72$), or had a medical contraindication ($n = 57$), or some combination of these, to established approaches.

Patients were included who had a diagnosis of episodic migraine with or without aura ($n = 59$) or chronic migraine ($n = 131$) [23]. Patients were excluded if their treating physician felt they were unsuitable, such as presence of metal in the upper body or history of epilepsy.

There were no stipulations placed on patients to change their use of medicines during the TMS treatment period, for those who were also using medicines, except that for the initial experience medication overuse [24] was actively discouraged. Patients could continue on preventives ($n = 64$). Thirty three patients used an anticonvulsant (topiramate $n = 17$; gabapentin $n = 8$; valproate $n = 3$; pregabalin $n = 2$; lamotrigine $n = 2$; topiramate and valproate $n = 1$) with one stopping topiramate 25 mg during the reporting period.

Patients had the option to discontinue device use at any point if they wished.

The data were compiled and analysed with the objective of carrying out a service evaluation that in UK practice does not require Research Ethics Committee review (http://www.hra-decisiontools.org.uk/research/).

### Patient selection

As a non-drug treatment in a specialist clinic setting, sTMS provided an alternative option for a patient group with unmet needs. Throughout the pilot program, participating clinicians selected sTMS specifically for patients with disabling migraine who could not successfully use established treatments for a variety of reasons.

- Lack of efficacy on current treatment.
- Poor tolerability for current acute or preventive treatments.
- Medical conditions that rendered established medications unsafe to use and where patients were trying to conceive.

During the later months of the program patients with medication overuse were included, using combination (Triptan with NSAID ± paracetamol (acetaminophen); $n = 53$), codeine ($n = 12$) or triptans ($n = 22$).

### Device distribution

Following receipt of the doctor's prescription, the portable device was delivered to the patient at home and within a week, a headache specialist nurse (RB or EK) made first contact with the patient. At the initial call, the patients were advised how to treat, based on the Medical Advisory Board (MAB) guidelines (Table 1). Their typical migraine pattern was documented, in terms of frequency, severity and duration of attacks.

### Data collection

Following a telephone (RB, EK) review with collection of historical baseline data over the previous 3 months, and a training call at the start of treatment, telephone surveys at weeks 6 and 12 were conducted during the treatment period. The questionnaire data at week 12 was anonymised and subsequently analysed. Upon completion, patients' progress with treatment was reported back to their prescribing doctor.

### Treatment

To treat migraine symptoms, the device is switched on and positioned on the occiput by the patient and the pulse is delivered with the press of a button. The device weighs 1.5 Kg with dimensions H: 81 mm; W: 220 mm; D: 134 mm. A brief sound is heard as the pulse is delivered. A second pulse may be delivered if required. At treatment, a single magnetic field pulse is delivered of nominally 0.9 T [20], measured 1 cm from the device surface, with a rise time of 180 μsec and a total pulse length of less than 1 ms.

**Table 1** Initiation strategy from Medical Advisory Board

- Initiate treatment as early as possible when patient first experiences symptoms of migraine, including pain and/or aura symptoms.
- Fill-out the headache diary immediately after treatment or at any time after the migraine attack subsides.
- Record all symptoms, triggers and medications used during each attack in a diary
- Increase the number of pulses delivered during an attack using the following systematic method as needed to improve pain and symptom relief.

To Begin:

- Encourage the patient to deliver 2 sequential pulses as early as possible at the beginning of the migraine attack.
- Continue with 2 pulses every 15 min for 1–2 h or until pain and symptoms resolve.
- Encourage patients to withhold using rescue medication for the first hour or two if possible.

Evaluate after the first month (3–4 attacks) - if needed increase the number of pulses delivered

- Encourage the patient to deliver 3 sequential pulses as early as possible at the beginning of the migraine attack.
- Continue with 3 pulses every 15 min for 1–2 h or until pain and symptoms resolve.

Evaluate again after the second month (3–4 attacks) - if needed increase the number of pulses delivered

- Encourage the patient to deliver 4 sequential pulses as early as possible at the beginning of the migraine attack.
- Continue with 4 pulses every 15 min for 1–2 h or until pain and symptoms resolve.

Patients were advised to treat as the guideline (Table 1) and to initiate early treatment where possible. They were advised to place the device over the back of the head (Fig. 1).

Patients commenced treatment by delivering two consecutive pulses (a double pulse), which they repeated after a minimum interval of 15 minutes on treatment days. A total number of 16 single pulses, or eight double pulses, per treatment day could be used with the option to use more if required during months two and three of the treatment period.

They could treat on as many acute migraine days as they wished.

Over time, some doctors advised patients with a frequent migraine pattern to start with daily sTMS treatment and review the effect of varying treatment patterns to reach an optimum individual level.

### Treatment in pregnancy

Three patients were prescribed sTMS during the second trimester of their pregnancy. They each suffered disabling

migraine attacks during the first trimester and the attacks continued into the second trimester. They had been treating with medications (paracetamol [acetaminophen] and codeine) without benefit. They each treated as per the guideline (Table 1).

### Analysis

Data were compiled from the patient survey responses into a spreadsheet (Excel 2010) in which summary measures were prepared. Our primary outcome measure was the migraine day. A migraine day was defined as, any day on which there was head pain of moderate or severe intensity, pain scale four or more out of a zero to ten scale, lasting at least 4 hours, and fulfilling current criteria [23]. Secondary measures included a migraine attack, defined as a succession of migraine days terminated by a non-migraine day, and a headache day, which was a day with any headache of any severity for more than an hour. Migraine days at 12 weeks was tested for normality (Kolmogorov-Smirnov Z test). To explore features that may be associated with a useful outcome for migraine prevention a generalized linear model was used with migraine days at 12 weeks as the dependent variable, co-factors: sex, episodic or chronic migraine, aura presence or absence, and covariates of age and baseline migraine days. The link function was identity. Migraine days at 12 weeks was compared to baseline using a Wilcoxon signed-rank test. A 5 % level of significance was used to assess outcomes (IBM SPSS Statistics 21).

### Results

#### Patient characteristics

A total of 449 patients were prescribed sTMS of which 331 completed initial training and first survey at 6 weeks. One hundred and ninety (42 %) used the device to treat

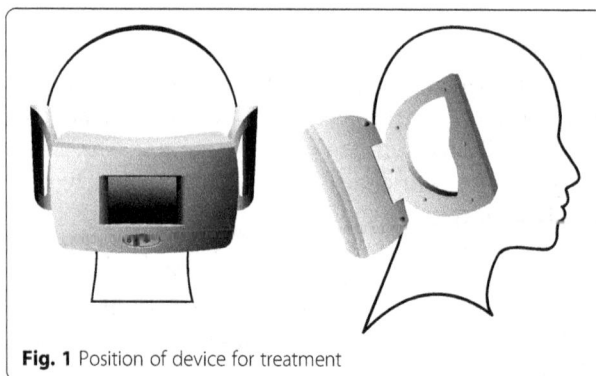

**Fig. 1** Position of device for treatment

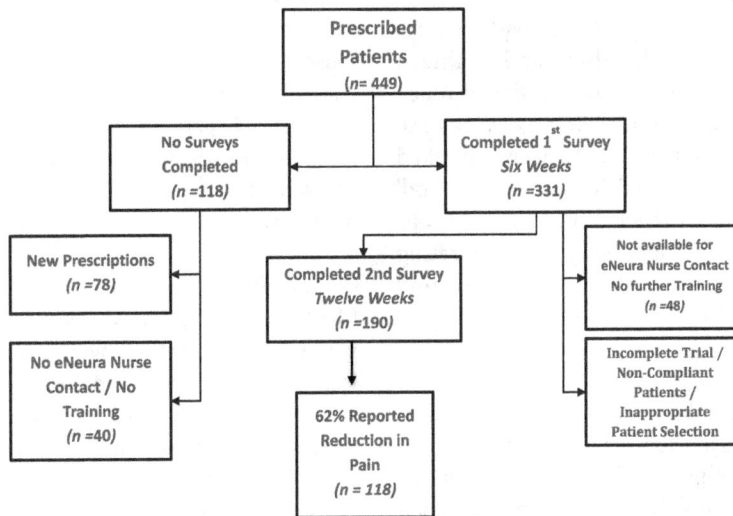

**Fig. 2** Patient disposition. *New patient- survey provided and no data at the time of the evaluation. **Data set for primary analysis

migraine attacks for 3 months and completed all surveys (Fig. 2). By the treating physician's choice, 40 were not available to us for any training or follow-up and without data these are not further reported. These patients returned their devices. Seventy-eight patients are newly prescribed and have not yet completed surveys. An additional 48 patients treated for 3 months but did not complete all surveys. At the time of writing one hundred and ninety (42 %, 140 females), aged $49 \pm 13$ (mean $\pm$ SD) completed questionnaires at the initial contact, 6- and 12-week time points. The report here focuses on the one hundred and ninety patients who treated for 3 months for efficacy and reports adverse events for all patients who have made any such reports (Table 2).

#### Frequency of migraine days
Patients treated an average of 13 attacks each month, with a baseline frequency of migraine days of 15 (median, 10–20 IQ range). This frequency was 11 [6, 16] at 6 weeks and 8 [3, 13] at 12 weeks. The frequency at 12 weeks was normally distributed ($Z = 1.13$, $P = 0.16$) and reduced compared to the baseline ($Z = 5.1$, $P < 0.001$). The baseline frequencies are set out in Table 3.

The migraine day outcome could be predicted by a model including presence or absence of aura and baseline frequency ($\chi_5^2 = 93.8$, $P < 0.001$). The 12 week frequency was lower in patients with aura ($\chi^2 = 8.1$, $P = 0.004$). Sex, age, or episodic versus chronic diagnosis did not predict the outcome at 12 weeks.

**Table 3** Migraines per month, pain severity and duration of attack by number of patients in each grouping over the reporting period

| Migraine days/month | Baseline | 6 weeks | 12 weeks |
|---|---|---|---|
| <5 | 8 | 11 | 27 |
| 5–9 | 19 | 35 | 33 |
| 10–14 | 35 | 42 | 45 |
| 15–20 | 56 | 36 | 32 |
| 21–25 | 14 | 12 | 9 |
| 26–30 | 58 | 52 | 44 |
| Pain severity[a] | Baseline | 6 weeks | 12 weeks |
| 0 | 0 | 3 | 2 |
| 1–3 | 0 | 44 | 63 |
| 4–6 | 32 | 85 | 75 |
| 7–9 | 140 | 54 | 47 |
| 10 | 18 | 4 | 3 |
| Duration in days | Baseline | 6 weeks | 12 weeks |
| <1 | 34 | 66 | 84 |
| 1 | 55 | 55 | 48 |
| 2 | 34 | 30 | 27 |
| 3 | 41 | 24 | 20 |
| 4 | 19 | 7 | 3 |
| >4 | 2 | 2 | 3 |

[a]Pain severity – 0 to 10 scale

**Table 2** Patient characteristics

| Migraine features | # of patients | # of attacks treated |
|---|---|---|
| Migraine with aura | 83 | 3802 |
| Migraine without aura | 107 | 5913 |
| Of these: | | |
| Episodic | 59 | 3470 |
| Chronic | 131 | 6245 |

## Pain

Data on one hundred and ninety patients with reports on pain were available. One hundred and eighteen (62 %) patients reported the device was effective at reducing or alleviating their migraine pain after 12-weeks use in over 9000 attacks. At each survey, patients were asked to rate their responses. They rated 'Good', 'Very Good' and'Excellent' as effective pain relief and a treatment option they would want to continue using. Patients rating the treatment 'No Effect' or 'Fair' ($n = 42$), did not find benefit or adequate benefit to continue the treatment.

## Associated symptoms

Of 190 patients reporting at 12 weeks, 174 provided data on at least one associated symptoms- nausea, photophobia or phonophobia. Sixteen reported they did not typically have any associated symptoms. Of the 174 who had such symptoms, 121 (64 %) reported an improvement, defined in their own terms by asking, was there improvement.

## Reduced attack duration

A reduction in the number of headache days per attack was reported in 102 of 185 patients reporting duration data at 12 weeks. The average reduction was a mean decrease from 2.2 days to 0.7 days per attack. Five of the 190 patients did not report duration data at 12 weeks.

A reduction in the number of headache days per attack was reported in 112 (59 %) of 190 patients reporting duration data at 12 weeks (Fig. 3). Forty-eight patients (25 %) reported no change in duration at 12 weeks.

## Dosing schedules

On average patients reported optimal dosing for their symptoms in the range from 10 to 12 pulses per treatment day. The majority of patients, 101 (53 %), treated

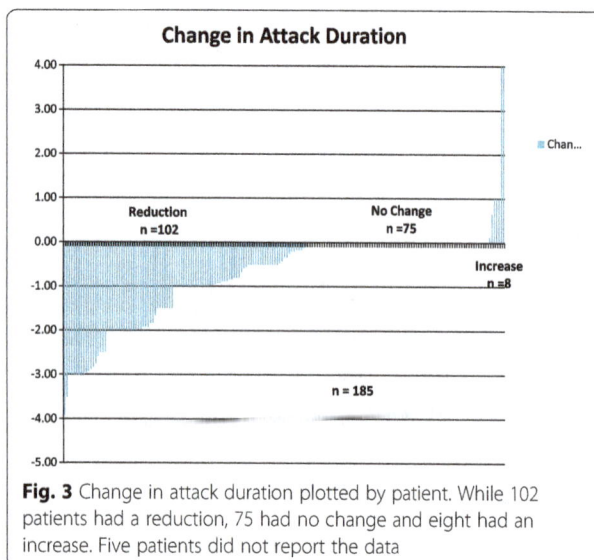

**Fig. 3** Change in attack duration plotted by patient. While 102 patients had a reduction, 75 had no change and eight had an increase. Five patients did not report the data

with two sequential pulses separated by 15-minute intervals, per treatment day. Eight patients preferred a single pulse repeated at 15 min intervals as they derived adequate benefit with this. During the second and third months, 53 patients treated with 3 sequential pulses separated by 15-minute intervals and 28 used 4 sequential pulses separated by 15-minute intervals per treatment day.

## Overall effect

Most patients (120 of 190) reported treating earlier worked better. Patients were not specifically asked but at least one half reported that when their attack was aborted, they felt clearer and did not have lingering 'mugginess' and tiredness. Some described that feeling the next day as 'crystal clear', which they would not typically experience at the end of an acute attack or when using medications.

## Disability: HIT-6 scoring

One hundred and thirty-nine patients provided pre-treatment scores (66, 62–70; median and interquartile range) and post- (61, 56–66) TMS HIT-6 scores. Of those patients, 19 (14 %) reported no change, 20 (14 %) reported a higher score post-TMS and 100 (72 %) reported a lower score post-TMS. Nineteen (14 %) reported scores below 50 points.

## Medication use

One hundred and sixty four of one hundred and ninety patients reported using acute medications for attacks at baseline. Of these, 119 patients reported a reduction in acute medication use, averaging ($8.5 \pm 7.7$) days reduction in medication use.

## Durability of response

Over the course of the 3 month treatment period, patients who found benefit at 6 weeks, maintained or saw greater improvement by week twelve. At 6 weeks 55 % ($n = 106$) of patients had had benefit and this rose to 62 % ($n = 118$) at 12 weeks.

## Tolerability

sTMS was well tolerated. No serious adverse events were reported. Thirty- eight of 190 (20 %) patients reported transient light-headedness for up to 20 min after pulse delivery. Nineteen reported side effects of either tinnitus, dizziness or tingling over the back of the head at the site of pulse delivery up to 30 min following stimulation. Thirteen reported worsening of migraine symptoms. One patient reported neck and upper shoulder pain that lasted 2 weeks although it is not clear whether this was related to sTMS treatment. The discontinuation rate was 55 % ($n = 105$): no benefit or inadequate benefit ($n = 49$), cost and lack of National Health Service coverage ($n = 17$), inconvenient ($n = 15$), migraine improved or resolved ($n = 12$), inadequate or incomplete trial (did not change dose when suggested; $n = 7$), side effects ($n = 2$) and none stated ($n = 3$).

### Pregnancy

All three patients treated their attacks throughout the pregnancy on a regular basis and reported benefit (Table 4). A reduction in pain severity, shorter attack duration and a reduction in severity of associated symptoms were reported. All three patients subsequently gave birth without complication to healthy children, and continued to treat in the post-partum period. No adverse effects were reported.

### Discussion

The data presented from an open-label experience with single pulse transcranial magnetic stimulation (sTMS) in a specialist headache clinic setting are broadly consistent with the randomised sham-control data that is available [20]. sTMS seems effective and is well tolerated. The open label data extends the treatment experience to patients with migraine without aura and chronic migraine, doing so based on preclinical data [15, 19], and interestingly the results seem broadly comparable. The data suggest there is a cumulative effect, in that patients do better the longer they are treated, that attacks are shortened, typically by about 1 day and that acute medication use is reduced. From a functional viewpoint, disability scores as recorded with HIT-6 are reduced. Importantly there were no serious or unanticipated adverse events, in keeping with the generally excellent tolerability of the

sTMS [21]. Taken together the data support the use of sTMS in migraine.

During the majority of this pilot programme, patients selected were typically those who could not use established acute migraine medications due to intolerable side effects, lack of efficacy or inadequate efficacy or they had medical contraindications to the medicines. Therefore, it was not an aim to look at the impact of sTMS on their medication use and reliance on acute treatments. However, as the programme evolved, patients were prescribed sTMS who also used acute medications regularly. This enabled an additional outcome where many patients reported a reduction in use of acute medicines. This may reflect a combination of factors such as shorter attack duration, reduced number of migraine days and effective pain relief from sTMS. This is a potential significant advantage for sTMS and requires further exploration.

Over time, it also became important to measure the impact of the benefit to patients [25]. An important goal of any treatment is to improve the quality of life for the sufferer. The impact of sTMS on alleviating migraine symptoms also had a significant impact on levels of disability. Reduced attack duration resulted in fewer headache days, less suffering and reduced migraine disability as reflected in HIT-6 scores [26]; HIT-6 is known to be sensitive to change [27]. Adherence to use is another surrogate for effect, since patients tend in general to abandon ineffective therapies. Patients responding to sTMS maintained use, which likely reflects its utility.

There are few safe medication treatments for patients during pregnancy and sTMS may be an option to consider for this patient group [21]. The three patients who

**Table 4** Patients treating during pregnancy

| Patient 1 | Patient 2 | Patient 3 |
|---|---|---|
| Age: 29. Episodic Migraine with Aura. | Age: 30. Chronic Migraine without aura. | Age: 32. Chronic Migraine without aura. |
| Pre-pregnancy migraine pattern: | Pre-pregnancy migraine pattern: | Pre-pregnancy migraine pattern: |
| Frequency: 12 days/month. Duration: 0.5–1 day. | Frequency: 10 days/month plus daily background pain. | Frequency: 15 days/month. Duration: 1–2 days. |
| Treatment: Triptan and sleep. | No effective treatment. | Treatment: frovatriptan, Syndol (paracetamol [acetaminopheno] + codeine + doxylamine + caffeine) and Naproxen, goes to bed. |
| During pregnancy: | During pregnancy: | During pregnancy: |
| Frequency: 2–4 days per week, Duration of 2–3 days, severe and in bed. Estimated 90 % reduced ability to function. | 16 days: acute attacks plus daily background pain. Duration: 1 day. Estimated 50 % reduced ability to function. | Treatment: Dihydocodeine during the early pregnancy with partial benefit. Estimated 60 % reduced ability to function. |
| TMS response: 2 consecutive pulses repeated after 15 min. Consistent reduced pain severity and duration. Could return to function and did not need to go to bed. | TMS response: 4 pulses per day (2 consecutive pulses repeated after 15 min). Stopped attack escalation and reduced the severity back down to a mild tolerable level within 1–2 h. Associated symptoms resolved or did not develop. | TMS response: a single pulse repeated after 15–30 min; up to 4 pulses per attack. Initially combined with dihydrocodeine. Subsequently used sTMS only and could abort the attack within an hour. Associated symptoms rarely developed. |

treated during pregnancy demonstrated safety and efficacy and derived adequate benefit, and may prove to be an additional treatment option for this patient group. We could not generalise these numbers to a blanket recommendation; suffice to say medical treatment of pregnant, disabled migraine sufferers is very challenging [28] and any new, apparently safe approach needs very serious consideration. In this vein it probably worth considering the TMS load that is offered in the treatment of depression with repetitive TMS (rTMS). A recent meta-analysis lists a range of stimuli from 1 to 2 Hz for 2–5 s with anywhere from 30 to 2,500 pulses per session for between 4 and 20 sessions [29], which is compared in sTMS to at most eight pulses in a day. Taken together with the estimated field strength at the apex of the fundus at term, which is about the same as three exposures to a microwave oven, and is shorter [21], sTMS is worth clinicians' consideration.

## Limitations

The study is an open-label patient experience without randomisation or allocation by protocol based on the licensed safety of the device and the data that exist. We sought to evaluate the device in practice. There will be a component of the placebo effect which for acute treatment would be between 10 and 25 %, depending on whether there was moderate/severe or mild pain at baseline. For a preventive treatment the placebo effect is assumed to be more substantial, although recent data suggests that may not be the case. The fact that the effect built up may be either a regression to the mean or a true evolution of the treatment effect. The botulinum toxin experience suggests that placebo can be seen over many weeks. Data are certainly missing, as one would expect from clinical practice, and this may have inflated the outcomes. It was a major issue that a substantial group could not be evaluated for logistic reasons of participation, although since this was limited to one site, the impact seems mitigated. Despite all the limitations, the outcomes are generally positive and the therapy very well tolerated.

## Conclusions

The sTMS device has demonstrated safety, efficacy and very good tolerability as an acute migraine treatment in open clinic settings. Our recent analysis suggests there may be a cost advantage to sTMS in the preventive setting [30], and such factors need to be considered as healthcare decisions are made going forward. It thus provided an effective treatment option for patients who could not treat, or treat adequately, with existing treatments. Further clinical use is warranted and careful follow-up will help determine its place in modern therapy.

## Competing interests

RB (rbhola@eneura.com) was employed part-time by eNeura Inc.
EK (ekinsella@eneura.com) was employed part-time by eNeura Inc.
NG (Nicola.Giffin@nhs.net) has nothing to declare.
SL (suelipscombe1@ntlworld.com) has nothing to declare.
FA (Fayyaz.Ahmed@hey.nhs.uk) is on advisory Boards for Allergan, Electrocore and Eneura. He has been consulted for Pfizer, Allergan, Menarini and received honorarium paid to the British Association for the Study of Headache from Allergan for conducting training workshops.
MW (mark.weatherall@doctors.co.uk) has served on Advisory Boards for Allergan, Eisai Pharmaceuticals, and UCB, and has received honoraria for lecturing from A Menarini Pharma and Janssen Cilag.
PJG is on the Advisory Board of eNeura, and has had grant support for experimental research. He is on Advisory Boards for Allergan, Colucid, MAP pharmaceuticals, Merck, Sharpe and Dohme, Autonomic Technologies Inc, Boston Scientific, Electrocore, Eli-Lilly, Medtronic, Linde gases, Arteaus, AlderBio and BristolMyerSquibb. He has consulted for Pfizer, Nevrocorp, Lundbeck, Zogenix, Impax, Zosano and DrReddy, and has been compensated for expert legal testimony. He has grant support from Allergan, Amgen, MAP, and MSD. He has received honoraria for editorial work from Journal Watch Neurology and for developing educational materials and teaching for the American Headache Society.

## Authors' contribution

RB & EK interviewed patients, compiled the data and prepared the first draft of the manuscript. NG contributed clinical data and revised the manuscript. SL contributed clinical data and revised the manuscript. FA contributed clinical data and revised the manuscript. MW contributed clinical data and revised the manuscript. PJG contributed clinical data, carried out all analyses and revised the manuscript. All authors read and approved the final manuscript.

## Acknowledgments

Drs B Davies, P Dorman, G Elrington, D Kernick, K Shields, S Silver, D Watson also prescribed to patients in the UK pilot programme.
Data was analysed by eNeura Inc and PJG.
The UK pilot programme was sponsored by eNeura Inc.

## Author details

[1]eNeura Therapeutics, Sunnyvale, CA, USA. [2]Department of Neurology, Royal United Hospital, Bath, UK. [3]Brighton and Sussex University Hospitals, Royal Sussex County, Brighton, UK. [4]Department of Neurology, Hull Royal Infirmary, Hull, UK. [5]Princess Margaret Migraine Clinic, Charing Cross Hospital, London, UK. [6]Headache Group, Basic & Clinical Neuroscience, King's College London, London, UK. [7]NIHR-Wellcome Trust Clinical Research Facility, King's College Hospital, London SE5 9PJ, UK.

## References

1. Goadsby PJ, Lipton RB, Ferrari MD (2002) Treatment of migraine. N Engl J Med 347:765–6
2. Murray CJ, Vos T, Lozano R, Naghavi M, Flaxman AD, Michaud C et al (2012) Disability-adjusted life years (DALYs) for 291 diseases and injuries in 21 regions, 1990–2010: a systematic analysis for the Global Burden of Disease Study 2010. Lancet 380:2197–223
3. Goadsby PJ, Sprenger T (2010) Current practice and future directions in the management of migraine: acute and preventive. Lancet Neurol 9:285–98
4. Akerman S, Holland P, Goadsby PJ (2011) Diencephalic and brainstem mechanisms in migraine. Nat Rev Neurosci 12:570–84
5. Goadsby PJ (2013) Therapeutic prospects for migraine: can paradise be regained? Ann Neurol 74:423–34
6. Bigal ME, Liberman JN, Lipton RB (2006) Obesity and migraine: a population study. Neurology 66(4):545–50, PubMed
7. Dodick D, Lipton RB, Martin V, Papademetriou V, Rosamond W, MaassenVanDenBrink A et al (2004) Consensus statement: cardiovascular safety profile of triptans (5-HT$_{1B/1D}$ Agonists) in the acute treatment of migraine. Headache 44:414–25
8. Barker AT, Jalinous R, Freeston IL (1985) Non-invasive magnetic stimulation of human motor cortex. Lancet 1(8437):1106–7, PubMed

Single-pulse transcranial magnetic stimulation (sTMS) for the acute treatment of migraine: evaluation...

175

9. Merton PA, Hill DK, Morton HB, Marsden CD (1982) Scope of a technique for electrical stimulation of human brain, spinal cord, and muscle. Lancet 2(8298):597–600, PubMed

10. Marsden CD, Merton PA, Morton HB (1976) Stretch reflex and servo action in a variety of human muscles. J Physiol 259(2):531–60, PubMed PMCID: 1309044

11. Marsden CD, Merton PA, Morton HB (1976) Servo action in the human thumb. J Physiol 257(1):1–44, PubMed PMCID: 1309342

12. Chen R, Cros D, Curra A, Di Lazzaro V, Lefaucheur JP, Magistris MR et al (2008) The clinical diagnostic utility of transcranial magnetic stimulation: report of an IFCN committee. Clin Neurophysiol 119(3):504–32, PubMed

13. Kobayashi M, Pascual-Leone A (2003) Transcranial magnetic stimulation in neurology. Lancet Neurol 2(3):145–56, PubMed

14. Mohammad YM, Kothari R, Hughes G, Krumah MN, Fischell S, Fischell R et al (2006) Transcranial magnetic stimulation (TMS) relieves migraine headache. Eur J Neurol 13(Suppl 2):23

15. Holland PR, Schembri C, Fredrick J, Goadsby PJ (2009) Transcranial magnetic stimulation for the treatment of migraine aura? Cephalalgia 29(Suppl 1):22

16. Lauritzen M (1994) Pathophysiology of the migraine aura. The spreading depression theory. Brain 117:199–210

17. Andreou AP, Summ O, Schembri C, Fredrick JP, Goadsby PJ (2010) Transcranial magnetic stimulation inhibits cortical spreading depression but not trigeminocervical activation in animal models of migraine. Headache 50(Suppl 1):58

18. Andreou AP, Sprenger T, Goadsby PJ (2012) Cortical spreading depression-evoked discharges on trigeminothalamic neurons. Headache 52:900

19. Andreou AP, Sprenger T, Goadsby PJ (2013) Cortical modulation of thalamic function during cortical spreading depression- unraveling a new central mechanism involved in migraine aura. J Headache Pain 14(Suppl 1):I6

20. Lipton RB, Dodick DW, Silberstein SD, Saper JR, Aurora SK, Pearlman SH et al (2010) Single-pulse transcranial magnetic stimulation for acute treatment of migraine with aura: a randomised, double-blind, parallel-group, sham-controlled trial. Lancet Neurol 9:373–80

21. Dodick DW, Schembri CT, Helmuth M, Aurora SK (2010) Transcranial magnetic stimulation for migraine: a safety review. Headache 50:1153–63

22. Bhola R, Lipscombe S, Giffin N, Elrington G, Weatherall M, Ahmed F et al (2013) Update of the UK post market pilot programme with single pulse transcranial magnetic stimulation (sTMS) for acute treatment of migraine. Cephalalgia 33:973

23. Headache Classification Committee of the International Headache Society (2013) The International Classification of Headache Disorders, 3rd edition (beta version). Cephalalgia 33:629–808

24. Silberstein SD, Olesen J, Bousser MG, Diener HC, Dodick D, First M et al (2005) The International Classification of Headache Disorders, 2nd Edition (ICHD-II)–revision of criteria for 8.2 Medication-overuse headache. Cephalalgia 25:460–5

25. Stewart WF, Lipton RB, Whyte J, Dowson A, Kolodner K, Liberman JN et al (1999) An international study to assess reliability of the Migraine Disability Assessment (MIDAS) score. Neurology 53:988–94

26. Bjorner JB, Kosinski M, Ware JE Jr (2003) Calibration of an item pool for assessing the burden of headaches: an application of item response theory to the headache impact test (HIT). Qual Life Res 12:913–33

27. Coeytaux RR, Kaufmann JS, Chao R, Mann JD, DeVellis RF (2006) Four methods of estimating the minimal important difference score were compared to establish a cliniclaly significant change in Headache Impact Test. J Clin Epidemiol 59:374–80

28. Goadsby PJ, Goldberg J, Silberstein SD (2008) Migraine in pregnancy. Br Med J 336:1502–4

29. Ren J, Li H, Palaniyappan L, Liu H, Wang J, Li C et al (2014) Repetitive transcranial magnetic stimulation versus electroconvulsive therapy for major depression: a systematic review and meta-analysis. Prog Neuropsychopharmacol Biol Psychiatry 51:181–9. doi:10.1016/j.pnpbp.2014.02.004, Epub 2014 Feb 18

30. Ahmed F, Goadsby PJ, Bhola R, Reinhold T, Bruggenjurgen B. Treatment cost analysis of refractory chronic migraine patients in a UK NHS setting [Abstract]. Cephalalgia. 2015;35:in press.

# Validation of potential candidate biomarkers of drug-induced nephrotoxicity and allodynia in medication-overuse headache

Elisa Bellei[1*], Emanuela Monari[1], Stefania Bergamini[1], Aurora Cuoghi[1], Aldo Tomasi[1], Simona Guerzoni[2], Michela Ciccarese[2] and Luigi Alberto Pini[2]

## Abstract

**Background:** Medication-overuse headache (MOH) is a chronic disorder that results from the overuse of analgesics drugs, triptans or other acute headache compounds. Although the exact mechanisms underlying MOH remain still unknown, several studies suggest that it may be associated with development of "central sensitization", which may cause cutaneous allodynia (CA). Furthermore, the epidemiology of drug-induced disorders suggests that medication overuse could lead to nephrotoxicity. The aim of this work was to confirm and validate the results obtained from previous proteomics studies, in which we analyzed the urinary proteome of MOH patients in comparison with healthy non-abusers individuals.

**Methods:** MOH patients were divided into groups on the basis of the drug abused: triptans, non-steroidal anti-inflammatory drugs (NSAIDs) and mixtures, (mainly containing indomethacin, paracetamol and, in some cases, caffeine). Healthy subjects, with a history of normal renal function, were used as controls. In this study, four proteins that were found differentially expressed in urine, and, on the basis of the literature review, resulted related to kidney diseases, were verified by Western Blot and Enzyme-linked Immunosorbent Assay (ELISA); Prostaglandin-H2 D-synthase (PTGDS), uromodulin (UROM), alpha-1-microglobulin (AMBP) and cystatin-C (CYSC).

**Results:** Western blot analysis allowed to validate our previous proteomics data, confirming that all MOH patients groups show a significant over-excretion of urinary PTGDS, UROM, AMBP and CYSC (excluding triptans group for this latter), in comparison with controls. Moreover, the expression of PTGDS was further evaluated by ELISA. Also by this assay, a significant increase of PTGDS was observed in all MOH abusers, according to 2-DE and Western blot results.

**Conclusions:** In this study, we confirmed previous findings concerning urinary proteins alterations in MOH patients, identified and demonstrated the over-expression of PTGDS, UROM, AMBP, and CYSC, particularly in NSAIDs and mixtures abusers. Over-expression of these proteins have been related to renal dysfunction and probably, PTGDS, to the development of CA. The detection and confirmation of this proteins pattern represent a promising tool for a better understanding of potential nephrotoxicity induced by drugs overuse and may enhance awareness related to the MOH-associated risks, even in absence of clinical symptoms.

**Keywords:** Medication-Overuse Headache; Prostaglandin-H2 D-synthase; Cystatin-C; Alpha-1-microglobulin; Uromodulin; Urine; Western blot; Proteomics

* Correspondence: elisa.bellei@unimore.it
[1]Department of Diagnostic Medicine, Clinic and Public Health, Proteomic Lab, University of Modena and Reggio Emilia, Via del Pozzo 71, 41124 Modena, Italy
Full list of author information is available at the end of the article

## Background

A specific condition observed in chronic migraine patients, classified as medication-overuse headache (MOH) and characterized by the frequent intake of antimigraine drugs, is assumed to increase the frequency and intensity of headache [1]. MOH may complicate every type of headache and, in principle, all acute drugs used for headache treatment could cause MOH (i.e. ergotamine derivatives, triptans, simple and combined analgesics, barbiturates and opioids) [2]. Although the specific mechanisms leading to MOH remain still unknown, several studies suggest that MOH may involve amplification processes, including descending facilitation and "central sensitization", and an increased excitability of spinal and medullary dorsal horn neurons resulting from a continuous input exerted by C-fiber nociceptors [3, 4]. This may lead to cutaneous allodynia (CA), a neurologic condition characterized by touch-evoked pain, elicited through ordinary non-nociceptive stimulation of the skin [5]. As a marker of central sensitization, allodynia has been proposed as a risk factor for progression to chronic migraine [6]. Recently, the development of MOH has been associated with long-lasting adaptive changes that occur within the peripheral and central nervous system. Preclinical studies have shown that repeated or continuous treatment with antimigraine drugs result in persistent up-regulation of neurotransmitters within the orofacial division of the trigeminal ganglia and in the development of CA in response to migraine triggers, even weeks after discontinuation of the antimigraine drug [7]. In our previous study we found elevated urinary levels of Prostaglandin-H2 D-synthase (PTGDS) in 3 MOH patient groups (triptans, NSAIDs and mixture abusers) in respect to healthy non-abusers individuals as control group [8]. Prostaglandin D2 is the most abundant prostanoid produced in the central nervous system of mammals, and is implicated in the modulation of neural functions, such as sleep induction, regulation of body temperature, nociception, pain responses and allodynia [9]. Some studies with animal models have demonstrated that prostaglandins play pivotal roles in central sensitization at spinal level, resulting in induction of hyperalgesia and CA (touch-evoked pain) [10]. Furthermore, elevated levels of PTGDS have been found in the serum of patients with renal impairment, so that the protein has even been suggested as a possible biochemical marker of renal insufficiency [11]. Therefore, PTGDS might contribute not only to the induction of allodynia [12], but also to the progression of chronic renal failure [13]. Based on the important functions assigned to PTGDS, the purpose of this study was the urinary quantification and validation in MOH abusers previously analyzed, by Western blotting and Enzyme-linked Immunosorbent Assay (ELISA). Moreover, in our previous works [8, 14] we identified, besides PTGDS, other proteins as potential biomarkers of nephrotoxicity, including Uromodulin (UROM), Alpha-1-microglobulin (AMBP) and Cystatin-C (CYTC). In recent years, proteomic researches have revealed numerous proteins as candidate biomarkers, but the lack of protein validation has represented a weakness for their application into clinical practice. The main purpose of the present work was to confirm and validate, by molecular biology techniques, proteins identified in earlier studies of our research group.

## Methods

### Subjects

Urine samples were taken from MOH patients, divided in 3 subgroups: triptans, NSAIDs and mixtures abusers. Moreover, urine of healthy non-abusers volunteers were collected and used as control. All patients groups and controls were matched for age and gender, and each subject gave informed consent to the study. Urinary routine parameters were measured in the clinical laboratory and resulted in the normal range. The exclusion criteria were renal insufficiency or kidney damage, ischemic heart disease, autoimmune disorders, oncologic or neurologic syndrome. The study received approval of the Ethical Committee of the University Hospital of Modena and was carried out in conformity with the Helsinki Declaration.

### Urine sample preparation

The second urine in the morning were collected into a sterile tube and centrifuged at 800 x g for 10 min at 4 °C, in order to remove cellular debris and contaminants. Then, urine samples were concentrated and desalted using filter devices with a 3 kDa MW cut-off (Millipore). The final total protein concentration was calculated by the Bradford method [15], using BSA as standard and rehydration buffer as blank.

### SDS-PAGE and two-dimensional gel electrophoresis

Sodium dodecyl sulphate-polyacrylamide gel electrophoresis (SDS-PAGE) was performed according to Laemmli's procedure under reducing conditions, as previously reported [14]. In brief, 5 µg of total urine proteins for each group were mixed with the Laemmli sample buffer with the addition of β-mercaptoethanol as reducing agent. Samples were then boiled at 95 °C for 5 min and subsequently loaded onto 12 % SDS polyacrylamide gel. At the end of the electrophoresis run, gel were stained with Coomassie Blue G-250. Urine samples were also subjected to two-dimensional gel electrophoresis (2-DE) analysis, as previously described [8]. Briefly, 100 µg of total protein were subjected to first dimension separation (isoelectric focusing) using 17 cm IPG strip pH range 3-10 (Ready Strip™, Bio-Rad). Later, the second dimension separation was performed employing 8-16 % polyacrylamide gradient gel and the spot were visualized with silver nitrate staining protocol [16]. All gel images were acquired by a calibrated densitometer (GS800, Bio-Rad) and both the bands and the spot of interest were excised and stored at -20 °C until mass spectrometry (MS) analysis.

## Mass spectrometry protein identification

Protein bands and protein spot were "in-gel" digested as previously reported [17]. Briefly, they were first subjected to a step of de-staining (with acetonitrile for protein bands and with a solution of potassium hexacyano-ferrate(III)/sodium thiosulphate for protein spot, respectively). In the next step, both samples were reduced with dithiotreitol and alkylated with iodoacetamide, followed by trypsin digestion at 37 °C overnight. The obtained peptides were extracted by a two-phase procedure, first with acetonitrile/ammonium bicarbonate and then using formic acid. Finally, the pooled peptides were concentrated in a vacuum dryer before MS analysis by a Nano LC-CHIP-MS system, composed of the 6520 ESI-Q-ToF coupled with a Nano HPLC-Chip microfluidic device (Agilent Technologies Inc., CA, USA), as previously described in detail [17]. The MASCOT search engine (version 2.4) was used for peptide sequence searching against the UniProt database, setting the following restrictions: *Homo sapiens* taxonomy (Human), parent ion tolerance ±20 ppm, MS/MS error tolerance ±0.1 Da, alkylation of cysteine residues (fixed modifications), oxidation of methionine (variable modifications), and two potentially missed trypsin cleavages. The highest score hits among MASCOT search results were selected. Protein identification was repeated at least once, using band/spot cut from replicated gel.

## Western blotting analysis

A total of 1.5 μg urine proteins were separated on 12 % SDS-PAGE and blotted onto nitrocellulose membranes, that were first blocked with 5 % non-fat milk and subsequently incubated overnight at 4 °C with the following primary antibodies (all from Abcam, Cambridge, UK): anti-Prostaglandin D Synthase (rabbit polyclonal, 1:500); anti-Uromucoid (rabbit polyclonal, 1:500); anti-Alpha-1-microglobulin (rabbit monoclonal, 1:1000); anti-Cystatin C (rabbit monoclonal, 1:500). Membranes were then incubated with a solution containing 1:2000 dilution of horseradish peroxidase (HRP)-conjugated goat anti-rabbit secondary antibody (DakoCytomation, Denmark). Target bands were visualized using a mix of peroxidase solution plus a luminol enhancer solution (WesternSure™ PREMIUM Chemiluminescent substrate). Results acquisition and band densitometric analysis (represented by arbitrary units, AU), were performed using the C-DiGit® Blot Scanner (LI-COR Biosciences, NE, USA) and the QuantityOne image analysis software (Bio-Rad). Human serum sample was used as positive (or negative) control.

## Measurement of PTGDS by ELISA

Immunoreactive PTGDS was determined by ELISA using a commercially available kit (BioVendor, NC, USA), on the basis of the manufacturer's instructions. Briefly, urine samples were diluted 100-fold with dilution buffer and then incubated for 1 h at room temperature with polyclonal anti-human L-PTGDS antibody immobilized to the surface of the plate wells. After three wash, 100 mL of conjugate solution (anti-PTGDS conjugated with horseradish peroxidase, HRP) were added and the plate incubated for 1 h at room temperature. Following 3 washing steps, the remaining HRP conjugate was allowed to react with the substrate solution (tetramethylbenzidine). Finally, the reaction was stopped by the addition of acidic solution and absorbance of the resulting yellow product was measured at λ 450 and 620 nm, using a microplate reader (Multiscan FC, Thermo Scientific, MA, USA). PTGDS concentrations were determined from a standard curve generated by the standards supplied with the kit.

## Data analysis

A statistical analysis of ELISA results (for urinary PTGDS), and of Western blot signal values (obtained from all proteins tested in each different group), was done with the Student $t$-test. A p-value $<0.05$ was considered as statistically significant. All data reported in Figs. 3 and 4 are provided as mean ± standard deviation (SD).

## Results

### SDS-PAGE, 2-DE and image analysis

Urine proteins were first separated according to their molecular weight by SDS-PAGE (Fig. 1) and gel images were acquired by a calibrated densitometer (GS800, Bio-Rad). The bands enclosed in rectangles were cut from each lane (corresponding to every group of patients and controls) and were subjected to MS analysis. As evident in Fig. 1, the result was the identification of the following proteins: UROM, expressed as a very intense band in all MOH patients (lane 2 = triptans, lane 3 = NSAIDs and lane 4 = mixtures abusers) respect to controls (lane 1); AMBP, particularly evident in NSAIDs group; PTGDS, an intensive band visible in NSAIDs and mixtures groups, which was much less observable in triptans abusers and even more in controls, and CYTC, with a perceptible band in NSAIDs group. To strengthen these results, we analyzed the same samples by 2-DE. Isolated and magnified differentially expressed spots obtained from 2D gels are reported in Fig. 2. The results overlapped those obtained by SDS-PAGE. In fact, analyzing the spot staining intensity by the PDQuest image analysis software (version 7.3.1, Bio-Rad), PTGDS was significantly over-excreted in NSAIDs (A3), mixtures (A4) and triptans groups (A2) in comparison to controls (A1);

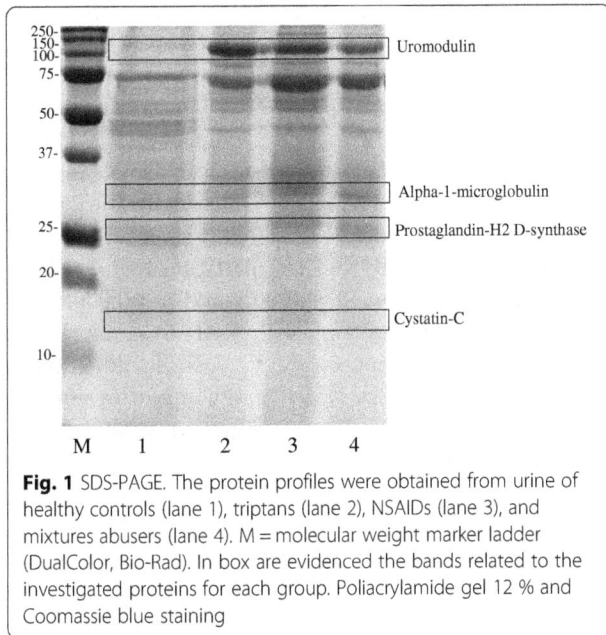

**Fig. 1** SDS-PAGE. The protein profiles were obtained from urine of healthy controls (lane 1), triptans (lane 2), NSAIDs (lane 3), and mixtures abusers (lane 4). M = molecular weight marker ladder (DualColor, Bio-Rad). In box are evidenced the bands related to the investigated proteins for each group. Poliacrylamide gel 12 % and Coomassie blue staining

## MS protein identification

MS analysis was performed using an Electrospray-Quadrupole-Time of Flight (ESI-Q-ToF) mass spectrometer (Agilent Technologies, CA, USA). Protein identification was achieved using the Agilent MassHunter Workstation software (version B.02.00) and the search was conducted by MASCOT search engine (version 2.4) against the UniProt database. During MASCOT search, the significant threshold was set up to maintain the False discovery Rate (FDR) below 1 %. The identification was done in duplicate, cutting bands and spot from replicate gels. The results obtained for each identified protein are listed in Table 1. Column 1 lists the protein entry names according to the UniProt knowledge database, while the others columns show the MS analysis data, such as the ion scores (column 2), expressed as the probability that the observed match between the experimental data and the database sequence could be due to a random event; queries (column 3), that is the total number of peptides that matched the identified proteins and the significant matches; the total number of sequences and the number of significant sequences (column 4) and the sequence coverage, namely the percentage of amino acids sequenced (final column).

UROM resulted over-expressed in triptans (B2), NSAIDs (B3) and mixtures abusers (B4), compared to controls (B1); AMBP spots were significantly increased only in NSAIDs (C3) and mixtures abusers (C4) respect to triptans (C2) and controls (C1); finally, CYTC resulted particularly elevated in NSAIDs abusers (D3). Furthermore, we illustrated the 3D views of PTGDS protein spot, developed with the PDQuest software, in order to provide a clearer vision of its expression change in the examined groups.

## Western blotting

In order to validate the results of electrophoresis (SDS-PAGE e 2-DE) and precisely verify the identity of proteins inferred from ESI-Q-ToF-MS analysis, we evaluated the levels of PTGDS, UROM, AMBP and CYTC by Western blot. The analysis was conducted with ten urine samples for each group. As shown in Fig. 3a, PTGDS protein

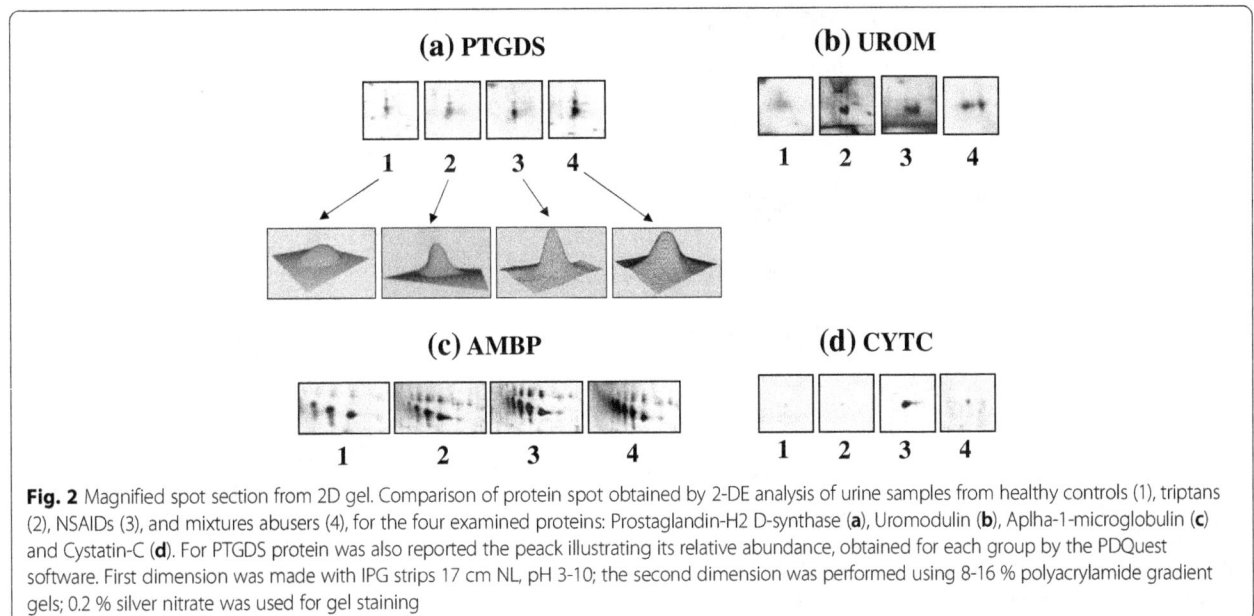

**Fig. 2** Magnified spot section from 2D gel. Comparison of protein spot obtained by 2-DE analysis of urine samples from healthy controls (1), triptans (2), NSAIDs (3), and mixtures abusers (4), for the four examined proteins: Prostaglandin-H2 D-synthase (**a**), Uromodulin (**b**), Aplha-1-microglobulin (**c**) and Cystatin-C (**d**). For PTGDS protein was also reported the peack illustrating its relative abundance, obtained for each group by the PDQuest software. First dimension was made with IPG strips 17 cm NL, pH 3-10; the second dimension was performed using 8-16 % polyacrylamide gradient gels; 0.2 % silver nitrate was used for gel staining

**Table 1** MS protein identification by ESI-Q-ToF-MS

| Protein name[a] | Score[b] | N° matches/sign.matches[c] | N° seq./sign.seq.[d] | Seq. cov.[e] |
|---|---|---|---|---|
| PTGDS | 158 | 25/14 | 3/2 | 33 % |
| UROM | 86 | 18/13 | 3/2 | 47 % |
| AMBP | 201 | 21/12 | 4/3 | 32 % |
| CYTC | 71 | 16/10 | 3/3 | 52 % |

[a]Protein entry name (UniProt knowledge database)
[b]The highest scores obtained using MASCOT search engine
[c]The total number of peptides matched and the significant matches
[d]The total number of sequences and the number of significant sequences
[e]Sequence coverage: the percentage of amino acids sequenced for the detected protein

was detected in all urine samples from every group, and precisely was found to have higher levels in mixtures ($p = 0.001$) and NSAIDs groups ($p = 0.01$), respect to triptans abusers ($p = 0.04$), when compared $vs$ healthy controls, similarly to the results of 2-DE analysis. UROM (Fig. 3b) showed a marked signal at 70 kDa and a significant increase in all MOH patients compared to control group. During Western Blot analysis, we used human serum sample as control; regarding UROM,

since it is exclusively produced in the kidney and secreted into the urine via proteolytic cleavage, no band was observed at UROM molecular weight. Therefore, serum sample can be considered as negative control, while it represents a positive control for PTGDS, AMBP and CYSC, that showed a clear signal; these 3 proteins, present in serum, are filtered by the kidney and excreted in urine. AMBP signal (Fig. 3c) was highly significant in all MOH abusers, particularly in NSAIDs and mixtures groups ($p = 0.0001$ and $p = 0.0005$, respectively) and also in triptans ($p = 0.006$) compared to controls. Finally, the increase of CYTC (Fig. 3d) showed its maximum signal in NSAIDs and mixtures abusers ($p = 0.001$ and $p = 0.04$ $vs$ control group), while triptans group showed no significativity.

### ELISA results

The expression level of PTGDS was estimated by ELISA assay (Fig. 4). When compared to control subjects, a significant increase in PTGDS immunoreactivity was observed in all MOH patients groups. Particularly, PTGDS level was highly significant in mixtures ($681 \pm 218$ ng/mL, $p < 1.00E-06$) and NSAIDs

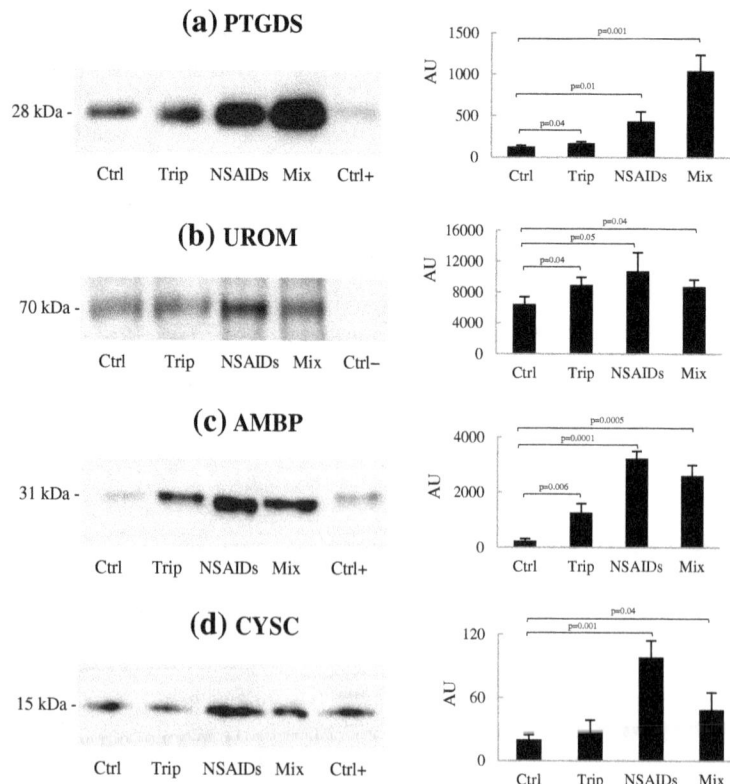

**Fig. 3** Protein expression by Western blot. The analysis for each protein was conducted on urine samples from the four groups. Serum sample was used as positive (or negative) control. The histograms show the quantitative representation of PTGDS (**a**), UROM (**b**), AMBP (**c**) and CYSC (**d**) obtained by densitometric analysis with QuantityOne image analysis software (the data represent mean ± SD). Ctrl, healthy control group; Trip, triptans abusers; NSAIDs abusers; Mix, mixtures abusers

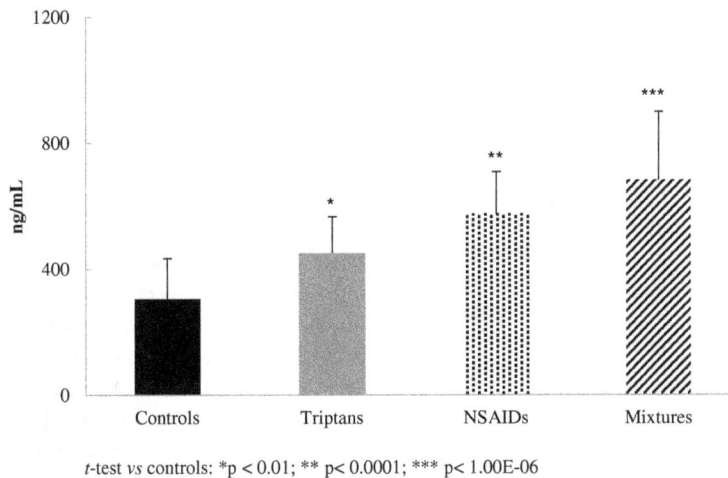

t-test vs controls: *p < 0.01; ** p< 0.0001; *** p< 1.00E-06

**Fig. 4** Immunoreactivity of PTGDS by ELISA assay. Results are expressed as mean ± SD. Significant differences were assessed by unpaired Student't t-test (*p < 0.01; **p < 0.0001; ***p < 1.00E-06 vs control group)

abusers ($572 \pm 135$ ng/mL, $p < 0.0001$) in respect to triptans abusers ($450 \pm 116$ ng/mL, $p < 0.01$), when compared to control group ($303 \pm 130$ ng/mL). These results are fully consistent with the data from 2-DE (Fig. 2-a) and Western blot analysis (Fig. 3a). The measured values of urinary PTGDS fell on the linear portion of the ELISA kit standard curve.

## Discussion

In the present study we carried out additional analysis, such as Western blot and ELISA assays, to validate our previous findings aimed to discover early biomarkers of drug-induced nephrotoxicity in MOH [8, 14], and to enhance its accuracy of prediction. Among the differentially expressed proteins previously identified, our study focused on UROM, AMBP and CYSC, since an ample literature provides evidence of their involvement in renal damage and nephropathy. The special role played by PTGDS, which is implicated in pain onset (particularly CA), was also investigated [13]. CA is defined as pain in response to non-nociceptive thermal and mechanical stimuli applied to normal skin, a very uncomfortable heightened sensitivity to touch [18, 19]. Some studies indicated that up to 80 % of migraine patients reported CA during an acute attack [6] or abnormal sensitivity of extracranial areas [20]; others showed that most migraine patients exhibit CA inside and outside their pain-referred areas when examined during a fully developed migraine attack [21]. CA in migraine is a clinical manifestation of central nervous system sensitization, and consequently several chronic pain syndromes and mood disorders are comorbid with migraine [22]. Given the complexity of pain and its arduous and not particularly effective treatment, there is an important need to define

who is susceptible to pain hypersensitivity, as well as to discover new molecules and mechanisms finalized to the identification of new therapeutic interventions with greater efficacy. Studies has been recently carried out to prove epigenetics role in the causation of chronic pain [23], trying to clarify a pain-specific protein interaction network [24, 25]. In the present study we focused on PTGDS, also known as β-trace protein, a lipocalin-type prostaglandin that is responsible for the conversion of prostaglandin $H_2$ ($PGH_2$) into prostaglandin $D_2$ ($PGD_2$), in the presence of sulfhydryl compounds [26]. PTGDS is actively produced in a variety of tissues and is involved in numerous physiological and pathological functions, such as vasodilatation, inhibition of platelet aggregation and nitric oxide release; moreover, it is a potent endogenous nociceptive modulator [9]. Western blot analysis (Fig. 3a) and ELISA test (Fig. 4) lead to the verification and validation of the proteomic data (Figs. 1 and 2-a), confirming that the MOH patients examined in this work show an over-expression of urinary PTGDS, especially NSAIDs and mixtures abusers, when compared with triptans group and more vs healthy controls. On the basis of these results, a clear indication arises directing to the involvement of PTGDS in the manifestation of CA, by decreasing pain threshold, as verified in MOH abusers and in migraineurs patients recruited in a previous study [27]. With the abuse of antimigraine drugs, migraineurs patients may develop MOH, a frequent and disabling condition characterized by increased headache frequency and intensity, inefficacy of medications and development of drug dependence [7]. Pain progression has been evaluated in MOH patients, suggesting the presence of a global alteration in the processing of noxious stimuli throughout the pain matrix and the occurrence of significant functional changes in the lateral pain pathway [28]. Only by understanding the molecular circuits complexity and the substances mediating pain, the development of increasingly specific tools for the identification of new markers, will be possible. In our study, MOH patients, showing high levels of PTGDS, suffer pain growth and progression, suggesting that PTGDS is indeed a potential urinary biomarker indicating CA development. Different types of prostaglandins play a key role in important physiological conditions, such as renal function and development. PTGDS is involved in the advancement of kidney diseases, and has been proposed in the past years as a potential diagnostic marker for renal injury [29]. Recently, animal studies have shown that the urinary excretion of PTGDS may predict the development of proteinuria and renal injury [30]. In our study, an elevated PTGDS level was determined in the urine of MOH patients (particularly in NSAIDs and mixture abusers) (Figs. 2-a, 3a and 4), suggesting the importance of monitoring MOH patients renal function that, at its turn, will enable the prevention of the drug-induced nephrotoxicity.

Other proteins involved in renal dysfunction, also tested in this study, were UROM, AMBP and CYSC. UROM (Tamm-Horsfall glycoprotein) is the most abundant protein excreted in the urine under physiological conditions, being exclusively synthesized by the cells of the thick ascending limb and early distal convoluted tubule of the kidney. UROM is produced in the endoplasmic reticulum, shuttled to the apical cell membrane, and released into the urine by proteolytic cleavage [31]. UROM has been known for more than 50 years and since its discovery several researches have been conducted, revealing novel roles for this protein [32]. Recently, genome-wide association studies identified UROM as a risk factor for chronic kidney disease (CKD) and hypertension, suggesting that the urinary level of UROM represents a useful biomarker for the development and progression of CDK [33, 34]. In our study, by Western blot analysis we confirmed a significant over-excretion of UROM (Fig. 3b) in all MOH patients compared to the control group; the same was also observed for AMBP (Fig. 3c). AMBP is a low molecular weight protein, also called protein HC, which is readily filtered by the glomerulus and reabsorbed and catabolised by the proximal tubular cells. Therefore, the presence of AMBP in urine is indicative of reduced resorptive capacity of the proximal tubule [35]; consequently, the urinary concentration of AMBP, which is stable at low pH, designate this protein as a useful marker of proximal tubular abnormalities and chronic asymptomatic renal tubular dysfunction [36]. Moreover, urinary AMBP can be considered as a useful marker for the early detection and monitoring of nephropathy in type 2 diabetes [37]. Finally, we found a significantly increased level of CYSC in NSAIDs and mixtures

abusers, but not in triptans abusers (Fig. 3d). Also CYSC has been used for many years as a clinical marker of kidney function [38]. This 15-kDa cysteine proteinase inhibitor is produced by all nucleated cells at a constant rate and constitutively secreted shortly after its synthesis. Following glomerular filtration, CYSC is reabsorbed by the proximal tubular cells, where it is almost completely catabolized, while the remaining uncatabolized protein is eliminated in the urine [39]. Thus, normal urinary CYSC concentration is very low, whereas in case of tubular diseases CYSC degradation is reduced, leading to an increase in its urinary elimination. Furthermore, a recent study reported that urinary CYSC levels and tubular proteinuria may predict the progression of type 2 diabetic nephropathy [40]. Accumulating evidence suggests CYSC as a reliable biomarker and predictor of impaired renal function, in particular of tubular damage [41]. In summary, we have now firmly established that PTGDS, UROM, AMBP and CYSC are proteins over-excreted in the urine of MOH patients, especially in NSAIDs and mixtures abusers, compared to healthy non-abusers individuals.

The debate on the association between nonphenacetin-containing combined analgesics and renal disease has been going on for a long time. Some years ago, an international ad hoc peer-reviewed committee of scientists concluded that there is no sufficient evidence to associate nonphenacetin combined analgesics with nephropathy [42]. A population-based case–control study with incident cases of end-stage renal disease (ESRD) demonstrated that the use of a high cumulative lifetime dose (3rd tertile) of analgesics up to five years before dialysis was not associated with ESRD [43]. Others case-controls studies have shown that caffeine-containing analgesics are associated with analgesic nephropathy (odds ratio = 4.9, 95 % CI 2.3 to 10.3) [44]. In the series observed in our studies, we did not register any case of clinical impairment of renal functions. The main NSAIDs used were indomethacin, paracetamol and, in some cases, compounds containing caffeine. However, if caffeine produces nephrotoxicity on its own, or increases analgesics-related nephrotoxicity is yet to be established [44]. In literature there is a lack of definite data regarding causative analgesics, including those concerning paracetamol. Hence, patients should not be withheld for paracetamol, an effective and commonly recommended agent, for fear of worsening renal function [45], but, at the same time, an increasing universal awareness about rational use of analgesics is important for MOH prevention.

## Conclusions

MOH has a prevalence of 1-2 % in the general population worldwide and it is likely to be the most costly neurological disorder known [46]. Even more significantly, MOH has similarities with traditional drug addiction.

Nonetheless, there is a lack of research into awareness, education and prevention of MOH [47, 48]. With the present work we firmly confirmed and strengthen our previous findings regarding the possibility of drug-induced nephrotoxicity in MOH patients, particularly in the case of NSAIDs and mixtures abuse. These results contribute to emphasize the importance in providing educational and preventive strategies concerning the risks linked to MOH, such as the probability of developing renal injuries. Therefore, the proteins under our scrutiny may represent a reliable and distinctive panel of prospective early target of kidney dysfunctions, useful to monitor over time renal function of MOH abusers, recognizing patients prone to progress toward nephropathy. Accordingly, these findings could enhance the awareness about the risks associated to MOH, helping to reduce morbidity. Moreover, the present results on PTGDS may be useful to provide a common target for advanced study, aimed to analyze pain mechanisms and pathways at the molecular level, particularly in the case of CA. The increase of urinary PTGDS observed also in patients taking triptans could be an early indicator of a nervous system driven up-regulation associated to chronic pain, as in the case of MOH. Even if there are no conclusive data showing a direct impact of NSAIDs on kidney functions in headache patients, these findings could represent an initial marker linked to a specific type of pain, such as CA.

## Abbreviations
AMBP: Alpha-1-microglobulin; CA: Cutaneous allodynia; CYTC: Cystatin-C; 2-DE: Two-dimensional gel electrophoresis; MS: Mass spectrometry; PTGDS: Prostaglandin-H2 D-synthase; UROM: Uromodulin.

## Competing interests
The authors declare that they have no competing interest.

## Authors' contributions
EB conceived the study, performed proteomics analysis and Western Blot, drafted the manuscript; EM carried out the immunoassays and participated in Western blot analysis; SB performed samples preparation for mass spectrometry analysis and participated in proteomic analysis; AC performed mass spectrometry analysis and participated in Western blot analysis; AT provided useful advices to improve performance of the work and revised the manuscript; SG participated in the design and coordination of the study, and was responsible of patients recruitment; MC participated in study design and helped during the selection of patients and controls; LAP supervised the work, participated in its design and coordination, helped to draft the manuscript. All authors read and approved the final version of the manuscript.

## Acknowledgments
We thank "Fondazione Cassa di Risparmio di Modena", Italy, for financial support in the purchase of the mass spectrometer used in this work. Moreover, we thank the technicians of the C.I.G.S., University of Modena and Reggio Emilia, Italy, for their assistance during mass spectrometry analysis.

## Author details
[1]Department of Diagnostic Medicine, Clinic and Public Health, Proteomic Lab, University of Modena and Reggio Emilia, Via del Pozzo 71, 41124 Modena, Italy. [2]Headache and Drug Abuse Study Center, University of Modena and Reggio Emilia, Via del Pozzo 71, 41124 Modena, Italy.

## References
1. Negro A, Martelletti P (2011) Chronic migraine plus medication overuse headache: two entities or not? J Headache Pain 12:593–601
2. Evers S, Marziniak M (2010) Clinical features, pathophysiology, and treatment of medication-overuse headache. Lancet Neurol 9:391–401
3. Dodick D, Silberstein S (2006) Central sensitization theory of migraine: clinical implications. Headache 46(Suppl 4):S82–S91
4. De Felice M, Ossipov MH, Porreca F (2011) Persistent medication-induced neural adaptations, descending facilitation, and medication overuse headache. Curr Opin Neurol 24:193–196
5. Bigal ME, Ashina S, Burstein R, Reed ML, Buse D, Serrano D, Lipton RB (2008) Prevalence and characteristics of allodynia in headache suffers: a population study. Neurology 70(17):1525–1533
6. Lipton RB, Bigal ME, Ashina S, Burstein R, Silberstein S, Reed ML, Serrano D, Stewart WF (2008) Cutaneous allodynia in the migraine population. Ann Neurol 63:148–158
7. De Felice M, Ossipov MH, Porreca F (2011) Update on medication-overuse headache. Curr Pain Headache Rep 15(1):79–83
8. Bellei E, Monari E, Cuoghi A, Bergamini S, Guerzoni S, Ciccarese M, Ozben T, Tomasi A, Pini LA (2013) Discovery by a proteomic approach of possible early biomarkers of drug-induced nephrotoxicity in medication-overuse headache. J Headache Pain 14:6
9. Urade Y, Hayaishi O (2000) Biochemical, structural, genetic, physiological, and pathophysiological features of lipocalin-type prostaglandin D synthase. Biochim Biophys Acta 1482:259–271
10. Ito S, Okuda-Ashitaka E, Minami T (2001) Central and peripheral roles of prostaglandins in pain and their interactions with novel neuropeptides nociceptin and nocistatin. Neurosci Res 41:299–332
11. Melegos DN, Grass L, Pierratos A, Diamandis EP (1999) Highly elevated levels of prostaglandin D synthase in the serum of patients with renal failure. Urology 53:32–37
12. Eguchi N, Minami T, Shirafuji N, Kanaoka Y, Tanaka T, Nagata A, Yoshida N, Urade Y, Ito S, Hayaishi O (1999) Lack of tactile pain (allodynia) in lipocalin-type prostaglandin D synthase mice. Proc Natl Acad Sci U S A 96:726–730
13. Maesaka JK, Palaia T, Fishbane S, Ragolia L (2002) Contribution of prostaglandin $D_2$ synthase to progression of renal failure and dialysis dementia. Semin Nephrol 22(5):407–414
14. Bellei E, Cuoghi A, Monari E, Bergamini S, Fantoni LI, Zappaterra M, Guerzoni S, Bazzocchi A, Tomasi A, Pini LA (2012) Proteomic analysis of urine in medication-overuse headache patients: possible relation with renal damages. J Headache Pain 13:45–52
15. Bradford MM (1976) A rapid and sensitive method for the quantitation of microgram quantities of protein utilizing the principle of protein-dye binding. Anal Biochem 72:248–254
16. Bellei E, Rossi E, Lucchi L, Uggeri S, Albertazzi A, Tomasi A, Iannone A (2008) Proteomic analysis of early urinary biomarkers of renal changes in type 2 diabetic patients. Proteomics Clin Appl 2:478–491
17. Bellei E, Bergamini S, Monari E, Fantoni LI, Cuoghi A, Ozben T, Tomasi A (2011) High-abundance proteins depletion for serum proteomic analysis: concomitant removal of non-targeted proteins. Amino Acids 40:145–156
18. Burstein R, Yarnitsky D, Goor-Aryeh I, Ransil BJ, Bajwa ZH (2000) An association between migraine and cutaneous allodynia. Ann Neurol 47:614–624
19. Sandkühler J (2009) Models and mechanisms of hyperalgesia and allodynia. Physiol Rev 89:707–758
20. Mathew NT, Kailasam J, Seifert T (2004) Clinical recognition of allodynia in migraine. Neurology 63:848–852
21. Burstein R, Cutrer MF, Yarnitsky D (2000) The development of cutaneous allodynia during a migraine attack. Brain 123:1703–1709
22. Tietjen GE, Brandes JL, Peterlin BL, Eloff A, Dafer RM, Stein MR, Drexler E, Martin VT, Hutchinson S, Aurora SK, Recober A, Herial NA, Utley C, White L, Khuder SA (2009) Allodynia in migraine: association with comorbid pain conditions. Headache 49:1333–1344
23. Denk F, McMahon SB (2012) Chronic pain: emerging evidence for the involvement of epigenetics. Neuron 73:435–444
24. Wuchty S (2014) Controllability in protein interaction networks. PNAS 111(19):7156–7160
25. Jamieson DG, Moss A, Kennedy M, Jones S, Nenadic G, Robertson DL, Sidders B (2014) The pain interactome: connecting pain-specific protein interactions. Pain 155(11):2243–2252
26. Urade Y, Hayaishi O (2000) Prostaglandin D synthase: structure and function. Vitam Horm 58:89–120

27. Zappaterra M, Guerzoni S, Cainazzo MM, Ferrari A, Pini LA (2011) Basal cutaneous pain threshold in headache patients. J Headache Pain 12:303–310

28. Ferraro S, Grazzi L, Mandelli ML, Aquino D, Di Fiore D, Usai S, Bruzzone MG, Di Salle F, Bussone G, Chiapparini L (2012) Pain processing in medication overuse headache: a functional magnetic resonance imaging (fMRI) study. Pain Med 13:255–262

29. Hoffmann A, Nimtz M, Conradt HS (1997) Molecular characterization of β-trace protein in human serum and urine: a potential diagnostic marker for renal diseases. Glycobiology 7(4):499–506

30. Ogawa M, Hirawa N, Tsuchida T, Eguchi N, Kawabata Y, Numabe A, Negoro H, Hakamada-Taguchi R, Seiki K, Umemura S, Urade Y, Uehara Y (2006) Urinary excretions of lipocalin-type prostaglandin D2 synthase predict the development of proteinuria and renal injury on OLETF rats. Nephrol Dial Transplant 21:924–934

31. Lhotta K (2010) Uromodulin and chronic kidney disease. Kidney Blood Press Res 33:393–398

32. Zhou J, Chen Y, Liu Y, Shi S, Wang S, Li X, Zhang H, Wang H (2013) Urinary uromodulin excretion predicts progression of chronic kidney disease resulting from IgA nephropathy. PLoS ONE 8(8), e71023

33. Rampoldi L, Scolari F, Amoroso A, Ghiggeri G, Devuyst O (2011) The rediscovery of uromodulin (Tamm-Horsfall protein): from tubulointerstitial nephropathy to chronic kidney disease. Kidney Int 80:338–347

34. Prajczer S, Heidenreich U, Pfaller W, Kotanko P, Lhotta K, Jennings P (2010) Evidence for a role of uromodulin in chronic kidney disease progression. Nephrol Dial Transplant 25:1896–1903

35. Shore N, Khurshid R, Saleem M (2010) Alpha-1-microglobulin: a marker for early detection of tubular disorders in diabetic nephropathy. J Ayub Med Coll Abbottabad 22(4):53–55

36. Yu H, Yanagisawa Y, Forbes MA, Cooper EH, Crockson RA, MacLennan ICM (1983) Alpha-1-microglobulin: an indicator protein for renal tubular function. J Clin Pathol 36:253–259

37. Hong CY, Hughes K, Chia KS, Ng V, Ling SL (2003) Urinary $\alpha_1$-microglobulin as a marker of nephropathy in type 2 diabetic asian subjects in Singapore. Diabetes Care 26:338–342

38. Shlipak MG, Mattes MD, Peralta CA (2013) Update on cystatin C: incorporation into clinical practice. Am J Kidney Dis 62(3):595–603

39. Conti M, Moutereau S, Zater M, Lallali K, Durrbach A, Manivet P, Eschwege P, Loric S (2006) Urinary cystatin C as a specific marker of tubular dysfunction. Clin Chem Lab Med 44(3):288–291

40. Kim SS, Song SH, Kim IJ, Jeon YK, Kim BH, Kwak IS, Lee EK, Kim YK (2013) Urinary cystatin C and tubular proteinuria predict progression of diabetic nephropathy. Diabetes Care 36:656–661

41. Westhuyzen J (2006) Cystatin C: a promising marker and predictor of impaired renal function. Ann Clin Lab Sci 36(4):387–394

42. Feinstein AR, Heinemann LAJ, Curhan GC, Delzell E, DeSchepper PJ, Fox JM, Graf H, Luft FC, Michielsen P, Mihatsch MJ, Suissa S, van der Woude F, Willich S (2000) Relationship between nonphenacetin combined analgesics and nephropathy: a review. Kidney Int 58:2259–2264

43. van der Woude FJ, Heinemann LA, Graf H, Lewis M, Moehner S, Assmann A, Kühl-Habich D (2007) Analgesics use and ESRD in younger age: a case-control study. BMC Nephrol 8:15–26

44. Zhang WY (2001) A benefit-risk assessment of caffeine as an analgesic adjuvant. Drug Saf 24(15):1127–1142

45. Waddington F, Naunton M, Thomas J (2015) Paracetamol and analgesic nephropathy: are you kidneying me? Int Med Case Rep J 8:1–5

46. Russell MB, Lundqvist C (2012) Prevention and management of medication overuse headache. Curr Opin Neurol 25:290–295

47. Lai JTF, Dereix JDC, Ganepola RP, Nightingale PG, Markey KA, Aveyard PN, Sinclair AJ (2014) Should we educate about the risks of medication overuse headache? J Headache Pain 15:10

48. Westergaard ML, Hansen EH, Glümer C, Jensen RH (2015) Prescription pain medications and chronic headache in Denmark: implications for preventing medication overuse. Eur J Clin Pharmacol DOI: 10.1007/s00228-015-1858-3

# The effects of acupuncture treatment on the right frontoparietal network in migraine without aura patients

Kuangshi Li[†], Yong Zhang[†], Yanzhe Ning, Hua Zhang, Hongwei Liu, Caihong Fu, Yi Ren[*] and Yihuai Zou[*]

## Abstract

**Background:** Functional and structural abnormalities in resting-state brain networks in migraine patients have been confirmed by previous functional magnetic resonance imaging (fMRI) studies. However, few studies focusing on the neural responses of therapeutic treatment on migraine have been conducted. In this study, we tried to examined the treatment-related effects of standard acupuncture treatment on the right frontoparietal network (RFPN) in migraine patients.

**Methods:** A total of 12 migraine without aura (MWoA) patients were recruited to undergo resting-state fMRI scanning and were rescanned after 4 weeks standard acupuncture treatment. Another 12 matched healthy control (HC) subjects underwent once scanning for comparison. We analyzed the functional connectivity of the RFPN between MWoA patients and HC subjects before treatment and that of the MWoA patients before and after treatment. Diffusion tensor images (DTI) data analyzing was also performed to detect fiber-related treatment responses.

**Results:** We observed significantly decreased FC in the RFPN and that the decreased FC could be reversed by acupuncture treatment. The changes of FC in MWoA patients was negatively correlated with the decrease of visual analogue scale (VAS) scores after treatment. This study indicated that acupuncture treatment for MWoA patients was associated with normalizing effects on the intrinsic decreased FC of the RFPN.

**Conclusions:** Our study provided new insights into the treatment-related neural responses in MWoA patients and suggested potential functional pathways for the evaluation of treatment in MWoA patients. Future studies are still in need to confirm the current results and to elucidate the complex neural mechanisms of acupuncture treatment.

**Keywords:** Acupuncture; Functional magnetic resonance imaging (fMRI); Migraine without aura (MWoA); Right frontoparietal network (RFPN); Resting-state

## Background

As the most prevalent neurological disorder, migraine is affecting more than 100 million people in Europe [1] and the USA [2]. Migraine ranks in the top 20 of the most disabling medical illnesses globally, and has substantial effects on the quality of life of patients and their families and on health costs [3]. It has attracted more and more attention worldwide as a public health issue because of its high prevalence, frequent attack history, significant medical burden, and a serious reduction in quality of life [4].

Migraine is typically associated with pain and its regulation. A series of multiple functional and structural abnormalities within pain related resting-state brain networks in migraine patients have been confirmed by previous functional magnetic resonance imaging (fMRI) studies [5-9]. Altered functional connectivity mainly distribute in the right frontoparietal network (RFPN), the default mode network (DMN), the sensorimotor network (SMN), the silence network, the periaqueductal gray networks, and so on. As a powerful tool to map intrinsic brain activities, fMRI also provides means to elucidate the possible neural mechanisms associated with

* Correspondence: rywendy1982@sina.com; zouyihuai2004@163.com
[†]Equal contributors
Department of Neurology and Stroke Center, Dongzhimen Hospital, The First Affiliated Hospital of Beijing University of Chinese Medicine, Beijing 100700, China

successful treatment for certain diseases. Previously, the neural responses of medical therapies on major depression [10], stroke [11] and some other diseases have been confirmed by fMRI studies. However, few studies focusing on the neural responses of therapeutic treatment on migraine have been conducted.

A large body of clinical researches [12-14] and systematic reviews [15] have confirmed the successful effects of acupuncture for migraine. Existing results suggest that acupuncture is able to alleviate headache degree and/or improve the quality of life and it is as effective, if not more effective, as prophylactic drug treatment. Converging evidence from recent fMRI studies have demonstrated that immediate acupuncture stimulation evoke certain neural activities of different brain regions and networks in both healthy subjects and patients [16,17]. Thus, we believe that acupuncture could be applied as a therapeutic treatment in fMRI studies investigating the neural responses associated with treatment in migraine patients.

To our knowledge, only one study reported the neural responses of acupuncture treatment in migraine patients [18]. Their results indicated that acupuncture treatment evoked cerebral response in the pain matrix, the lateral pain system, the medial pain system, the DMN, and some cognitive components of the pain processing system. However, changes of functional connectivity between pain related brain regions and networks were not well explored in this study. Moreover, the acupuncture treatment involved only four acupoints which could not be regarded as comprehensive acupuncture treatment for migraine patients.

Given the fact that multiple functional and structural abnormalities exist in migraine patients and that acupuncture is an effective treatment for migraine, we hypothesized that acupuncture treatment would modulate the altered brain function of specific brain regions and networks. This hypothesis is of particular interest in respect of elucidating the mechanisms of treatment related neural responses in migraine patients. To test our hypothesis, we examined the effects of 4 weeks standard acupuncture treatment on acupuncture-naive migraine without aura patients. We focused on changes of functional connectivity in the RFPN, an important and dominant brain network strongly related to the processing and regulating of pain [19]. Relationships between functional changes and migraine symptom improvements were also examined. We also performed diffusion tensor images (DTI) data analyzing to detect fiber-related treatment responses.

## Methods
### Ethics statement
Written informed consents were obtained from all subjects. The data was analyzed anonymously. All research procedures were approved by the ethical committee of Dongzhimen Hospital affiliated to Beijing University of

Chinese medicine and conducted in accordance with the Declaration of Helsinki.

### Subjects
A total of 12 MWoA patients (10 females, mean age: $28.1 \pm 6.8$ years) were recruited from Dongzhimen Hospital. All 12 patients met the following inclusion criteria: diagnosed of MWoA according to the classification criteria of the International Headache Society; between 18 and 60 years old; right-handed; 2 to 6 migraine attacks per month during the last 3 months; with a history of migraine longer than 1 year; without history of prophylactic or therapeutic medicine during the last 3 months; without history of acupuncture treatment; without history of smoking, alcohol or drug abuse; without history of long-term analgesics consumption; without history of dysmenorrhea or other chronic painful disease; with education background of more than 10 years; without any MRI contraindications; the informed consent form signed. Patients were excluded if they met any of the criteria below: other types of migraine; the first occurrence of migraine attack appeared after 50 years old; concurrence of neurological disease or psychiatric disorder; with diseases of the cardiovascular system, liver, kidney, or hematopoietic system; pregnant or lactating women; participation in other clinical trials.

Another 12 right-handed normal subjects matched in age, gender and education level were recruited to serve as healthy control (HC). All 12 HC subjects passed normal neurological examination and had no history of migraine or other neurological disease, psychiatric disorder or any MRI contraindications. The demographic and clinical information of MWoA patients and HC subjects was summarized in Table 1.

### Acupuncture treatment
All MWoA patients received standard acupuncture treatment for 4 weeks. The acupuncture treatment course was established according to Chinese guidelines of acupuncture for migraine patients. The following acupoints were selected for needling: bilateral Sizhukong (SJ23), Shuaigu (GB8), Fengchi (GB20), Taiyang (EX-HN5), Hegu (LI4), Taichong (LR3), Waiguan (SJ5), Yanglingquan (GB34), and Zulinqi (GB41). All acupoints were located according to the WHO standard acupuncture point locations in the Western Pacific Region. The disposable stainless steel acupuncture needles ($0.25 \times 40$ mm, Ande Co., Guizhou, China) were inserted in an appropriate angle to a depth of 1.5-2.5 cm. Each acupuncture needle was twisted until the patient felt a de-qi sensation and retained for 30 min. Acupuncture treatment was performed by an independent practitioner with 7 years of clinical experience. The acupuncture treatment took place 5 times per week (form Monday to Friday) and lasted for 30 min every time.

**Table 1 The demographic and clinical information of MWoA patients and HC subjects**

| Items | Healthy control (N=12) | MWoA patients before treatment (N=12) | MWoA patients after treatment (N=12) |
|---|---|---|---|
| Gender (male/female) | 2/10 | 2/10 | 2/10 |
| Age (years) | 29.8 ± 7.2 | 28.1 ± 6.8[#] | 28.1 ± 6.8 |
| migraine history (months) | / | 47.3 ± 42.1 | 47.3 ± 42.1 |
| Educational level (years) | 14.8 ± 5.5 | 15.2 ± 4.4[#] | 15.2 ± 4.4 |
| VAS scores | / | 5.5 ± 1.3 | 2.7 ± 0.7[*] |
| Frequency of migraine attacks (times/month) | / | 4.5 ± 1.1 | 1.9 ± 0.7[*] |
| Duration of migraine attacks (days/month) | / | 6.1 ± 3.2 | 4.3 ± 1.8[*] |

Note: [#]results from independent sample t-test of the comparison between MWoA patients and HC subjects, P > 0.05.
[*]results from paired t-test of the comparison in MWoA patients before and after treatment, P < 0.05.

To ensure the pure effect of acupuncture treatment, all MWoA patients were told not to take any medication or preventive treatment during the whole study. In case of intolerable migraine attacks, patients could take analgesics they commonly used without the effect of migraine prevention and should record the doses and effects.

### fMRI data acquisition

All MWoA patients received two separate resting-state fMRI scanning, before and after the acupuncture treatment course respectively. The HC subjects participated in one resting-state scanning as control.

FMRI images were acquired using a 3.0 T MRI scanner (Siemens, Sonata, Germany). During scanning, subjects remained in the supine position with their heads immobilized by a custom-built head holder to prevent head movements. Subjects wore earplugs throughout the experiment to attenuate MRI gradient noise. Thirty-two axial slices (field of view = 225 mm × 225 mm, matrix = 64 × 64, thickness = 3.5 mm) parallel to the anterior-posterior commissure plane and covering the whole brain were obtained using a T2-weighted single-shot, gradient-recalled echo planar imaging sequence (repetition time = 2000 ms, echo time = 30 ms, flip angle = 90°). Prior to the functional run, high-resolution structural information on each subject was also acquired using 3D MRI sequences with a voxel size of 1 mm3 for anatomical localization (repetition time = 1900 ms, echo time = 2.52 ms, flip angle = 90°, matrix = 256 × 256, field of view = 250 mm × 250 mm, slice thickness = 1 mm).

The DTI data were obtained with a single-shot, echo-planar imaging sequence. The diffusion sensitizing gradients were applied along 30 non-collinear directions (b = 1000 s/mm$^2$) with an acquisition without diffusion weighting (b = 0 s/mm$^2$). The imaging parameters were 80 contiguous axial slices (repetition time = 18000 ms, echo time = 94 ms, flip angle = 90°, matrix = 160 × 160, field of view = 256 mm × 256 mm, slice thickness = 1.5 mm).

In the current fMRI study, for the MWoA patients, we set a rule that the acupuncture treatment should begin within 3 days after the first fMRI scanning and the second scanning should be done within 3 days after the acupuncture treatment course ended. It has to be emphasized that if there was a migraine attack during the due date of scanning, the fMRI scan should be postponed for 72 hours. Another rule for female subjects in both the migraine and control groups was that all fMRI scanning should be done at least 3 day away from their menstrual period.

### FMRI data processing and analyzing

The fMRI data included resting scans of HC subjects and MWoA patients. The HC subjects were scanned once and the scans of MWoA patients were collected before and after the acupuncture treatment. The first 10 time points of all datasets were discarded to avoid unstable magnetization and to ensure the participants adapted the scanning circumstance. All data was preprocessed using the DPARSFA 2.3 software [20]. The images were firstly corrected for acquisition delay between slices by aligning to the first image of each session for motion correction using method of voxel specific head motion [21]. Afterwards, fMRI data was registered to the templates created by T1 images segmented by DARTEL method. Data was further processed with spatial normalization based on the MNI space and resampled at 2 mm × 2 mm × 2 mm. All subjects' had less than 1.5 mm head motions and less than 1.5° rotation in any direction. In addition, a Gaussian kernel with a full width at half-maximum of 6 mm was used to smooth the images in order to reduce noise and residual differences. Finally, we detrended the data to minimize the influence of magnetic machine temperature rise.

Data after preprocessing was analyzed by independent component analysis using the GIFT software. Then, the best goodness-of-fit score to the frontoparietal network template [19,22] was calculated by the way of goodness-of-fit [23] after removing the components not related to the spectrum of resting-state networks (spectrum of resting state networks was 0.01-0.08Hz). The images of component with best goodness-of-fit score were normalized to Z-scores with Fisher's r-to-z transformation to acquire the entire brain Z-score map of each subject.

For group-level analyses, the functional connectivity was conducted by two-sample T-test and paired T-test using SPM8 software (two-tailed, $p < 0.05$, Monte Carlo Simulations correction). The reported statistics were color-coded and mapped in Talairach space. Finally, for the regions of interest in which MWoA patients showed decreased functional connectivity before acupuncture treatment in contrast with HC and significant increased functional connectivity after acupuncture, the Z values of each patient in these regions were extracted, averaged and regressed against patients' visual analogue scale (VAS) scores.

### DTI data processing and analyzing

The data processing and analyzing were mainly carried out using FMRIB Software Library (FSL) and Analysis of Functional NeuroImage (AFNI) software. Firstly, the original DTI data was deobliqued to ensure the images were accord with anterior-posterior commissure line. Then, the Brain Extraction Tool in FSL software was used for brain extraction. And the eddy current distortion and head motion of raw diffusion data were corrected using FSL software. After that, b-vectors was rotated to accord with the results of eddy-correct [24]. Finally, tensor was computed using AFNI software.

We used the DTITK and DTI VISTA software in this procession. The details of DTITK processing steps were as follows [25,26]: firstly, initial template was bootstrapped from each subject's tensor and IIT3 mean template image to achieve the optimal spatial normalization. Secondly, tensors were affinely registered to the initial template using a similarity metric known as Euclidean Distance Squared. Thirdly, each subject's tensor after affine registration was deform ably aligned to the initial template to improve alignment quality by removing size or shape differences in the local structures. Then, a matrix combining the affine transformation and deformable transformation was applied on the original tensors. At last, tensors after the above processing were combined to produce a final average template with characteristics of all subjects. After producing the average template, mean DTI data was transformed from average template by using the AFNI software. After that, DTI VISTA processing was applied.

We defined the following brain regions as regions of interest (ROI): brain regions that showed decreased functional connectivity in MWoA patients compared with HC before treatment (ROI1); brain regions that showed increased functional connectivity in MWoA patients after treatment compared with that before (ROI2); and the left precentral gyrus (ROI3). Fibers from the left

thalamus to the above mentioned three ROIs were calculated by ConTrack algorithm [27]. The fibers that not corresponding with anatomical position were cut by the Quench software. Finally, we applied Brain Voyager QX to present the results.

## Results

### Treatment response

A total of 12 MWoA patients were involved in the acupuncture treatment and finished the treating course as planned. All patients reported the sensation of de-qi and no adverse invents happened. Compared with baseline assessments, the results of VAS scores, duration and frequency of migraine attacks showed significant decrease ($P < 0.05$) after 4 weeks acupuncture treatment (see Table 1).

### Resting-state results

To investigate differences of functional connectivity with the RFPN between MWoA patients and HC subjects, we compared the data of HC subjects and MWoA patients before acupuncture treatment. MWoA patients revealed significantly decreased functional connectivity with the RFPN in the left precentral gyrus, the left supramarginal gyrus, the left inferior parietal lobule, and the left postcentral gyrus (Figure 1). And the decreased functional connectivity of brain regions in MWoA patients was negatively correlated with their VAS scores before treatment (Figure 2, $P = 0.0494$, $R = -0.6289$). No brain regions with increased functional connectivity in the MWoA patients were observed before treatment.

For the MWoA patients, a comparison between before and after the acupuncture treatment was done to detect the changes of functional connectivity with the RPFN induced by acupuncture treatment. This was to evaluate the neural responses of acupuncture treatment in MWoA patients. After the acupuncture treatment, compared with that before, MWoA patients showed significantly increased functional connectivity with the RFPN in the left precentral gyrus, the left inferior parietal lobule, and the left postcentral gyrus (Figure 3). And the increased functional connectivity of brain regions in MWoA patients was negatively correlated with the decrease of VAS scores after treatment (Figure 4, $P = 0.0370$, $R = -0.6633$). No brain regions showed decreased functional connectivity with the RFPN when comparing the results after treatment with that before.

### DTI results

Three probabilistic fibers were shown in Figure 5. The red, yellow and cyan fibers indicated fibers from the left thalamus to ROI1, ROI2 and RIO3 respectively. These three kind of fibers basically coincided with anatomical location. Moreover, these fibers passed the external capsule and posterior limb of the internal capsule which are

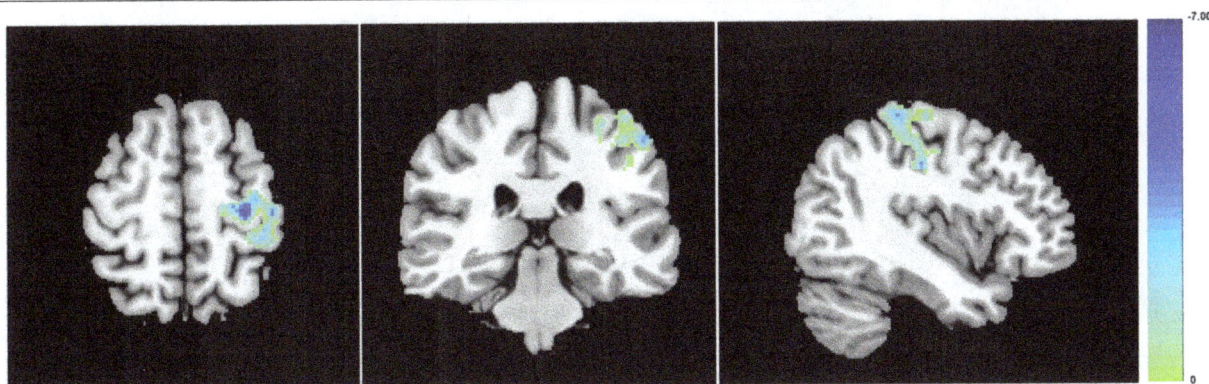

**Figure 1** Compared with HC subjects, MWoA patients showed decreased functional connectivity in the left precentral gyrus, the left supramarginal gyrus, the left inferior parietal lobule, and the left postcentral gyrus. Results from two-tailed, p < 0.05, corrected by Monte Carlo Simulations, iterated 1000 times, and cluster size > 349 voxels.

in accord with the pathways of thalamic radiation. Most fibers passing through the posterior limb of the internal capsule terminated at the dorsal thalamus and fibers passing through the external capsule ended at the thalamus ventralis.

## Discussion

This is the first study to investigate the neural effects of standard acupuncture treatment on the functional connectivity of the RFPN in MWoA patients. We found decreased functional connectivity in the left precentral gyrus, the left supramarginal gyrus, the left inferior parietal lobule, and the left postcentral gyrus and that the decreased functional connectivity could be reversed by acupuncture treatment. Our results indicated that 4 weeks standard acupuncture treatment had normalizing effects on abnormally decreased functional connectivity in the RFPN in MWoA patients. We propose that the reversal of

functional connectivity in the RFPN may lead to further interpretation of treatment-related neural responses in MWoA patients.

The RFPN is recognized as an important brain network that corresponds to perception, somesthesis, and pain [19]. The frontoparietal region played a dominant role in the formation and transmission of sensation. This region connected the primary sensory area with the secondary sensory area [28]. Other studies demonstrated that the frontoparietal lobe is closely related to cognitive processing, memory working and attention keeping [29,30]. Accordingly, chronic continually pain suffers in MWoA patients, invariably causing human attention, might change the functional connectivity of the RFPN. Some recent researches also indicated that the functional connectivity of the RFPN exist abnormality in patients suffering from chronic pain [31,32]. Our results revealed decreased functional connectivity between the RFPN

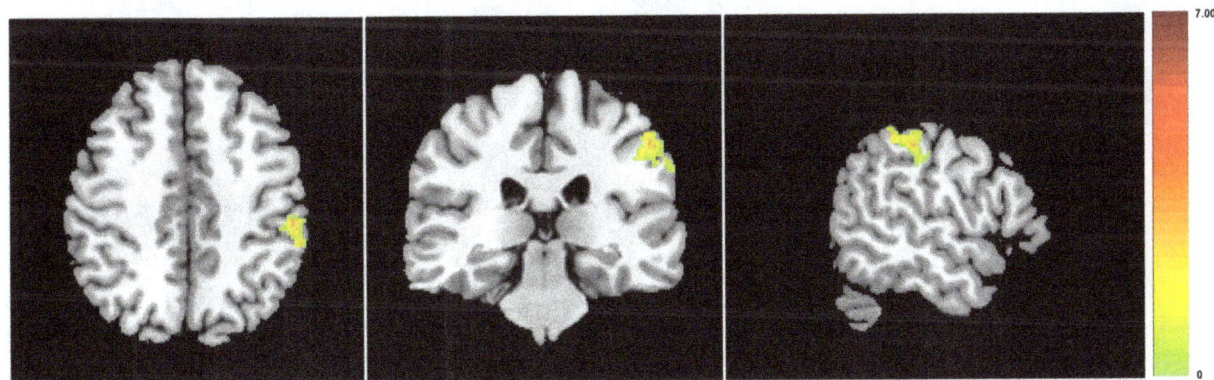

**Figure 2** Compared with before acupuncture treatment, MWoA patients showed increased functional connectivity in the left precentral gyrus, the left inferior parietal lobule, and the left postcentral gyrus, after acupuncture treatment. Results from two-tailed, p < 0.05, corrected by Monte Carlo Simulations, iterated 1000 times, and cluster size > 349 voxels.

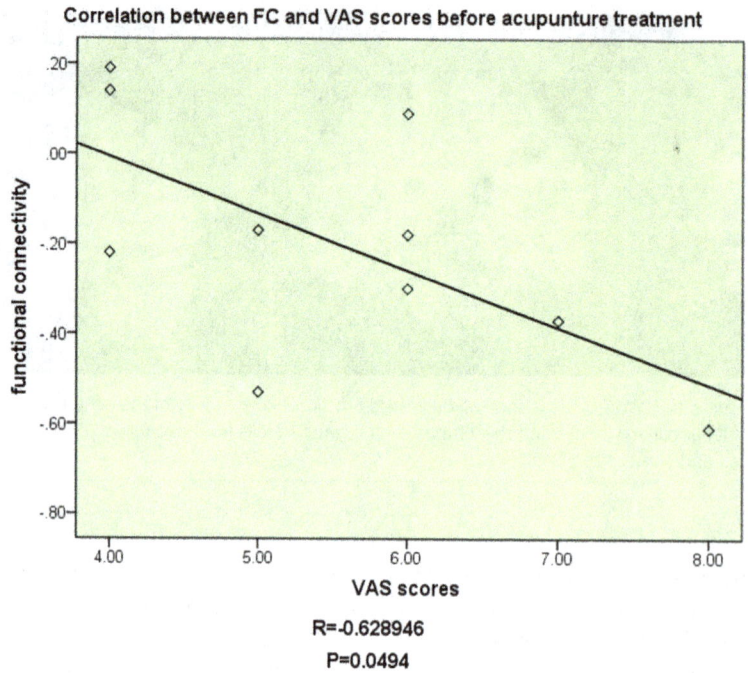

**Correlation between FC and VAS scores before acupuncture treatment**

R=-0.628946
P=0.0494

**Figure 3** The decreased functional connectivity of brain regions in MWoA patients was negatively correlated with their VAS scores before treatment.

and some other brain regions. These brain regions are involved in direct or indirect relation with pain. The postcentral gyrus, which is usually called the primary somatosensory cortex (SI), is included in the pain matrix and accepts pain signals straightly [33]. The precentral gyrus, which is called the primary sensorimotor cortex (MI), is typically associated with voluntary movement. Recent studies have found links between the SI and MI indicating that some sensory signals could transmit from the SI to MI [34]. Other studies also revealed abnormal

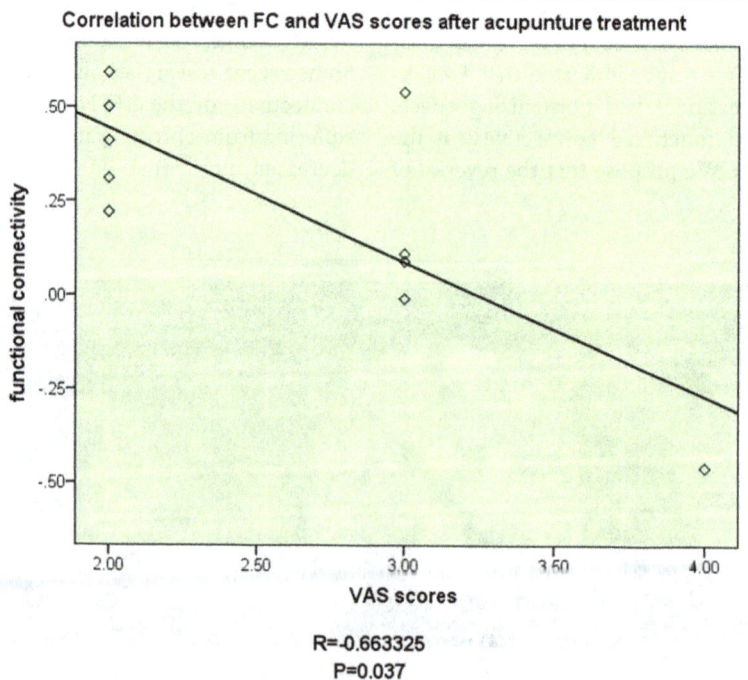

**Correlation between FC and VAS scores after acupunture treatment**

R=-0.663325
P=0.037

**Figure 4** The increased functional connectivity of brain regions in MWoA patients was negatively correlated with the decrease of VAS scores after treatment.

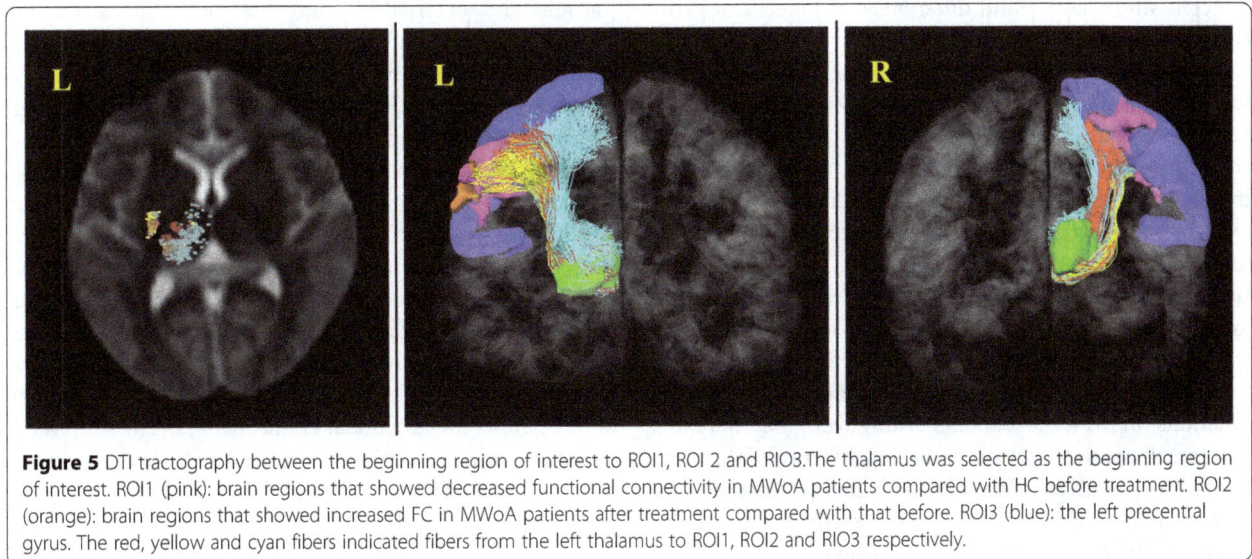

**Figure 5** DTI tractography between the beginning region of interest to ROI1, ROI 2 and RIO3.The thalamus was selected as the beginning region of interest. ROI1 (pink): brain regions that showed decreased functional connectivity in MWoA patients compared with HC before treatment. ROI2 (orange): brain regions that showed increased FC in MWoA patients after treatment compared with that before. ROI3 (blue): the left precentral gyrus. The red, yellow and cyan fibers indicated fibers from the left thalamus to ROI1, ROI2 and RIO3 respectively.

nodal centrality in the MI in MWoA patients when compared with HC subjects [35,36]. The changes of functional connectivity in the supramarginal gyrus and the MI were also reported in nociception [7]. Taken together, the brain regions showed decreased functional connectivity with the RFPN in our study played important roles in pain processing and regulating. The decreased functional connectivity in these brain regions probably caused by hyperexcitability of pain pathway which led to disorders between the RFPN and its related external regions [37,38]. In addition, the average functional connectivity value of the brain regions which showed decreased functional connectivity negatively correlated with VAS scores of MWoA patients. This suggested that these pain related brain regions became more hypo-connected with the RFPN as the pain intensity increase. The decreased functional connectivity in MWoA patients revealed the modulations of brain functions associated with ongoing nociceptive stimulus. From the perspective of brain network, our current findings provided a conceptualization of MWoA as the dysfunctions of brain networks [7,8,39,40].

In the comparison study before and after acupuncture treatment, we found that acupuncture treatment had normalizing effects on abnormally decreased functional connectivity between the RFPN and its external eareas in MWoA patients. After a 4-week acupuncture treatment, MWoA patients showed increased functional connectivity in the left precentral gyrus, the left inferior parietal lobule, and the left postcentral gyrus with the RFPN. From the perspective of transformation, we assumed that the normalizing effects might be associated with the changes of relation among different brain networks. The RFPN and DMN are considered as two main components of human brain resting-state networks [19]. The RFPN is strongly involved in perception, somesthesis, and pain [19]. While the DMN is involved in self-referential processing, conscious, awareness, mind wandering, manipulation of episodic memories and semantic knowledge [41,42]. The right insula was considered as an important node of the RFPN in previous studies [43]. And the inferior parietal lobule relating to the processing of pain was regarded as an important part of the DMN [19,44]. The right insula and left inferior parietal lobule revealed strong functional connectivity in resting-state in a recent research [45]. Some study also stated that the higher functional connectivity of the RFPN within the region of the intraparietal sulcus would lead to greater intrinsic DMN connectivity to insula, which was outside of the classical boundaries of the DMN [46]. Fibers connecting the inferior parietal lobe and the insula have also been found [47]. In our study, the functional connectivity of inferior parietal lobule after acupuncture treatment significantly increased when compared with that before acupuncture treatment. While this area of MWoA patients showed decreased functional connectivity before acupuncture compared with HC subjects. Thus, we speculated that the DMN was connected with the RFPN through certain nodes and that the left inferior parietal lobule probably was included in these nodes. The theory that some treatment methods were able to change the functional connectivity of nodes in brain networks had been confirmed in recent researches [48,49]. Our study confirmed that the abnormally decreased functional connectivity of the RFPN could be reversed by acupuncture treatment. The functions of the precentral gyrus and the postcentral gyrs in the rehabilitation of migraine are still unclear. However, a recent study have found differences of precentral gyrus cortical thickness between migraine patients and HC subjects [50]. Besides, the precentral gyrus was also found as an abnormal nodal centrality which related to pain-processing [35]. Other researchers have revealed increased metabolism in migraine patients after acupuncture treatment by PET-CT [51]. Therefore, the therapeutic effects of acupuncture might be associate with the adjustment in these brain regions as well their related functions. In combination with the current knowledge of physiological functions of the RFPN, we propose that such reversal in the functional connectivity of the RFPN may lead to a beneficial impact on pain processing and regulating functions in MWoA patients. Moreover, the increased functional connectivity of brain regions in MWoA patients was negatively correlated with the decrease of VAS scores after treatment. The symptomatic improvement suggested that the changes of functional connectivity of the RFPN may act as objective indicators of the clinical responses of MWoA patients to different treatment. Accordingly, our study indicated that acupuncture could improve the functional connectivity of nodes between the RFPN and DMN to promote the rehabilitation of migraine. Besides, successful acupuncture treatment was associated with a normalizing effects on the functional connectivity of the left precentral gyrus, left inferior parietal lobule and left postcentral gyrus in MWoA patients.

A large number of studies have been conducted to investigate the structural changes in multiple DTI-derived indices in MWoA patients [52-55]. However, microstructural studies could not support the functional studies in anatomy. Therefore, we tracked the fibers' path to support the results of fMRI in the current study. According to the anatomical position, thalamic radiation distributed in the broad cortex including the frontal lobe, the parietal lobe, the occipital lobe and the temporal lobe. At the same time, the thalamus was also an important structure in researches of acupuncture [56,57]. Therefore, the thalamus was selected as the beginning region of interest based on the anatomical structure and the effects of acupuncture. Then we defined brain regions that showed decreased functional connectivity in MWoA patients compared with HC before treatment as ROI1, brain regions that showed increased functional connectivity in MWoA patients after treatment compared with that before as ROI2, and the left precentral gyrus as ROI3. The results showed central thalamic radiation (showed in Figure 5, Cyan fibers), which started from the left thalamus to ROI3, corresponded to existing anatomy. Besides, fibers which started from the left thalamus to ROI2 overlapped with the central thalamic radiation. The fibers which started from the left thalamus to ROI1 also coincided with the central thalamic radiation. The fibers entirely passed though the posterior limb of the internal

capsule and external capsule. Previous studies showed that the superior and posterior thalamic radiation, which directly related to sensory, joined the posterior limb of the internal capsule [58,59]. Moreover, fibers passed through external capsule were generally considered to be involved in movement and coordination of movement [60,61]. In our studies, the fibers mostly terminated in the lower part of the sensory region and motor region in cerebral cortex. According to anatomy, the distribution of sensory region and motor region in cerebral cortex were inverted human form. Dominant region of sensorimotor in head and face were mostly in the lower part of the motor cortex and sensory cortex. Therefore, we considered that the regions showed different functional connectivity, between MWoA patients and HC subjects, were related to the sensorimotor of head and face according to the anatomical location. Besides, the fibers, which started from the left thalamus to ROI3, also joined the thalamic radiation and ended at the MI and SI. Previous study showed that a conduction loop which could execute movement according to the sense existed between the motor cortex and sensory cortex [62]. To sum up, we speculate that the differences of functional connectivity between MWoA patients and HC subjects are related to the disorder of the sensorimotor pathways, and that changes of these pathways are possible one aspect of interpretations of treatment-related neural mechanisms. We also speculate that these pathways probably are the substance basis of functional connectivity in brain networks.

Our study has several limitations. First, we didn't clearly confirm whether the changes of functional connectivity after treatment were due to the specific effects of acupuncture treatment, changes related to the natural course of the illness, a placebo effect, or some combination of these possibilities. Moreover, the DTI results only showed the contribution of fibers, but couldn't explain the differences of fibers property between HC subjects and MWoA patients. Thus, comparing scores of fibers need to be applied on the follow-up studies. Finally, Further studies with larger sample size are still needed to confirm these results.

## Conclusions

In conclusion, the current study indicated that acupuncture treatment for MWoA patients was associated with normalizing effects on the intrinsic decreased functional connectivity of the RFPN. This study provided new insights into the treatment-related neural responses in MWoA patients and suggested potential functional pathways for the evaluation of treatment in MWoA patients. Future studies are still in need to confirm the current results and to elucidate the complex neural mechanisms of acupuncture treatment.

## Abbreviations

DMN: Default mode network; DTI: Diffusion tensor images; fMRI: Functional magnetic resonance; HC: Healthy control; MwoA: Migraine without aura; RFPN: Right frontoparietal network; ROI: Regions of interest; SMN: Sensorimotor network..

## Competing interests

The authors declare that they have no competing interests.

## Authors' contributions

KSL, YZ, YR and YHZ conceived and designed the study. KSL, YZ and HZ analyzed the data. YZ, YZN, HWL and CHF performed the experiment. KSL, YZ, YR and YHZ drafted the manuscript and gave final approval of the manuscript

## Acknowledgment

This study was supported by the National Natural Science Foundation of China (No. 81473667), the Beijing Young Talent program of Beijing Education Committee (No. YETP0823).

## References

1. Olesen J, Gustavsson A, Svensson M, Wittchen HU, Jönsson B, on behalf of the Csg and the European Brain C (2012) The economic cost of brain disorders in Europe. Eur J Neurol 19:155–162

2. Lipton RB, Bigal ME, Diamond M, Freitag F, Reed ML, Stewart WF and Group obotAA (2007) Migraine prevalence, disease burden, and the need for preventive therapy. Neurology 68:343–349

3. Jensen R, Stovner LJ (2008) Epidemiology and comorbidity of headache. Lancet Neurol 7:354–361

4. Buse DC, Lipton RB (2013) Global perspectives on the burden of episodic and chronic migraine. Cephalalgia 33:885–890

5. Jin C, Yuan K, Zhao L, Zhao L, Yu D, von Deneen KM, Zhang M, Qin W, Sun W, Tian J (2013) Structural and functional abnormalities in migraine patients without aura. NMR Biomed 26:58–64

6. Maleki N, Becerra L, Brawn J, Bigal M, Burstein R, Borsook D (2012) Concurrent functional and structural cortical alterations in migraine. Cephalalgia 32:607–620

7. Mainero C, Boshyan J, Hadjikhani N (2011) Altered functional magnetic resonance imaging resting-state connectivity in periaqueductal gray networks in migraine. Ann Neurol 70:838–845

8. Tessitore A, Russo A, Giordano A, Conte F, Corbo D, De Stefano M, Cirillo S, Cirillo M, Esposito F, Tedeschi G (2013) Disrupted default mode network connectivity in migraine without aura. J Headache Pain 14:89

9. Zhao L, Liu J, Dong X, Peng Y, Yuan K, Wu F, Sun J, Gong Q, Qin W, Liang F (2013) Alterations in regional homogeneity assessed by fMRI in patients with migraine without aura stratified by disease duration. J Headache Pain 14:85

10. Yang R, Zhang H, Wu X, Yang J, Ma M, Gao Y, Liu H, Li S (2014) Hypothalamus-anchored resting brain network changes before and after sertraline treatment in major depression. Biomed Res Int 2014:915026

11. Yang S, Jiang C, Ye H, Tao J, Huang J, Gao Y, Lin Z, Chen L (2014) Effect of integrated cognitive therapy on hippocampal functional connectivity patterns in stroke patients with cognitive dysfuction: A resting-state fMRI study. Evid-Based Complent Alternat Med 2014:962304

12. Li Y, Zheng H, Witt CM, Roll S, Yu SG, Yan J, Sun GJ, Zhao L, Huang WJ, Chang XR, Zhang HX, Wang DJ, Lan L, Zou R, Liang FR (2012) Acupuncture for migraine prophylaxis: a randomized controlled trial. CMAJ 184:401–410

13. Wang LP, Zhang XZ, Guo J, Liu HL, Zhang Y, Liu CZ, Yi JH, Wang LP, Zhao JP, Li SS (2011) Efficacy of acupuncture for migraine prophylaxis: a single-blinded, double-dummy, randomized controlled trial. Pain 152:1864–1871

14. Diener HC, Kronfeld K, Boewing G, Lungenhausen M, Maier C, Molsberger A, Tegenthoff M, Trampisch HJ, Zenz M, Meinert R (2006) Efficacy of acupuncture for the prophylaxis of migraine: a multicentre randomised controlled clinical trial. Lancet Neurol 5:310–316

15. Linde K, Allais G, Brinkhaus B, Manheimer E, Vickers A, White AR (2009) Acupuncture for migraine prophylaxis. Cochrane Database Syst Rev 1, CD001218

16. Huang W, Pach D, Napadow V, Park K, Long X, Neumann J, Maeda Y, Nierhaus T, Liang F, Witt CM (2012) Characterizing acupuncture stimuli using brain imaging with FMRI–a systematic review and meta-analysis of the literature. PLoS One 7, e32960

17. Bai L, Tian J, Zhong C, Xue T, You Y, Liu Z, Chen P, Gong Q, Ai L, Qin W, Dai J, Liu Y (2010) Acupuncture modulates temporal neural responses in wide brain networks: evidence from fMRI study. Mol Pain 6:73

18. Zhao L, Liu J, Zhang F, Dong X, Peng Y, Qin W, Wu F, Li Y, Yuan K, von Deneen KM, Gong Q, Tang Z, Liang F (2014) Effects of long-term acupuncture treatment on resting-state brain activity in migraine patients: a randomized controlled trial on active acupoints and inactive acupoints. PLoS One 9, e99538

19. Smith SM, Fox PT, Miller KL, Glahn DC, Fox PM, Mackay CE, Filippini N, Watkins KE, Toro R, Laird AR, Beckmann CF (2009) Correspondence of the brain's functional architecture during activation and rest. Proc Natl Acad Sci U S A 106:13040–13045

20. Chao-Gan Y, Yu-Feng Z (2010) DPARSF: A MATLAB Toolbox for "Pipeline" Data Analysis of Resting-State fMRI. Front Syst Neurosci 4:13

21. Yan CG, Cheung B, Kelly C, Colcombe S, Craddock RC, Di Martino A, Li Q, Zuo XN, Castellanos FX, Milham MP (2013) A comprehensive assessment of regional variation in the impact of head micromovements on functional connectomics. NeuroImage 76:183–201

22. Pendse GV, Borsook D, Becerra L (2011) A simple and objective method for reproducible resting state network (RSN) detection in fMRI. PLoS One 6, e27594

23. White T, Gilleen JK, Shergill SS (2013) Dysregulated but not decreased salience network activity in schizophrenia. Front Hum Neurosci 7:65

24. Leemans A, Jones DK (2009) The B-matrix must be rotated when correcting for subject motion in DTI data. Magn Reson Med 61:1336–1349

25. Zhang S, Arfanakis K (2013) Role of standardized and study-specific human brain diffusion tensor templates in inter-subject spatial normalization. J Magn Reson Imaging 37:372–381

26. Adluru N, Zhang H, Fox AS, Shelton SE, Ennis CM, Bartosic AM, Oler JA, Tromp DPM, Zakszewski E, Gee JC, Kalin NH, Alexander AL (2012) A diffusion tensor brain template for Rhesus Macaques. NeuroImage 59:306–318

27. Sherbondy AJ, Dougherty RF, Ben-Shachar M, Napel S, Wandell BA (2008) ConTrack: Finding the most likely pathways between brain regions using diffusion tractography. J Vis 8:15

28. Lobanov OV, Quevedo AS, Hadsel MS, Kraft RA, Coghill RC (2013) Frontoparietal mechanisms supporting attention to location and intensity of painful stimuli. Pain 154:1758–1768

29. Seeley WW, Menon V, Schatzberg AF, Keller J, Glover GH, Kenna H, Reiss AL, Greicius MD (2007) Dissociable intrinsic connectivity networks for salience processing and executive control. J Neurosci 27:2349–2356

30. Corbetta M, Shulman GL (2002) Control of goal-directed and stimulus-driven attention in the brain. Nat Rev Neurosci 3:201–215

31. Seminowicz DA, Davis KD (2007) Pain enhances functional connectivity of a brain network evoked by performance of a cognitive task. J Neurophysiol 97:3651–3659

32. Seifert F, Schuberth N, De Col R, Peltz E, Nickel FT, Maihofner C (2013) Brain activity during sympathetic response in anticipation and experience of pain. Hum Brain Mapp 34:1768–1782

33. May A (2006) A review of diagnostic and functional imaging in headache. J Headache Pain 7:174–184

34. Frot M, Magnin M, Mauguiere F, Garcia-Larrea L (2013) Cortical representation of pain in primary sensory-motor areas (S1/M1)–a study using intracortical recordings in humans. Hum Brain Mapp 34:2655–2668

35. Liu J, Zhao L, Li G, Xiong S, Nan J, Li J, Yuan K, von Deneen KM, Liang F, Qin W, Tian J (2012) Hierarchical alteration of brain structural and functional networks in female migraine sufferers. PLoS One 7, e51250

36. Liu J, Qin W, Nan J, Li J, Yuan K, Zhao L, Zeng F, Sun J, Yu D, Dong M, Liu P, von Deneen KM, Gong Q, Liang F, Tian J (2011) Gender-related differences in the dysfunctional resting networks of migraine suffers. PLoS One 6, e27049

37. Wang X, Xiang J, Wang Y, Pardos M, Meng L, Huo X, Korostenskaja M, Powers SW, Kabbouche MA, Hershey AD (2010) Identification of abnormal neuromagnetic signatures in the motor cortex of adolescent migraine. Headache 50:1005–1016

38. Hoffken O, Stude P, Lenz M, Bach M, Dinse HR, Tegenthoff M (2009) Visual paired-pulse stimulation reveals enhanced visual cortex excitability in migraineurs. Eur J Neurosci 30:714–720

39. Hadjikhani N, Ward N, Boshyan J, Napadow V, Maeda Y, Truini A, Caramia F, Tinelli E, Mainero C (2013) The missing link: enhanced functional connectivity between amygdala and visceroceptive cortex in migraine. Cephalalgia 33:1264–1268

40. Russo A, Tessitore A, Giordano A, Corbo D, Marcuccio L, De Stefano M, Salemi F, Conforti R, Esposito F, Tedeschi G (2012) Executive resting-state network connectivity in migraine without aura. Cephalalgia 32:1041–1048

41. Li W, Han T, Qin W, Zhang J, Liu H, Li Y, Meng L, Ji X, Yu C (2013) Altered functional connectivity of cognitive-related cerebellar subregions in well-recovered stroke patients. Neural Plast 2013:452439

42. Bush G, Luu P, Posner MI (2000) Cognitive and emotional influences in anterior cingulate cortex. Trends Cogn Sci 4:215–222

43. Menon V, Uddin LQ (2010) Saliency, switching, attention and control: a network model of insula function. Brain Struct Funct 214:655–667

44. Ferraro S, Grazzi L, Mandelli ML, Aquino D, Di Fiore D, Usai S, Bruzzone MG, Di Salle F, Bussone G, Chiapparini L (2012) Pain processing in medication overuse headache: a functional magnetic resonance imaging (fMRI) study. Pain Med 13:255–262

45. Stern ER, Fitzgerald KD, Welsh RC, Abelson JL, Taylor SF (2012) Resting-state functional connectivity between fronto-parietal and default mode networks in obsessive-compulsive disorder. PLoS One 7, e36356

46. Xue T, Yuan K, Zhao L, Yu D, Zhao L, Dong T, Cheng P, von Deneen KM, Qin W, Tian J (2012) Intrinsic brain network abnormalities in migraines without aura revealed in resting-state fMRI. PLoS One 7, e52927

47. Uddin LQ, Supekar K, Amin H, Rykhlevskaia E, Nguyen DA, Greicius MD, Menon V (2010) Dissociable connectivity within human angular gyrus and intraparietal sulcus: evidence from functional and structural connectivity. Cereb Cortex 20:2636–2646

48. You Y, Bai L, Dai R, Cheng H, Liu Z, Wei W, Tian J (2013) Altered hub configurations within default mode network following acupuncture at ST36: a multimodal investigation combining fMRI and MEG. PLoS One 8, e64509

49. Bai L, Cui F, Zou Y, Lao L (2013) Acupuncture de qi in stable somatosensory stroke patients: relations with effective brain network for motor recovery. Evid Based Complement Alternat Med 2013:197238

50. Schwedt TJ, Chong CD (2014) Correlations between brain cortical thickness and cutaneous pain thresholds are atypical in adults with migraine. PLoS One 9, e99791

51. Yang J, Zeng F, Feng Y, Fang L, Qin W, Liu X, Song W, Xie H, Chen J, Liang F (2012) A PET-CT study on the specificity of acupoints through acupuncture treatment in migraine patients. BMC Complement Altern Med 12:123

52. Jung RE, Grazioplene R, Caprihan A, Chavez RS, Haier RJ (2010) White matter integrity, creativity, and psychopathology: disentangling constructs with diffusion tensor imaging. PLoS One 5, e9818

53. Beaulieu C (2002) The basis of anisotropic water diffusion in the nervous system - a technical review. NMR Biomed 15:435–455

54. Alexander AL, Lee JE, Lazar M, Field AS (2007) Diffusion tensor imaging of the brain. Neurotherapeutics 4:316–329

55. Song SK, Sun SW, Ramsbottom MJ, Chang C, Russell J, Cross AH (2002) Dysmyelination revealed through MRI as increased radial (but unchanged axial) diffusion of water. NeuroImage 17:1429–1436

56. Napadow V, Dhond R, Park K, Kim J, Makris N, Kwong KK, Harris RE, Purdon PL, Kettner N, Hui KK (2009) Time-variant fMRI activity in the brainstem and higher structures in response to acupuncture. NeuroImage 47:289–301

57. Zyloney CE, Jensen K, Polich G, Loiotile RE, Cheetham A, LaViolette PS, Tu P, Kaptchuk TJ, Gollub RL, Kong J (2010) Imaging the functional connectivity of the Periaqueductal Gray during genuine and sham electroacupuncture treatment. Mol Pain 6:80

58. Chowdhury F, Haque M, Sarkar M, Ara S, Islam M (2010) White fiber dissection of brain; the internal capsule: a cadaveric study. Turk Neurosurg 20:314–322

59. Mamata H, Mamata Y, Westin CF, Shenton ME, Kikinis R, Jolesz FA, Maier SE (2002) High-resolution line scan diffusion tensor MR imaging of white matter fiber tract anatomy. AJNR Am J Neuroradiol 23:67–75

60. Rosenbloom MJ, Sassoon SA, Pfefferbaum A, Sullivan EV (2009) Contribution of Regional White Matter Integrity to Visuospatial Construction Accuracy, Organizational Strategy, and Memory for a Complex Figure in Abstinent Alcoholics. Brain Imaging Behav 3:379–390

61. Sullivan EV, Rosenbloom MJ, Rohlfing T, Kemper CA, Deresinski S, Pfefferbaum A (2011) Pontocerebellar contribution to postural instability and psychomotor slowing in HIV infection without dementia. Brain Imaging Behav 5:12–24

62. Hoon AH Jr, Stashinko EE, Nagae LM, Lin DD, Keller J, Bastian A, Campbell ML, Levey E, Mori S, Johnston MV (2009) Sensory and motor deficits in children with cerebral palsy born preterm correlate with diffusion tensor imaging abnormalities in thalamocortical pathways. Dev Med Child Neurol 51:697–704

# Permissions

All chapters in this book were first published in TJHP, by BioMed Central; hereby published with permission under the Creative Commons Attribution License or equivalent. Every chapter published in this book has been scrutinized by our experts. Their significance has been extensively debated. The topics covered herein carry significant findings which will fuel the growth of the discipline. They may even be implemented as practical applications or may be referred to as a beginning point for another development.

The contributors of this book come from diverse backgrounds, making this book a truly international effort. This book will bring forth new frontiers with its revolutionizing research information and detailed analysis of the nascent developments around the world.

We would like to thank all the contributing authors for lending their expertise to make the book truly unique. They have played a crucial role in the development of this book. Without their invaluable contributions this book wouldn't have been possible. They have made vital efforts to compile up to date information on the varied aspects of this subject to make this book a valuable addition to the collection of many professionals and students.

This book was conceptualized with the vision of imparting up-to-date information and advanced data in this field. To ensure the same, a matchless editorial board was set up. Every individual on the board went through rigorous rounds of assessment to prove their worth. After which they invested a large part of their time researching and compiling the most relevant data for our readers.

The editorial board has been involved in producing this book since its inception. They have spent rigorous hours researching and exploring the diverse topics which have resulted in the successful publishing of this book. They have passed on their knowledge of decades through this book. To expedite this challenging task, the publisher supported the team at every step. A small team of assistant editors was also appointed to further simplify the editing procedure and attain best results for the readers.

Apart from the editorial board, the designing team has also invested a significant amount of their time in understanding the subject and creating the most relevant covers. They scrutinized every image to scout for the most suitable representation of the subject and create an appropriate cover for the book.

The publishing team has been an ardent support to the editorial, designing and production team. Their endless efforts to recruit the best for this project, has resulted in the accomplishment of this book. They are a veteran in the field of academics and their pool of knowledge is as vast as their experience in printing. Their expertise and guidance has proved useful at every step. Their uncompromising quality standards have made this book an exceptional effort. Their encouragement from time to time has been an inspiration for everyone.

The publisher and the editorial board hope that this book will prove to be a valuable piece of knowledge for researchers, students, practitioners and scholars across the globe.

# List of Contributors

**Stefan Evers**
Department of Neurology, University of Münster, Münster, Germany
Department of Neurology, Krankenhaus Lindenbrunn, Coppenbrügge, Germany

**Lorenzo Pinessi and Lidia Savi**
Department of Neurology, University of Turin, Turin, Italy

**Stefano Omboni**
Italian Institute of Telemedicine, Varese, Italy

**Carlo Lisotto**
Department of Neurology, Hospital of Pordenone, Pordenone, Italy

**Giorgio Zanchin**
Department of Neurology, University of Padova, Padova, Italy

**Mark Braschinsky and Sulev Haldre**
Estonian Headache Society, L Puusepa str 8H, Tartu, Estonia
Clinic of Neurology, University of Tartu, L Puusepa str 8H, Tartu, Estonia

**Mart Kals**
Estonian Genome Centre, University of Tartu, Riia 23b, Tartu, Estonia

**Anna Iofik, Ave Kivisild, Jaanus Korjas and Silvia Koljal**
Faculty of Medicine, University of Tartu, Ravila 19, Tartu, Estonia

**Zaza Katsarava**
Department of Neurology, University of Duisburg-Essen, Essen, Germany

**Timothy J. Steiner**
Department of Neuroscience, Norwegian University of Science and Technology, Edvard Griegs Gate, Trondheim NO-7489, Norway
Division of Brain Sciences, Imperial College London, London, UK

**Malgorzata Pihut, Ewa Ferendiuk and Michal Szewczyk**
Department of Dental Prosthetics, Jagiellonian University in Krakow, College of Medicine, Institute of Dentistry, 4 Montelupich St., 31-155 Krakow, Poland

**Katarzyna Kasprzyk**
Department of Neurology, Jagiellonian University in Krakow, College of Medicine, 3 Botaniczna St., 31-503 Krakow, Poland

**Mieszko Wieckiewicz**
Department of Prosthetic Dentistry, Faculty of Dentistry, Wroclaw Medical University, 26 Krakowska St., 50-425 Wroclaw, Poland

**Mattias Gjelset**
Orofacial Pain and Jaw Function, Department of Dental Medicine, Karolinska Institutet, SE-141 04 Huddinge, Sweden

**Amal Al-Khotani and Nikolaos Christidis**
Scandinavian Center for Orofacial Neurosciences (SCON), Huddinge, Sweden
Orofacial Pain and Jaw Function, Department of Dental Medicine, Karolinska Institutet, SE-141 04 Huddinge, Sweden

**Aron Naimi-Akbar**
Cariology, Department of Dental Medicine, Karolinska Institutet, SE-141 04 Huddinge, Sweden

**Emad Albadawi**
Dental Speciality Center, Ministry of Health, Jeddah, Saudi Arabia

**Lanre Bello**
Pediatric Dentistry and Orthodontics Department, College of Dentistry, King Saud University, Riyadh, Saudi Arabia

**Britt Hedenberg-Magnusson**
Department of Clinical Oral Physiology at the Eastman Institute, Stockholm Public Dental Health (Folktandvården SLL AB), SE-113 24 Stockholm, Sweden

Scandinavian Center for Orofacial Neurosciences (SCON), Huddinge, Sweden
Orofacial Pain and Jaw Function, Department of Dental Medicine, Karolinska Institutet, SE-141 04 Huddinge, Sweden

**Sırma Geyik, Aylin Akçalı and Ayşe Münife Neyal**
Department of Neurology, Faculty of Medicine, University of Gaziantep, Gaziantep, Turkey

**Sercan Ergun**
Ulubey Vocational Higher School, Ordu University, Ordu, Turkey

**Samiye Kuzudişli**
Department of Neurology, Emine-Bahaeddin Nakiboglu Medical Faculty, Zirve University, Gaziantep, Turkey

**Figen Şensoy**
Neurology Clinics, Medical Park Hospital, Gaziantep, Turkey

**Murat Korkmaz, Ebru Temiz and Hasan Dağlı**
Department of Medical Biology, Faculty of Medicine, University of Gaziantep, Gaziantep, Turkey

**Erman Altunışık**
Division Of Neurology, Turkish Ministry Of Health Siirt State Hospital, Siirt, Turkey

**Seval Kul**
Department of Biostatistics, Faculty of Medicine, University of Gaziantep, Gaziantep, Turkey

**James Morris and Simon Walker**
Cogentia Healthcare Consulting Ltd., Richmond House, 16-20 Regent Street, Cambridge CB2 1DB, UK

**Andreas Straube**
Ludwig Maximilian University of Munich, Marchioninistr 15, Munich D81377, Germany

**Hans-Christoph Diener**
Department of Neurology and Headache Center, University Hospital Essen, Hufelandstrasse 55, 45122 Essen, Germany

**Fayyaz Ahmed**
Hull and Yorkshire Hospitals, Hull Royal Infirmary, Anlaby Road, Hull HU3 2JZ, UK

**Nicholas Silver**
The Walton Centre for Neurology and Neurosurgery, Lower Lane, Liverpool L9 7LJ, UK

**Eric Liebler**
electroCore, LLC, 150 Allen Road, Suite 201, Basking Ridge, NJ 07920, USA

**Charly Gaul**
Migraine and Headache Clinic Königstein, Ölmühlweg 31, 61462 Königstein im Taunus, Germany
Department of Neurology and Headache Center, University Hospital Essen, Hufelandstrasse 55, 45122 Essen, Germany

**Michail Vikelis**
Headache Clinic, Mediterraneo Hospital, Glyfada, Greece
Headache Outpatient Clinic, 1st Department of Neurology, National and Kapodistrian University of Athens, Athens, Greece
Glyfada Headache Clinic, 8 Lazaraki Str, Glyfada 16675, Greece

**Dimos D. Mitsikostas**
Headache Outpatient Clinic, 1st Department of Neurology, National and Kapodistrian University of Athens, Athens, Greece

**Andreas A. Argyriou**
Neurology Department of the Saint Andrew's State General Hospital of Patras, Patras, Greece

**Emmanouil V. Dermitzakis**
Department of Neurology, "Geniki Kliniki" Euromedica, Thessaloniki, Greece

**Konstantinos C. Spingos**
Corfu Headache Clinic, Corfu, Greece

**Shanil Ebrahim**
Department of Clinical Epidemiology & Biostatistics, McMaster University, Hamilton, ON, Canada

**Edward J. Mills and Kristian Thorlund**
Redwood Outcomes, 302-1505 2nd Ave. West, Vancouver, BC, Canada
Department of Clinical Epidemiology & Biostatistics, McMaster University, Hamilton, ON, Canada

**Christina Sun-Edelstein**
Department of Medicine, St. Vincent's Hospital, The University of Melbourne, Melbourne, Australia

**Eric Druyts**
Department of Medicine, Faculty of Medicine, University of British Columbia, Vancouver, BC, Canada

**Steve Kanters**
School of Population and Public Health, Faculty of Medicine, University of British Columbia, Vancouver, BC, Canada

**Rahul Bhambri and Elodie Ramos**
Pfizer Ltd, New York, NY, USA

**Stewart Tepper**
Geisel School of Medicine at Dartmouth, Hanover, NH, USA

**Michel Lanteri-Minet**
INSERM U1107, Neuo-Dol, Trigeminal Pain and Migraine Université Auvergne, Clermont-Ferrand, France
Pain Department, CHU Nice, France - FHU InovPain, Université Nice Côte d'Azur, Nice, France

**I. Aicua-Rapun, A. Hernando, E. Porqueres and F. Iglesias**
Neurology Department, Hospital Universitario de Burgos, Burgos, Spain

**A. L. Guerrero, E. Martínez-Velasco and M. Ruiz**
Neurology Department, Hospital Clínico Universitario de Valladolid, Avda. Ramón y Cajal 3, 47005 Valladolid, Spain

**S. Herrero, A. Rojo and A. Carreres**
Neurology Department, Hospital Clínico Universitario, Valladolid, Spain

**Zhiye Chen**
Department of Neurology, Chinese PLA General Hospital, Beijing 100853, China
Department of Radiology, Chinese PLA General Hospital, Beijing 100853, China
Department of Radiology, Hainan Branch of Chinese PLA General Hospital, Beijing 100853, China

**Shuangfeng Liu and Lin Ma**
Department of Radiology, Chinese PLA General Hospital, Beijing 100853, China

**Shengyuan Yu and Xiaoyan Chen**
Department of Neurology, Chinese PLA General Hospital, Beijing 100853, China

**Mengqi Liu**
Department of Radiology, Hainan Branch of Chinese PLA General Hospital, Beijing 100853, China
Department of Radiology, Chinese PLA General Hospital, Beijing 100853, China

**S. Louca Jounger, N. Christidis and M. Ernberg**
Section for Orofacial Pain and Jaw Function, Department of Dental Medicine, Karolinska Institutet, SE 14104, Huddinge, Sweden
Scandinavian Center for Orofacial Neurosciences (SCON), Huddinge, Sweden

**P. Svensson**
Section of Orofacial Pain and Jaw Function, School of Dentistry and Oral Health, Aarhus University, Vennelyst Boulevard 9, DK-8000 Aarhus C, Denmark
Scandinavian Center for Orofacial Neurosciences (SCON), Huddinge, Sweden
Section for Orofacial Pain and Jaw Function, Department of Dental Medicine, Karolinska Institutet, SE 14104, Huddinge, Sweden

**T. List**
Scandinavian Center for Orofacial Neurosciences (SCON), Huddinge, Sweden
Faculty of Odontology, Malmö University, Malmö, Sweden

**Sagar Munjal, Elimor Brand-Schieber and Kent Allenby**
Dr. Reddy's Laboratories Ltd., 107 College Road East Princeton, Princeton, NJ 08540, USA

**Egilius L.H. Spierings**
Dental Medicine Headache & Face Pain Program Tufts Medical Center, Craniofacial Pain Center Tufts University School, 800 Washington Street Boston, Boston, MA 02111, USA

**Roger K. Cady**
Clinvest/A Division of Banyan Inc., 3805 S Kansas Expy Springfield, Springfield, MO 65807, USA

**Alan M. Rapoport**
David Geffen School of Medicine at UCLA, Los Angeles, CA, USA

**Songlin He and Jinhua Wang**
College of Stomatology, Chongqing Medical University, No. 426 Songshibei Road, Chongqing 401147, China

Chongqing Key Laboratory of Oral Diseases and Biomedical Sciences, Chongqing, China
Chongqing Municipal Key Laboratory of Oral Biomedical Engineering of Higher Education, Chongqing, China

**Cristina Tassorelli**
Headache Science Center, National Neurological Institute C. Mondino, Pavia, Italy
Department of Brain and Behavioral Sciences, University of Pavia, Via Mondino 2, 27100 Pavia, Italy

**Marco Aguggia**
Headache Center, Neurology Department, Asti Hospital, Asti, Italy

**Marina De Tommaso**
Applied Neurophysiology and Pain Unit, SMBNOS Department, Polyclinic General Hospital, Bari Aldo Moro University, Bari, Italy

**Pierangelo Geppetti**
Headache Center, Department of Health Sciences, University of Florence, Florence, Italy

**Licia Grazzi**
Headache and Neuroalgology Unit, Neurological Institute "C. Besta" IRCCS Foundation, Milan, Italy

**Luigi Alberto Pini**
Center for Neuroscience and Neurotechnology, Polyclinic Hospital, University of Modena and Reggio Emilia, Modena, Italy

**Paola Sarchielli**
Neurology Clinic, University Hospital of Perugia, Perugia, Italy

**Gioacchino Tedeschi**
Department of Medical, Surgical, Neurological, Metabolic and Aging Sciences, University of Campania "Luigi Vanvitelli", Naples, Italy

**Paolo Martelletti**
Department of Clinical and Molecular Medicine, Sapienza University of Rome and Regional Referral Headache Center, Sant'Andrea Hospital, Rome, Italy

**Pietro Cortelli**
Department of Biomedical and Neuromotor Sciences, University of Bologna, Bologna, Italy
IRCCS Institute of Neurological Sciences of Bologna, Bellaria Hospital, Bologna, Italy

**Kai Le, Dafan Yu, Jiamin Wang, Abdoulaye Idriss Ali and Yijing Guo**
Department of Neurology, Affiliated ZhongDa Hospital, School of Medicine, Southeast University, Nanjing, Jiangsu 210009, People's Republic of China

**Manjit Matharu**
University College London (UCL) Institute of Neurology and The National Hospital for Neurology and Neurosurgery, Queen Square, London WC1N3BG, UK

**Rashmi Halker**
Mayo Clinic, Department of Neurology, 5777 East Mayo Blvd, Phoenix, AZ 85054, USA

**Patricia Pozo-Rosich**
Headache and Pain Research Group, Institut de Recerca, Universitat Autònoma de Barcelona, Barcelona, Spain
Neurology Department, Vall d'Hebron University Hospital, P.de la Vall d'Hebron, 119-129 08035 Barcelona, Spain

**Ronald DeGryse and Aubrey Manack Adams**
Allergan plc, 2525 Dupont Dr, Irvine, CA, USA

**Sheena K. Aurora**
Formerly of the Department of Neurology, Stanford University, 300 Pasteur Dr. Room A301 MC 5325, Stanford, CA, USA

**Carlo Baraldi, Lanfranco Pellesi, Simona Guerzoni, Maria Michela Cainazzo and Luigi Alberto Pini**
Medical Toxicology - Headache and Drug Abuse Centre, University of Modena and Reggio Emilia, Via del Pozzo 71, 41124 Modena, Italy

**Francesca Puledda and Peter J. Goadsby**
Headache Group, Department of Basic and Clinical Neuroscience, King's College London, and NIHR-Wellcome Trust King's Clinical Research Facility, Wellcome Foundation Building, King's College Hospital, London SE5 9PJ, UK

**Prab Prabhakar**
Department of Paediatric Neurology, Great Ormond Hospital for Children NHS Foundation Trust, London, UK

**Christian Lampl and Mirjam Rudolph**
Headache Medical Center, Ordensklinikum Linz Barmherzige Schwestern, Linz, Austria

**Elisabeth Bräutigam**
Headache Medical Center, Department of Radio-Oncology, Ordensklinikum Linz Barmherzige Schwestern, Linz, Austria

**Thijs H. T. Dirkx, Danielle Y. P. Haane and Peter J. Koehler**
Department of Neurology, Zuyderland Medical Center Heerlen, 6401, CX, Heerlen, The Netherlands

**Rosaria Greco, Chiara Demartini, Antonina Stefania Mangione and Giuseppe Nappi**
Laboratory of Neurophysiology of Integrative Autonomic Systems, Headache Science Centre, "C. Mondino" National Neurological Institute, Pavia, Italy

**Mariapia Vairetti and Andrea Ferrigno**
Department of Internal Medicine and Therapeutics, Pharmacology and Toxicology Unit, University of Pavia, Pavia, Italy

**Annamaria Zanaboni and Cristina Tassorelli**
Department of Brain and Behavioural Sciences, University of Pavia, Pavia, Italy

**Fabio Blandini**
Laboratory of Functional Neurochemistry, Center for Research in Neurodegenerative Diseases, "C. Mondino" National Neurological Institute, Pavia, Italy

**Ria Bhola and Evelyn Kinsella**
eNeura Therapeutics, Sunnyvale, CA, USA

**Nicola Giffin**
Department of Neurology, Royal United Hospital, Bath, UK

**Sue Lipscombe**
Brighton and Sussex University Hospitals, Royal Sussex County, Brighton, UK

**Fayyaz Ahmed**
Department of Neurology, Hull Royal Infirmary, Hull, UK

**Mark Weatherall**
Princess Margaret Migraine Clinic, Charing Cross Hospital, London, UK

**Peter J Goadsby**
Headache Group, Basic & Clinical Neuroscience, King's College London, London, UK
NIHR-Wellcome Trust Clinical Research Facility, King's College Hospital, London SE5 9PJ, UK

**Elisa Bellei, Emanuela Monari, Stefania Bergamini, Aurora Cuoghi and Aldo Tomasi**
Department of Diagnostic Medicine, Clinic and Public Health, Proteomic Lab, University of Modena and Reggio Emilia, Via del Pozzo 71, 41124 Modena, Italy

**Luigi Alberto Pini, Simona Guerzoni and Michela Ciccarese**
Headache and Drug Abuse Study Center, University of Modena and Reggio Emilia, Via del Pozzo 71, 41124 Modena, Italy

**Kuangshi Li, Yong Zhang, Yanzhe Ning, Hua Zhang, Hongwei Liu, Caihong Fu, Yi Ren and Yihuai Zou**
Department of Neurology and Stroke Center, Dongzhimen Hospital, The First Affiliated Hospital of Beijing University of Chinese Medicine, Beijing 100700, China

# Index

**A**

Allodynia, 44, 70, 76, 176-177, 183

Almotriptan, 1-5

Alpha-1-microglobulin, 176-177, 179, 183-184

Analgesics, 2, 51-59, 61, 65, 71, 77, 80, 112, 146-147, 176-177, 182, 184, 186-187

Asymmetric Dimethylarginine, 160, 166-167

**B**

Biopsychosocial Model, 19, 27, 90

Botox, 13-15, 18, 46-47, 49-50, 62-63, 92, 101-102, 145-146, 150

Botulinum Toxin Type A, 13, 17-18, 102, 150

**C**

Celecoxib, 121, 123-125, 128-130, 132, 136-137

Cerebrospinal Fluid, 71, 77

Chronic Migraine, 36, 45-47, 49-50, 59-60, 62-63, 92-93, 95, 97, 100-103, 110, 112-113, 116, 119-120, 137, 139-144, 150, 168-170, 173, 175, 177, 183, 193

Cluster Headache, 37-39, 43-45, 81, 101, 121, 134-136, 138-139, 143-145, 149-153, 158-159

Cortical Spreading Depression, 169, 175

Cystatin-c, 176-177, 179, 183

**D**

Diffusion Tensor Images, 186, 193

Dihydroergotamine, 38, 44, 52

Dimethylarginine Dimethylaminohydrolase, 160-161, 166-167

Dysgeusia, 79, 84-85

**E**

Enzyme-linked Immunosorbant Assays, 162

Episodic Migraine, 45-46, 50, 54, 58, 65, 68, 79-80, 85, 98, 113, 120, 168, 173

**F**

Frovatriptan, 1-5, 173

**G**

Gabapentin, 16, 121, 123-124, 126, 129-137, 169

Gamma-aminobutyric Acid, 149

Glomerular Filtration Rate, 30

Glyceryl Trinitrate, 86, 160, 162-167

Greater Occipital Nerve, 137, 139-144

**H**

Headache Disorders, 5-8, 12, 14, 18, 35-36, 43, 45, 50-51, 58-59, 62, 65, 69, 79-80, 99-101, 105-106, 112, 114, 119-121, 134-135, 138-140, 143-144, 149-150, 159, 175

Headache Impact Test, 113, 115-116, 118-120, 146, 149, 175

Hemicrania Continua, 121-124, 132, 134-136, 143

**I**

Indomethacin, 121, 123-126, 128-136, 176, 182

Interleukin, 71, 73-74, 76-78

Intranasal Sumatriptan, 79-80, 85

**L**

Lidocaine, 72, 121, 126-127, 129-131, 133-134, 136-137, 139-140

**M**

Magnetic Resonance Imaging, 64, 68, 184-185, 194

Masseter Muscle Pain, 13-17

Medication-overuse Headache, 12, 45, 51, 59, 64-66, 68-69, 102, 175-177, 183

Mesencephalon, 161-164

Methylprednisolone, 123, 126, 129-130, 133-134, 136, 138-140

Migraine Disability Assessment Scale, 30-31, 35

Migraine Prophylaxis, 47, 50, 92-93, 100, 111-113, 116, 119, 133, 146, 149, 193

Migraine With Aura, 1, 4, 134, 141, 143, 168-169, 173

Minor Occipital Nerve Blockade, 123, 134

Myalgia, 6, 9-10, 70-78, 83, 117

Myasthenia Gravis, 14, 146

**N**

Nitric Oxide, 77, 160-161, 166-167, 181

Non-invasive Vagus Nerve Stimulation, 37-38, 40, 42, 44-45, 135

**O**

Onabotulinumtoxina, 47, 50, 60, 101-102, 113-120, 123, 125, 134, 145-146, 148-150

Opioids, 51-58, 64, 177

**P**

Paroxysmal Hemicranias, 135

Periaqueductal Gray, 64, 68, 193-194

Pharmacokinetic, 5, 80, 165

Phonophobia, 31-32, 46, 168, 172

Photophobia, 31-32, 46, 168, 172

Piroxicam, 121, 123-126, 128-129, 132-133, 135, 137

Placebo, 43-44, 47, 50, 59, 62, 85, 93, 100-120, 122, 134, 137, 143-144, 149-150, 159, 174, 192

Pressure-pain Thresholds, 70-71

Prophylactic Treatment, 18, 30, 37, 42, 44, 59-60, 100, 102, 111, 116, 119-120, 145-146, 149, 158

Prostaglandin-h2 D-synthase, 176, 179, 183

## R

Refractoriness, 145

Right Frontoparietal Network, 185, 193

Rizatriptan, 1-5

Rostral Ventromedial Medulla, 64

## S

Short Lasting Neuralgiform Headache Attacks, 121

Single Nucleotide Polymorphisms, 30

Somatic Complaints, 20, 22-24, 26

Sumatriptan, 4-5, 37-38, 40-41, 52, 79-81, 85-86, 123-125, 129, 132, 135-136, 153, 167

## T

Temporomandibular Joint Dysfunction, 13-15, 17, 28, 90

Tension-type Headache, 2, 9-10, 13-17, 139-141, 144, 166

Topiramate, 38, 42, 48, 59-62, 100, 102-112, 121, 123-126, 128-136, 144, 147, 169

Transcranial Magnetic Stimulation, 168, 173, 175

Trigeminal Autonomic Cephalalgias, 45, 121, 134-137, 141

Trigeminocervical Complex, 104, 140

Triptan, 1-4, 38, 41, 45, 52-53, 80, 84-85, 173

Tumor Necrosis Factor, 44, 73-74, 76

## U

Uromodulin, 176-177, 179, 183-184

Urotensin-2, 29, 31-32, 35

## V

Valproate, 104, 127-129, 169

Verapamil, 38, 41, 44, 125, 127-137, 147, 153-154, 157-158

Verbal Numerical Rating Scale, 13

Visual Analogue Scale, 13, 15, 17, 65-66, 188

## W

Western Blot, 176, 178, 180-181, 183

## Z

Zolmitriptan, 1-5, 37, 40-41, 44, 59, 80, 86, 112